Cafer's Antipsychotics:

Visualize to Memorize drug interactions and trade/generic name pairings

First Edition, 2020

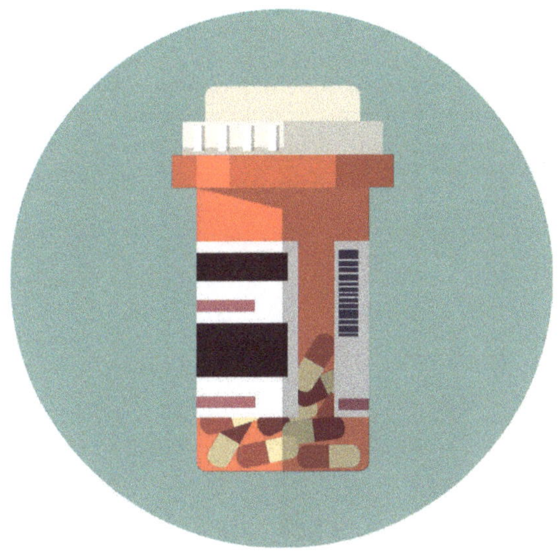

Author: Jason Cafer, MD

Editor: Julianna Link, PA-C

Cafer's Antipsychotics: Visualize to Memorize drug interactions and trade/generic name pairings

First Edition

Author: Jason Cafer, MD

Editor: Julianna Link, PA-C

Illustrations: Coccus from 99Designs

Cover design: BengsWorks from 99Designs

Licensed images: Shutterstock and Wikimedia Commons

ISBN: 978-1-7350901-1-5

Contact: jason@cafermed.com

This book includes a subset of 40 medication mascots from *Cafer's Psychopharmacology*, which contains 270. Medications chosen for this edition include:

- **First generation antipsychotics (FGAs)** – the "typicals"
- **Second generation antipsychotics (SGAs)** – the "atypicals"
- **Pimavanserin (Nuplazid)** – non-dopaminergic antipsychotic for hallucinations and delusions associated with Parkinson's disease
- **Dopamine depleting agents** used to treat tardive dyskinesia and Huntington's disease; These have antipsychotic properties.
- **Dopamine blocking antiemetics** including metoclopramide (Reglan), which is a common cause of tardive dyskinesia
- **Cannabidiol (CBD oil)** – cannabinoid receptor antagonist that is an effective off-label treatment for schizophrenia
- **Anticholinergics** used as adjuncts to antipsychotics to treat extrapyramidal symptoms (EPS) and clozapine-induced hypersalivation
- **Amantadine (Symmetrel)** – dopaminergic approved for EPS, as an alternative to anticholinergics
- **Metformin (Glucophage)** – diabetes medication used to counter antipsychotic-induced weight gain

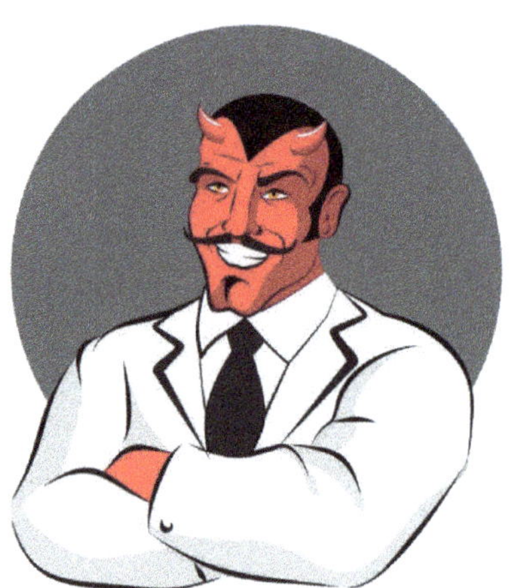

Antipsychotics are represented by spooky mascots.

The scope of drug interaction information is limited to what can be digested and applied to routine clinical practice. There are countless unmentioned drug-drug interactions that could be relevant for some patients but are omitted because the amount of material would be overwhelming.

This book is focused on medications, not overarching psychiatric care. Although chemicals are necessary for treatment of mania or acute psychosis, pharmacologic treatment of depression/anxiety/insomnia/etc is not always the best medicine. Always consider interventions including cognitive behavioral therapy, diet, exercise, mindfulness, sleep hygiene, etc.

Dosing recommendations are for healthy adults, and <u>may differ from FDA prescribing guidelines</u>. Refer to other sources for treatment of children, older adults, pregnancy/breastfeeding and renal/hepatic insufficiency.

Table of Contents

Antipsychotics are substrates of 1A2, 2D6 and 3A4. Antipsychotics are not enzyme inducers or inhibitors.

Lumateperone (Caplyta) is a UGT substrate.

Antipsychotics are antidopaminergic.

Compare/contrast NMS with serotonin syndrome.

The "typicals" – more likely to cause EPS and elevate prolactin

Loxapine (Loxitane) has atypical properties.

Prochlorperazine (Compaze) is approved for schizophrenia, but today is used almost exclusively as an antiemetic.

Metoclopramide (Reglan) poses a major risk of tardive dyskinesia.

The "atypicals" are a heterogenous group. Generalizations (low EPS, weight gain, diabetes risk) do not apply to all 2nd gens.

At high doses, risperidone and paliperidone behave like typical antipsychotics.

Pimavanserin (Nuplazid) is a $5\text{-}HT_{2A}$ inverse agonist, not an antidopaminergic. It is approved for Parkinson's psychosis.

Diphenhydramine, benztropine, and trihexyphenidyl are used to treat antipsychotic-induced dystonia.

PO Glycopyrrolate or sublingual atropine (eye)drops can be used for clozapine-induced hypersalivation.

Dopamine depleting agents have antipsychotic properties.

Austedo and Ingrezza are approved for the treatment of tardive dyskinesia.

Metformin can counter antipsychotic-induced weight gain.

High dose CBD oil is an effective antipsychotic.

Amantadine is a dopaminergic approved for the treatment of EPS.

Medication Monographs

#40 most prescribed US
1993
$4–$250

Chemical structure

Generic Name (TRADE NAME)
[pronunciation]
mnemonic phrase

❖ Class of medication
❖ Mechanism of action

100
200
400
mg

Year the drug was introduced to the U.S. market

Monographs focus on the unique aspects of the individual drug, to be taken in context of the medication class. Most of the medications in this book are psychotropic, i.e., capable of affecting the mind, emotions and behavior.

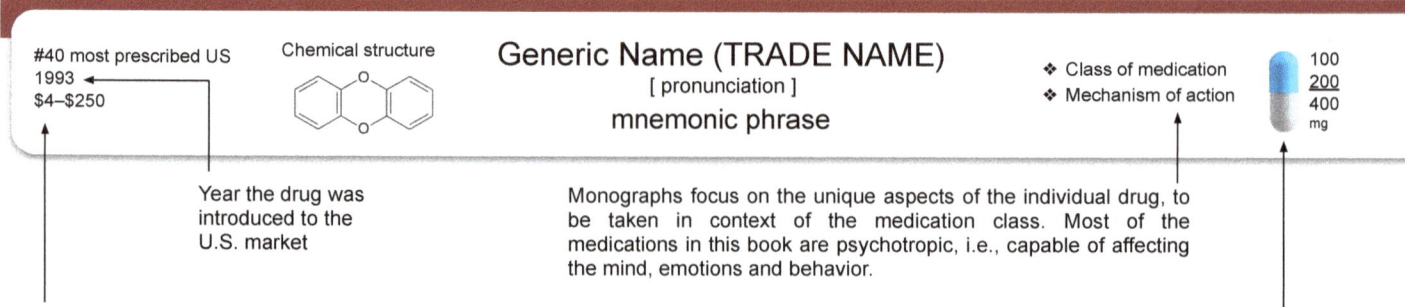

Price range for a month's supply of the generic (if available) version of the drug. The price is generally applicable to the most common prescription, which would be #30 for drugs usually dosed QD, #60 for those dosed BID, and #90 for those usually dosed TID. The applicable milligram strength is the number underlined in the upper righthand corner. The bottom dollar value is the lowest GoodRx price, available with a coupon at select pharmacies. The high dollar value is the average retail price in mid-late 2019. The wide price range from pharmacy to pharmacy shows the importance of checking a source like GoodRx before filling a script for cash.

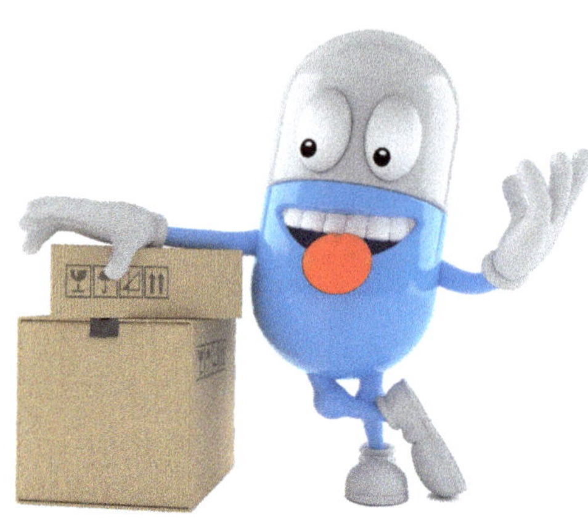

Each monograph features a mascot designed to pair the drug's generic name with the most common U.S. trade name.

A representative pill of the underlined strength, either a branded or generic version. The main purpose is to show whether we're talking capsules or tablets. For tablets, we try to show the side with score lines. If no score lines are shown, assume that the pill is not intended to be split. For any splittable psychotropic medication, giving a half dose for the first two days may be a good idea, depending on acuity of symptoms.

Dosing: When provided, dosing recommendations are applicable to healthy adults. Refer to other sources for pediatric recommendations. Older adults should generally be given lower doses. Doses may need to be modified when considering kinetic/dynamic interactions, pharmacogenetics, body weight, and renal/hepatic insufficiency.

Boxes like this contain contextual information about the drug.

A link to a page with relevant content looks like this: 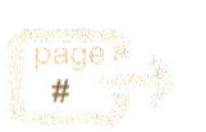

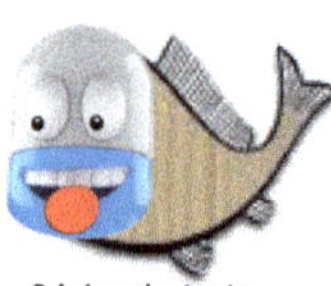

3A4 substrate

The box with rounded corners contains a visual hybrid of the mascot and CYP interaction mnemonic(s). Over half of prescription drugs are metabolized by 3A4, so there are plenty of fish.

Recurring Visuals

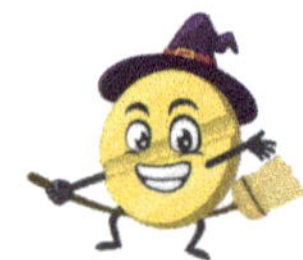

Antipsychotic (various spooky characters)

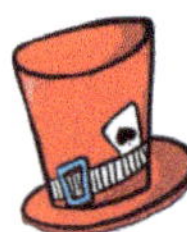

Anticholinergic with CNS effects (Mad as a hatter)

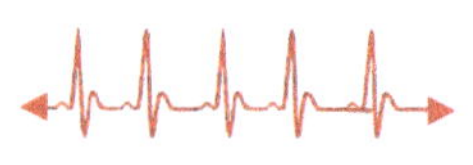

QT interval-prolonging medication

PHARMACODYNAMICS VS PHARMACOKINETICS

Drug-drug interactions fall into two main categories: **pharmacokinetic** and **pharmacodynamic**.

Pharmacodynamics is what a drug does to the body. Pharmacodynamic interactions are based on the drugs' mechanisms of action and do not involve alteration in blood levels of either interacting drug.

Pharmacokinetics is what the body does to a drug. Kinetic derives from the Greek verb *kinein*, "to move". In this case we're talking movement into and out of the body, for instance absorbing the chemical from the gut and processing it for excretion in urine or feces. Pharmacokinetic (PK) interactions are generally manifested by alteration of blood levels of one of the interacting drugs.

For simplicity's sake, let's drop the *pharmaco-* prefix and refer to these concepts as **kinetic** interactions and **dynamic** interactions.

PHARMACODYNAMIC INTERACTIONS

Dynamic interactions are intuitive if you understand how the interacting drugs work. Although dynamic interactions are understandable without silly pictures, here are a couple anyhow.

Dynamic interactions can be **additive/synergistic**, with enhanced effects brought about by combining medications with similar or complementary effects.

Like-minded "dynos" ganging up to reduce blood pressure, which is an additive/synergistic effect.

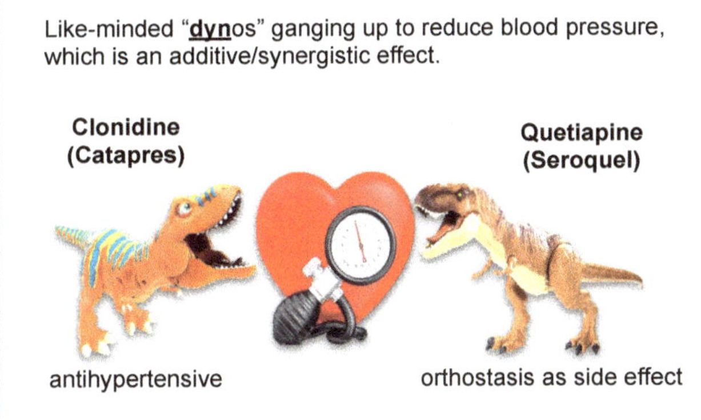

Other dynamic interactions are **antagonistic**, for instance combining a dopaminergic such as pramipexole (for restless legs) with an antidopaminergic like haloperidol (antipsychotic). Either medication can make the other ineffective.

Fighting "dynos" involved in an antagonistic interaction.

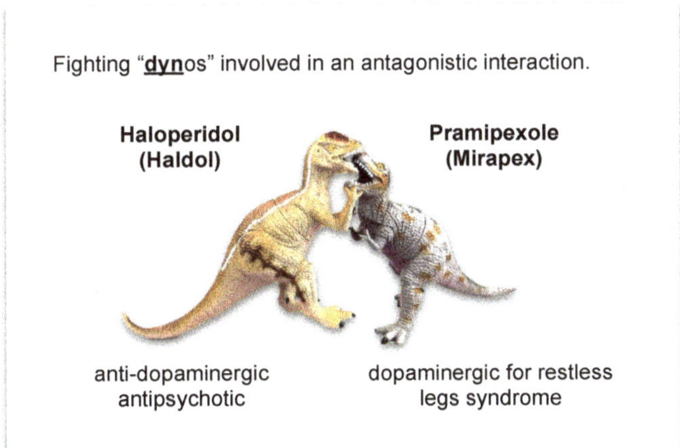

PHARMACOKINETIC INTERACTIONS

Kinetics involves the rate at which a drug gets into or out of the body or brain.

Drug-drug Interactions involving absorption are generally straightforward. For instance, anticholinergics slow gut motility and delay gastrointestinal absorption of other medications.

Kinetic interactions involving rate of elimination from the body are challenging to learn and daunting to memorize. It is important to consider these interactions to avoid underdosing or overdosing certain medications. This book tackles these tricky elimination interactions by illustrating:

❖ Phase I metabolism involving the six most important cytochrome P450 (CYP450) enzymes

❖ Phase II metabolism involving UGT enzymes, as applicable to lamotrigine (Lamictal)

❖ Renal clearance of lithium (in *Cafer's Mood Stabilizers* book)

A mysterious type of kinetic interaction involves drugs getting across the blood-brain barrier, as is necessary for a psychiatric medication to take effect. If such an interaction is occurring, the effect will not be detectable in serum drug levels. This will be discussed in the context of P-glycoprotein (page 9).

CYTOCHROME P450 ENZYMES

In the liver, kinetic interactions predominantly involve **CYtochrome P450 enzymes**, **CYP** enzymes for short, which can be pronounced "sip". Instead of concerning yourself with the origin of P450 nomenclature, take a moment to contemplate this picture of Ken (kinetic) taking a "sip" (CYP).

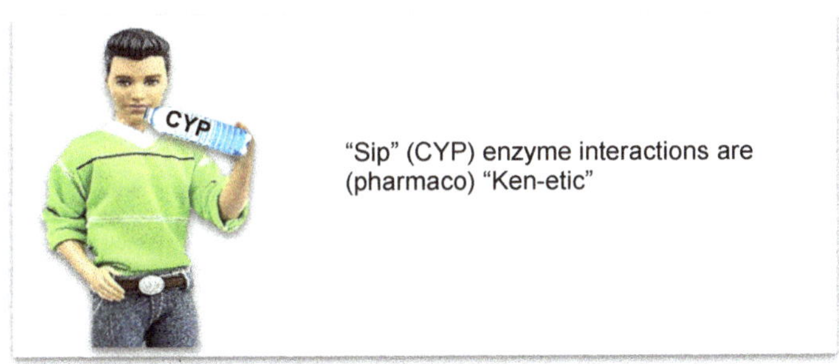

"Sip" (CYP) enzyme interactions are (pharmaco) "Ken-etic"

CYP enzymes, which reside primarily in the liver, make chemicals less lipid-soluble so they can be more easily excreted in urine or bile. Of over 50 CYP enzymes, six play a major role in the biotransformation of medications: 1A2, 2B6, 2C9, 2C19, 2D6 and 3A4. Our visual mnemonics will be built on the following phraseology:

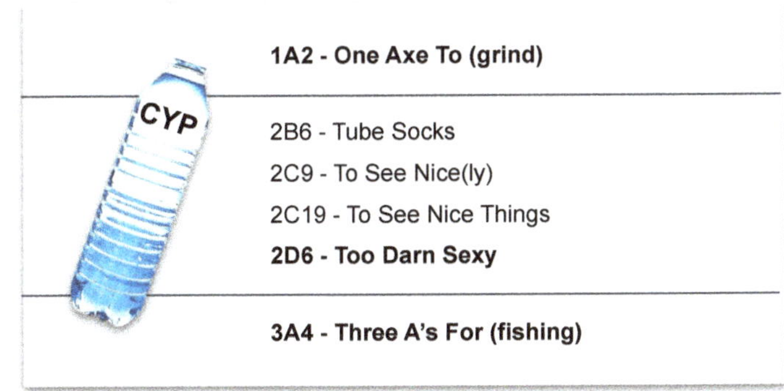

1A2 - One Axe To (grind)

2B6 - Tube Socks
2C9 - To See Nice(ly)
2C19 - To See Nice Things
2D6 - Too Darn Sexy

3A4 - Three A's For (fishing)

The three CYPs involved in metabolism of antipsychotics are **1A2, 2D6** and **3A4**. The other three enzymes are included for context.

SUBSTRATES

A drug that is biotransformed by a particular enzyme is referred to as a **substrate** of that enzyme. When the substrate is biotransformed (metabolized) it is then referred to as a **metabolite**.

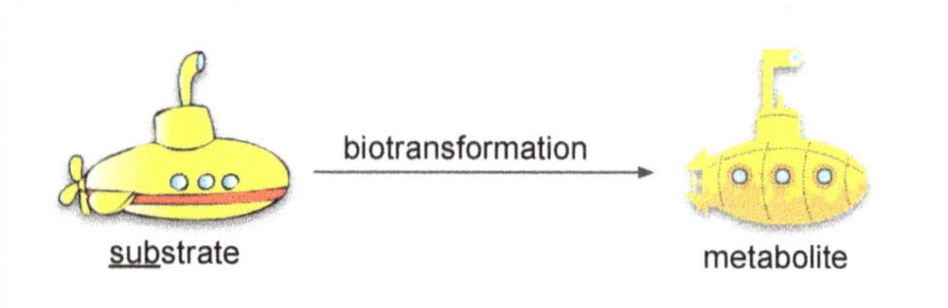

Each CYP enzyme can metabolize several substrates and most substrates can be metabolized by several CYP enzymes. Substrates are the "victims" of the interactions described in this chapter. Throughout this book we use the following visuals for CYP substrates:

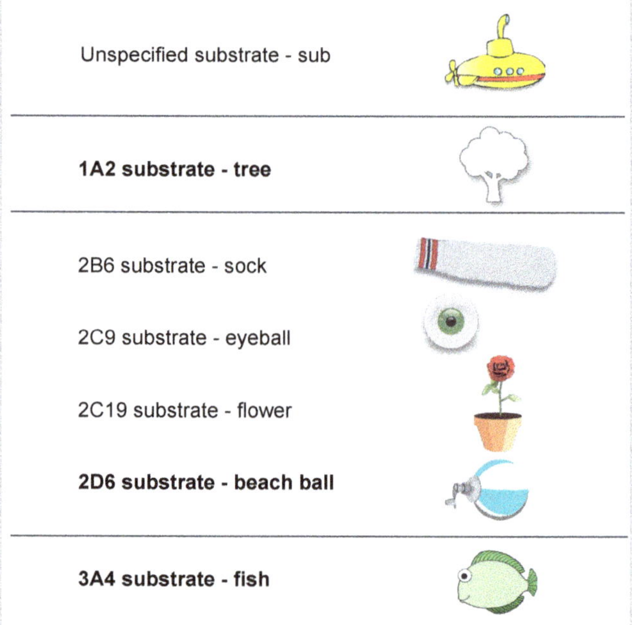

Unspecified substrate - sub
1A2 substrate - tree
2B6 substrate - sock
2C9 substrate - eyeball
2C19 substrate - flower
2D6 substrate - beach ball
3A4 substrate - fish

"Aggressor" medications affect how long victim substrates linger in the blood, and the relative serum concentration of parent drug (substrate) to metabolite. For a given enzyme, interfering medications (aggressors) are either inDucers or inHibitors. **InDucers** stimulate (inDuce) production of metabolic enzymes. **InHibitors** interfere with an enzyme's ability to metabolize other medications. Most antipsychotics are victim substrates, while none are inducers or inhibitors.

ENZYME INHIBITION

InHibition of an enzyme occurs when one drug (the inHibitor) binds more tightly to the enzyme than the victim substrate binds. The inHibitor itself may be metabolized by the enzyme, or act as a non-competitive inhibitor. When an inhibitor is bound to an enzyme, the victim substrate must find another enzyme to metabolize it, or hope that it can eventually be excreted unchanged. Strong inhibitors may cause the victim substrate to linger longer, prolonging the victim's half-life and elevating its concentration in the blood. For victim substrates that cross the blood brain barrier (as is necessary to be psychoactive), inhibition leads to increased drug concentration in the central nervous system.

Why is H being emphasized? Well, when an inHibitor is added to an individual's medication regimen, levels of victim drugs can escalate (H for High). InHibition takes effect quickly, within Hours (H for Hurried), although the effect may not be clinically evident for 2 to 4 days, until the victim substrate accumulates.

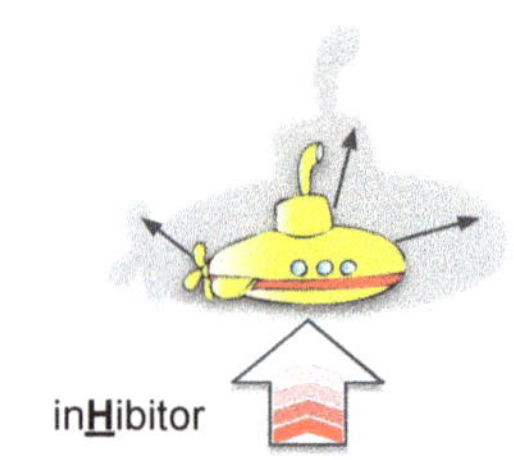

Increased concentration of substrate (and increased ratio of serum substrate:metabolite)

H for High and Hurried, within 2- 4 hours, although the effect may not be clinically evident for 2 - 4 days

InHibitors of CYP enzymes will be represented by:

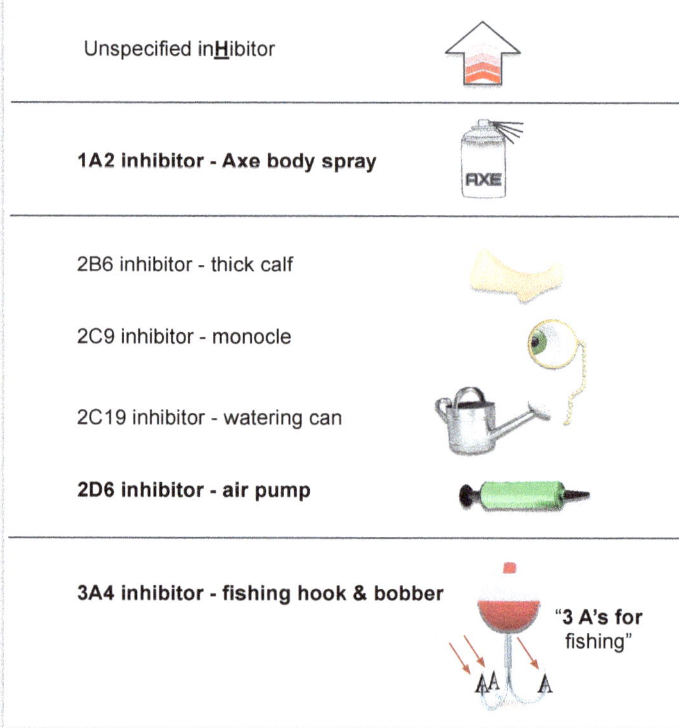

The medications in this book are not clinically significant inHibitors. The only exception is cannabidiol. When involved in kinetic interactions, antipsychotics and other dopaminergic medications almost always play the role of victim (substrate).

The magnitude to which an inHibitor increases the serum concentration of a specific substrate depends on the number of alternative pathways available to metabolize the substrate. If the drug is a substrate of, e.g., 1A2, 2D6 *and* 3A4, then inhibiting one of the three pathways should be of no consequence. Such substrates may be described as multi-CYP.

For a substrate metabolized by a single pathway, the effect of inhibition (and induction) will be dramatic. An example is lurasidone (Latuda), which is contraindicated with strong 3A4 inhibitors or inducers.

Some inhibitors are stronger than others. In general, expect blood levels of susceptible substrates to increase in the ballpark of:

- mild inhibitor ~ 25% - 50% increase
- moderate inhibitor ~ 50% - 100% increase
- strong inhibitor > 100% increase

Expect these numbers to vary widely between substrates and individuals, often unpredictably.

The "fluffers" – notorious strong inHibitors:

- **fluvoxamine** (Luvox) - SSRI
- **fluoxetine** (Prozac) - SSRI
- **fluconazole** (Diflucan) - antifungal
- **ketoconazole** (Nizoral) - antifungal

The last two are "cone"-azole antifungals.

ENZYME INDUCTION

The opposite of inHibition is **inDuction**. InDuction occurs when an inDucer stimulates the liver to produce extra enzymes, leading to enhanced metabolism and quicker clearance of victim drugs. More often than not, an inducer is itself a substrate of the enzyme.

The D is for Down, i.e., Decreased serum concentrations of victim substrates. Unlike inHibition (H for Hurried), inDuction is Delayed, not taking full effect for 2 to 4 weeks while we… wait for the liver to ramp up enzyme production.

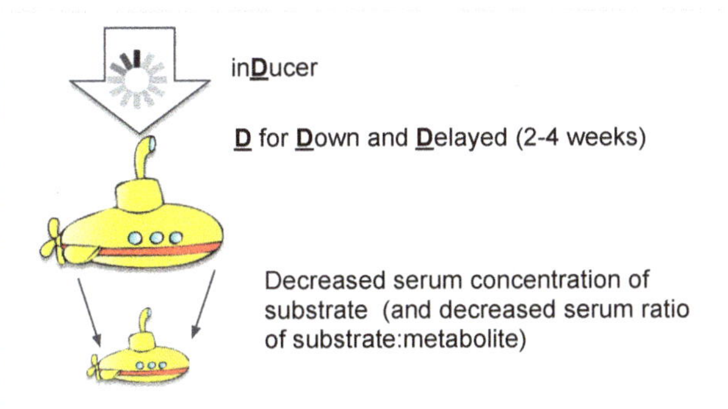

inDucer
D for Down and Delayed (2-4 weeks)
Decreased serum concentration of substrate (and decreased serum ratio of substrate:metabolite)

InDucers will be depicted by:

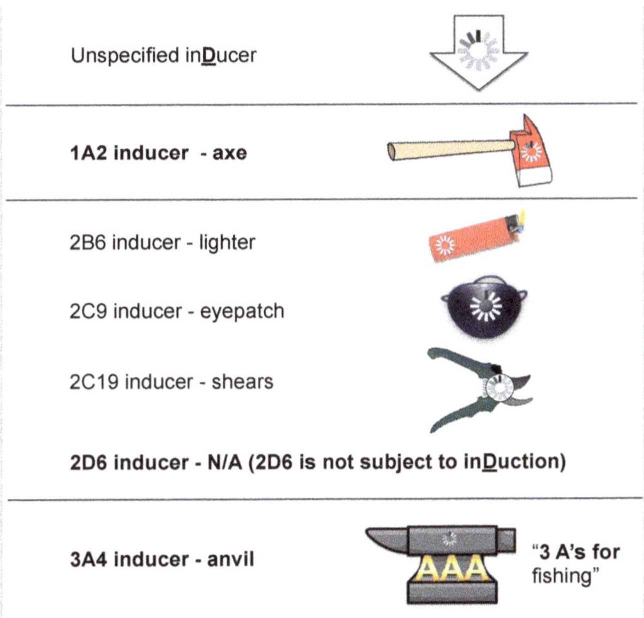

None of the medications featured in this book are clinically significant inDucers.

THE SHREDDERS

The **"shredders"** are four **strong inDucers** of several CYPs, which cause countless chemicals to be quickly expelled from the body:

- **carbamazepine** (Tegretol) – antiepileptic
- **phenobarbital** (Luminal) – barbiturate
- **phenytoin** (Dilantin) – antiepileptic
- **rifampin** (Rifadin) – antimicrobial

Dr. Jonathan Heldt refers to the shredders as **"Carb & Barb"** in his book *Memorable Psychopharmacology*.

St John's Wort (herbal antidepressant) also inDuces several CYPs, but does so with less potency than the four shredders.

Can shredding be problematic even if the patient is not taking a victim medication? Consider this:

Long-term use of a shredder leads to decreased bone mineral density. This is presumably due to inDuction of enzymes that inactivate 25(OH) vitamin D.

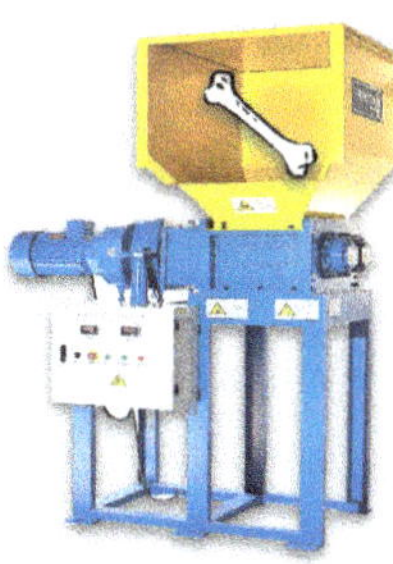

bone shredding machine

REVERSAL OF INHIBITION/ INDUCTION

All things being equal, it is best to avoid prescribing strong inducers or inhibitors. Even if there is no problematic interaction at the time, having a strong inhibitor or inducer on board may complicate future medication management.

Consider an individual on an established medication regimen who stops taking an inducer or inhibitor. The serum concentration of victim substrate(s) will change due to the **reversal** of induction/inhibition.

After an inDucer is withdrawn, the concentration of a victim substrate will increase gradually (D for Delayed) over a few weeks because the extra CYP enzymes are degraded without being replenished.

When an inHibitor is stopped, levels of a victim substrate will decrease as soon as the aggressor exits the body. "Hurriedly" does not mean immediately, because it takes about **five half-lives** for the inhibitor to be completely cleared.

For a patient on several psychotropic medications, reversal of inhibition or induction can really throw things out of whack.

While ePrescribe systems may warn the doctor when starting an interacting medication, there will be **no warning** when stopping a medication will lead to a reversal situation.

An example of **reversal of inDuction** involves tobacco, which is a 1A2 inDucer. A patient taking clozapine (1A2 substrate) stops smoking, reversing inDuction and causing clozapine levels to potentially double over the first week (which is faster than occurs with other inducers). The individual may become obtunded, hypotensive, or even have a seizure. To avoid this, the recommendation is to decrease clozapine dose by 10% daily over the first four days upon smoking cessation, and to check clozapine blood levels before and after the dose adjustment. Note that nicotine products (gum, patches, e-cigs) do not induce 1A2.

Consider a patient taking alprazolam (Xanax, 3A4 substrate) who suddenly stops **flu**voxamine (Luvox, 3A4 inHibitor). In absence of the inhibitor, alprazolam levels drop (from double) to normal. Since fluvoxamine has a short elimination half-life of 15 hours, it should be out of the body at 75 hours (15 hr x 5). So, you would expect the patient on Xanax to become more anxious 3 days after stopping Luvox. It may be difficult to discern whether the patient's emerging distress is due to serotonin withdrawal or decreased alprazolam levels.

Although reversal of inHibition is typically faster than reversal of induction, this does not apply to inhibitors with extremely long half-lives. For instance, **flu**oxetine (Prozac) has a long elimination half-life of about 7 days, keeping itself around for about 35 days (7 days x 5). Consider a patient with schizophrenia on aripiprazole (Abilify, 2D6 substrate) who stops Prozac (2D6 inHibitor). The patient is doing well at one month, but becomes paranoid two months out. Unless the prescriber anticipated this possibility, no one will realize what happened.

PRODRUGS

Phase I metabolism typically involves biotransformation of an active drug to an inactive (or less active) chemical.

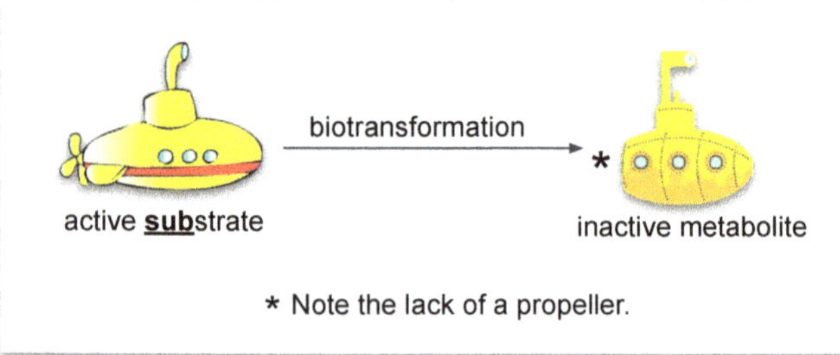

For a few medications, the parent drug has low therapeutic activity until it is biotransformed by a CYP enzyme. In such cases, the substrate is called a **prodrug**, and the biotransformation process can be referred to as **bioactivation**.

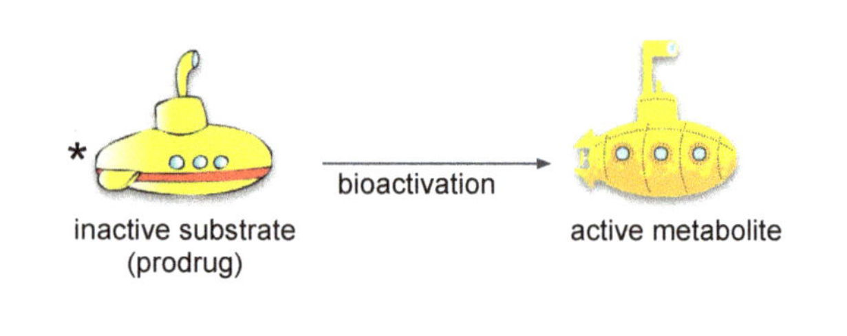

For most medications (active parent drug to inactive metabolite) inDuction decreases (D for Down) effect of the drug and inHibition (H for High) amplifies the therapeutic effect and/or side effects.

With prodrugs, the opposite effect is observed clinically. Induction increases and inhibition decreases the medication's effect(s).

Don't let prodrugs confuse you. InHibitors increase and InDucers decrease the levels of substrate regardless of whether the parent drug is pharmacologically active.

The following are **prodrugs** activated by 2D6:

- **Codeine** – metabolized to morphine
- **Tramadol** (Ultram) – weak opioid
- **Tamoxifen** – anti-estrogen for breast cancer

The bowling ball is explained on page 15.

PHASE II METABOLISM

Phase II metabolism occurs in the liver and is subject to kinetic interactions. CYP enzymes are not involved.

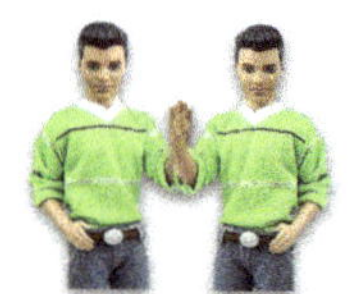

Two Kens without a bottle to "CYP" (sip)

Phase II reactions typically involve **conjugation** of a substrate with **glucuronic acid**. This makes the drug water-soluble and prepped for renal excretion.

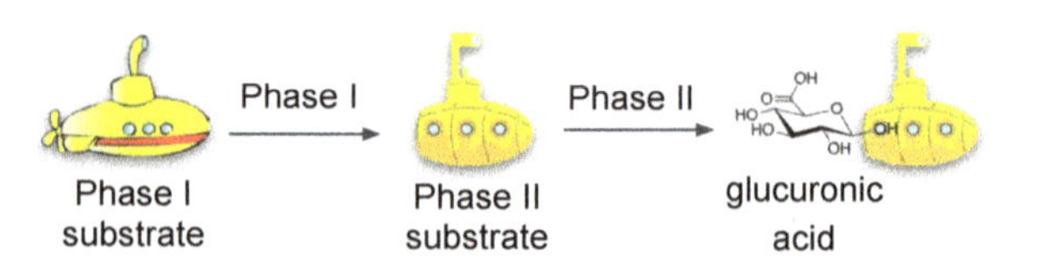

The responsible enzyme is UDP-glucuronosyltransferase, abbreviated **UGT**, as in "U Got Tagged" with glucuronic acid.

Medications metabolized primarily by Phase II are relatively immune to drug interactions. The most clinically relevant Phase II interactions are those involving the mood stabilizer lamotrigine (Lamictal) and the antipsychotic lumateperone (Caplyta) as substrates.

RENAL CLEARANCE

A few medications are excreted in urine without being metabolised. Such drugs are not subject to Phase I or II interactions, but may be victims of kinetic interactions. Renal "aggressors" act by slowing or hastening the rate of excretion of the victim drug in urine.

Interactions affecting renal clearance of victim drugs are also considered (pharmaco)"Ken"etic.

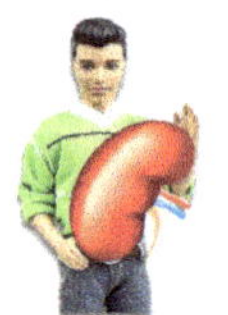

The aggressor in a renal interaction is not referred to as an inducer or inhibitor, because no enzyme is involved. Nor is the victim called a substrate, because it is not being biotransformed.

Lithium, excreted unchanged in urine, is the most vulnerable viction of kinetic interactions involving renal clearance.

CYP GENETIC PROFILES

Genetic polymorphisms can influence an individual's medication kinetics, which is most relevant for 2D6 and 2C19. Let's talk about 2D6, arguably the most consequential example.

Most individuals are genetically equipped with 2D6 genes that produce normal 2D6 enzymes that metabolize 2D6 substrates at the usual rate. These normal individuals are said to have a 2D6 **extensive metabolizer** (EM) genotype, resulting in a 2D6 EM phenotype.

Here is a cute representation of how a normal individual, i.e., 2D6 **extensive metabolizer** (EM), processes 2D6 substrates. The air inside the beach ball represents the substrate, which is being expelled from the ball as metabolite at the usual rate. 2D6 substrates will have typical elimination half-lives.

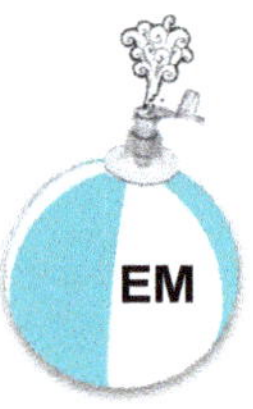

About 5% of the population have extra copies of 2D6 genes, resulting in an **ultrarapid metabolizer** (UM) phenotype. These individuals clear 2D6 substrates quickly.

For 2D6 **ultrarapid metabolizers** (UM), the air (2D6 substrate) flows out of the ball quickly as metabolite. 2D6 substrates could be ineffective for these individuals (with the exception of 2D6 prodrugs, which could be be too strong).

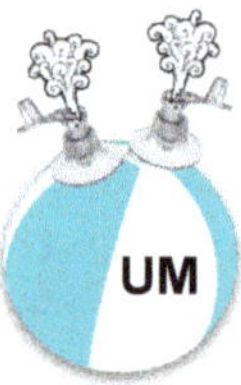

About 10% of individuals have defective 2D6 enzymes resulting in a 2D6 **poor metabolizer** (PM) phenotype. This condition may be found on a diagnosis list as "Cytochrome P450 2D6 enzyme deficiency".

For 2D6 "**POOR ME**"tabolizers (PM), air accumulates, resulting in unexpectedly long half-lives for 2D6 substrates. These individuals are more likely to report side effects.

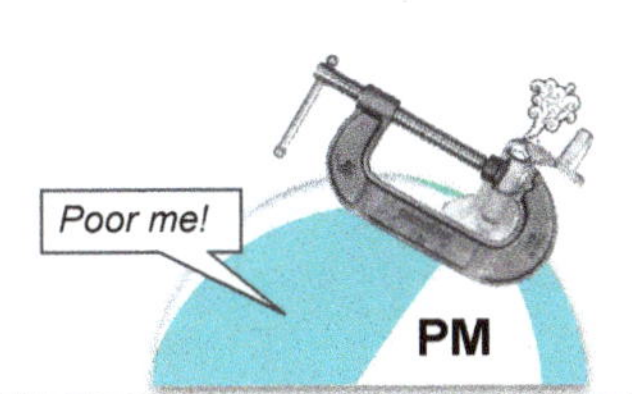

An individual taking a strong 2D6 in**H**ibitor (pump as illustrated on page 15) will metabolize 2D6 substrates **as if** the individual had a 2D6 PM genotype.

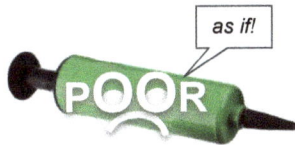

In summary, genetic testing of CYP polymorphisms will interpret the metabolizer profile for a given enzyme as either:

- Extensive metabolizer (EM) – normal
- Ultrarapid metabolizer (UM) – fast clearance of substrates
- Poor metabolizer (PM) – slow clearance of substrates

A genetic test result of **intermediate metabolizer** (IM) means that enzyme activity is likely to be a bit lower than that of an EM, i.e., an intermediate between EM and PM. Generally, IM individuals can be clinically managed normally, like an EM individual.

Standalone 2D6 genotyping costs at least $200. GeneSight or Genecept panels cost about $4,000 and report the six relevant CYPs and two UGT enzymes (UGT1A4 and UGT2B15). 23andMe ($199) reports 1A2, 2C9, and 2C19, among 100s of other genes. 23andMe does not report the most relevant CYP genotype, 2D6, because the genetics of 2D6 metabolism is more complicated.

Genotyping may be useful when choosing which medication to prescribe an individual patient. With GeneSight, about 1 in 5 patients have a genetic variation relevant to their treatment. For an individual already established on a medication, serum drug levels may be more useful than genotyping. There are situations when knowing the actual blood levels of clozapine, risperidone, olanzapine, aripiprazole, haloperidol, lamotrigine, etc. are clinically relevant. Unfortunately, these tests usually must be sent to an outside lab, and it may take a week to see the results. Levels of lithium, carbamazepine, phenytoin, and valproic acid are usually reported the same day.

P-GLYCOPROTEIN

P-glycoprotein (P-gp) is a gatekeeper at the gut lumen and the blood-brain barrier. P-gp pumps P-gp substrates out of the brain—"Pumpers gonna pump".

"Pumpers gonna pump" P-gp substrates out of the brain

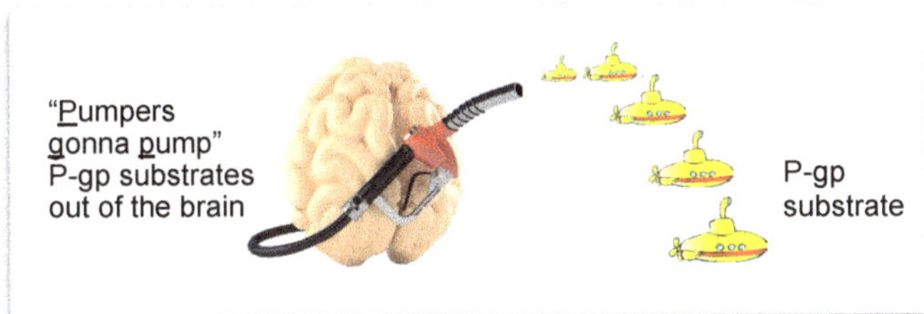

P-gp substrate

An example of a relevant P-gp interaction involves the OTC opioid antidiarrheal loperamide (Imodium). Loperamide does not cause central opioid effects under normal circumstances. If the individual takes a potent P-gp inhibitor, megadose loperamide can stay in the brain long enough to cause euphoria. The P-gp inhibitor typically used the achieve this recreational effect is omeprazole (Prilosec).

THE NATURE OF THIS INFORMATION

The information presented in the remainder of this chapter is a synthesis of sources including the OpeRational ClassificAtion (ORCA) system (as presented in *The Top 100 Drug Interactions* by Hansten & Horn, 2019), Lexicomp, Flockhart Table, ePocrates, Carlat Medication Fact Book, Stahl's Essential Psychopharmacology, The Medical Letter, Current Psychiatry, GeneSight, Genecept, various research papers and FDA prescribing information for the individual drugs.

Reputable sources are often at odds with each other regarding the strength of specific inducers/inhibitors, the vulnerability of specific substrates to induction/inhibition, or even which CYPs are relevant to a specific medication. CYP interactions are continuously being discovered and clarified. Even with the freshest information and full knowledge of a patient's genotype, the magnitude of a specific CYP interaction is difficult to predict.

HOW TO APPLY THIS INFORMATION

Refer to the tables on pages 20 and 21. Highlight the medications that you prescribe. First acquaint yourself with the in**D**ucers because the list is short. Memorize the bolded inducers (shredders) and those that you highlighted. After you know the inducers, move to the in**H**ibitor column. Memorize the bolded inhibitors (fluffers) and your highlighted medications. Antipsychotics and other medications featured in this book are highlighted for you.

When it comes to substrates, memorization is less important. Substrates are only relevant when an inducer or inhibitor is on board, or if the patient has a special metabolizer genotype. Of the medications you prescribe, be aware of the more susceptible substrates.

Consider running an interaction check whenever a patient is taking a shredder, fluffer, systemic antifungal, HIV medication, or cancer medication. ePocrates.com and the ePocrates app are adequate, and free.

Keep things simple. When choosing new medications, avoid major inducers and inhibitors if suitable alternatives are available. For the complicated psychiatric patient on several medications, try to avoid carbamazepine (shredder inducer) and the **flu**ffer SSRIs (**flu**oxetine and **flu**voxamine). Among SSRIs, escitalopram (Lexapro) and sertraline (Zoloft) are good choices—they are 2C19 substrates but do not affect the metabolism of other medications.

Also think about choosing less vulnerable substrates. Each drug on pages 18 and 19 is depicted in box/bubble because it is generally not involved in clinically significant kinetic interactions (although dynamic interactions almost always apply). You don't have to worry much about benzodiazepine interactions if you stick to the "LOT" benzos—lorazepam, oxazepam and temazepam. Most antipsychotics are susceptible substrates, but not so much for ziprasidone, loxapine and paliperidone.

This book uses picture association as a memorization technique. Pages 10 through 17 establish a visual mnemonic framework for various kinetic interactions that will be reinforced by a "mascot" for each medication. The mascots serve a double purpose of helping you remember US trade name / generic name pairings.

Since you probably won't be mentioning CYP nomenclature in casual conversation, you might want to bypass the technical naming system altogether. Instead of keeping a list of "3A4 substrates" in your memory bank, you could just learn the school of "fish".

I hope this book empowers you to understand and memorize topics that are otherwise daunting, so you can to use your knowledge to improve patient care. Without further ado, let's start our journey to becoming a superhero of psychotropic medication management.

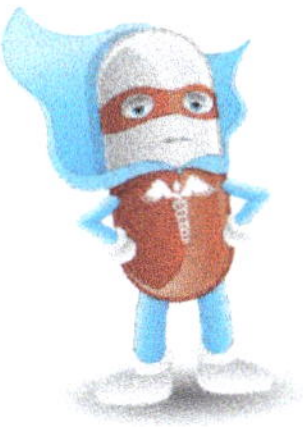

Cytochrome P450 1A2 (CYP1A2)

"One Axe to Grind; One Axe to Grow"

52% of individuals are 1A2 ultrarapid metabolizers;
< 1% are poor metabolizers

"1 Axe to 2 Grind"

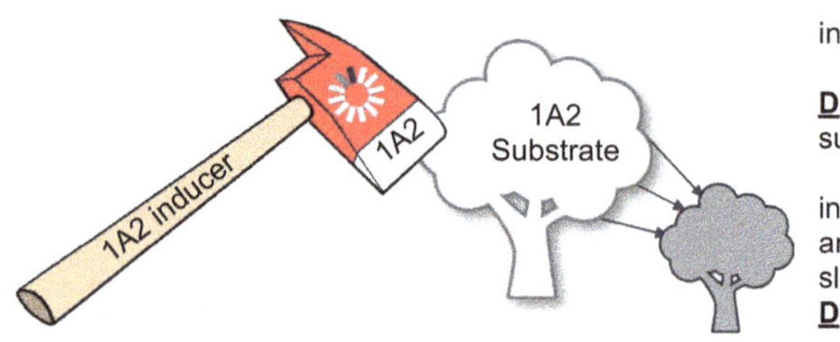

inDucer = Down

Decreased substrate levels

induction onsets and reverses slowly = Delayed *

Hydrocarbons from smoked herbs such as tobacco and cannabis are moderate potency 1A2 inducers. All other 1A2 inducers are weak.

"1 Axe 2 Grow"

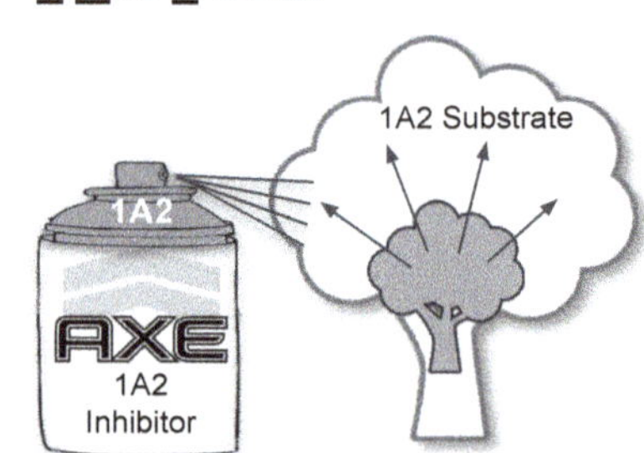

inHibitor = High

Increased substrate levels

inHibition happens within Hours = Hurried and reverses as soon as the inhibitor is cleared from the body (five half-lives of the inhibitor)

Fluvoxamine (Luvox) is the only strong 1A2 inhibitor.

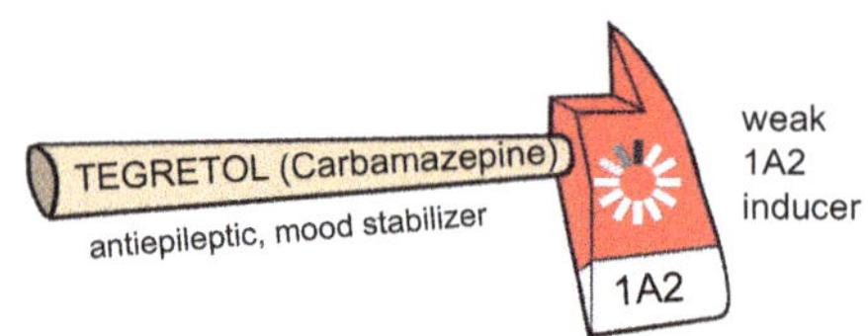

weak 1A2 inducer

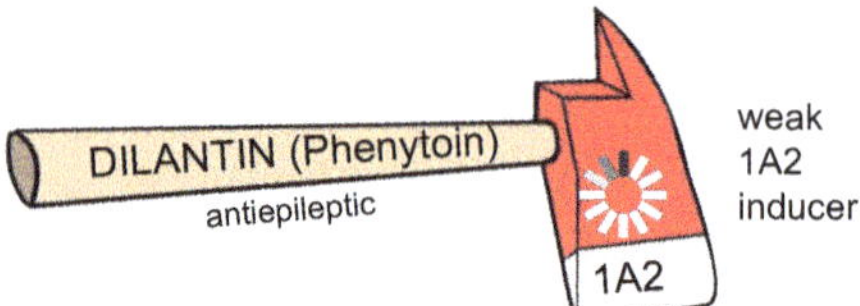

weak 1A2 inducer

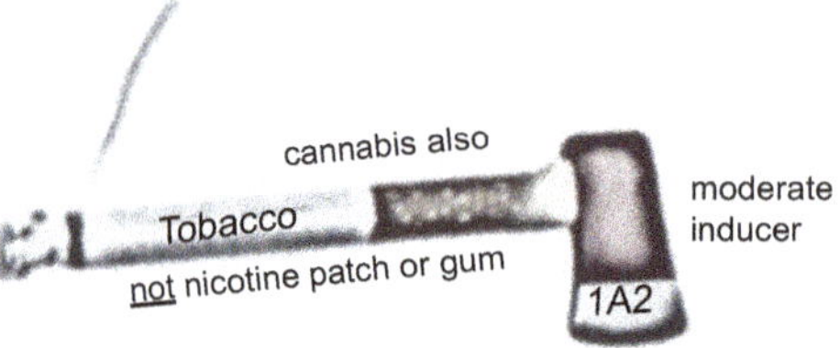

moderate inducer

* Induction by smoking takes about 3 days to start—notice the ax has no spinning wheel like the other axes. Upon cessation of smoking, induction reverses over the first week. This is much faster than with other inducers. 10 cigarettes daily is sufficient for maximum induction effect.

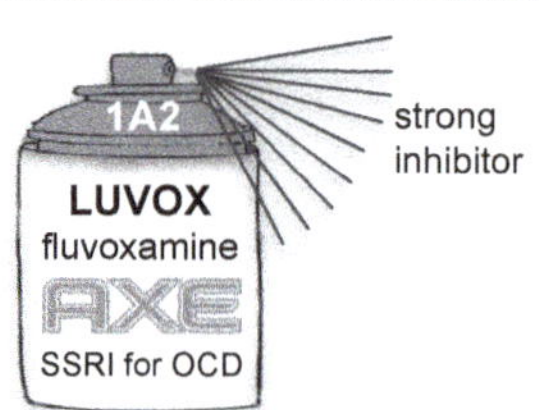

strong inhibitor

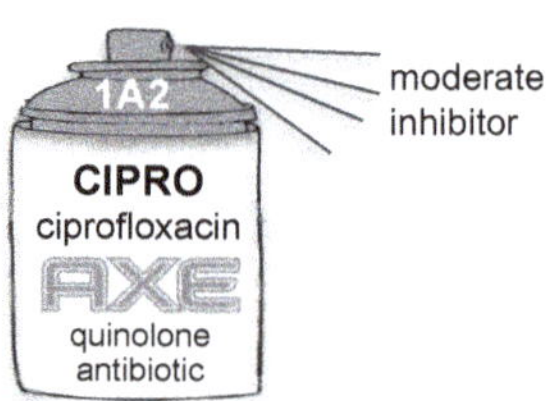

moderate inhibitor

1st Generation Antipsychotics

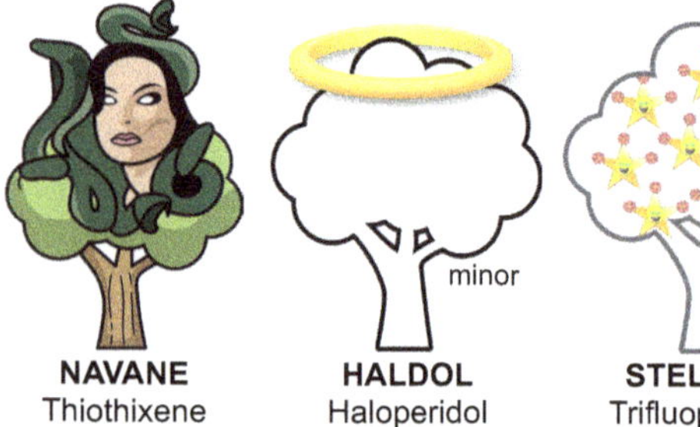

NAVANE Thiothixene

HALDOL Haloperidol (minor)

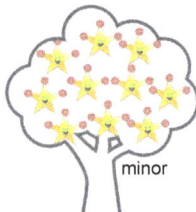

STELAZINE Trifluoperazine (minor)

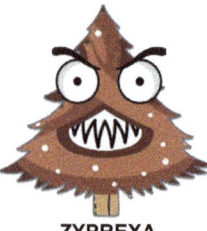

2nd Gen Antipsychotics "-pine" trees

ZYPREXA Olanzapine
~50% increase by Luvox

CLOZARIL Clozapine
3-fold increase by Luvox

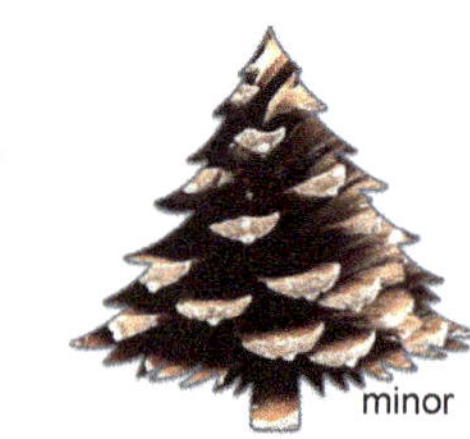

SAPHRIS Asenapine
Negligible decrease by tobacco

Antidepressant

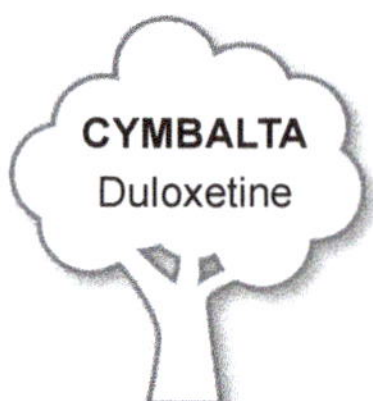

3-fold increase by Luvox

Melatonin agonists

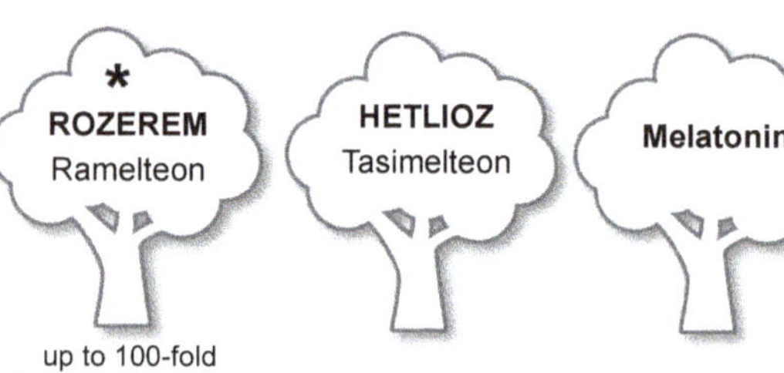

Rozerem: up to 100-fold increase by Luvox

Methylxanthines

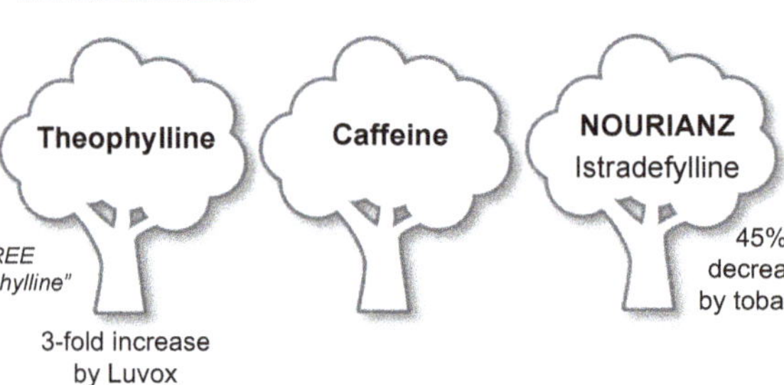

Theophylline: 3-fold increase by Luvox

Spasmolytic

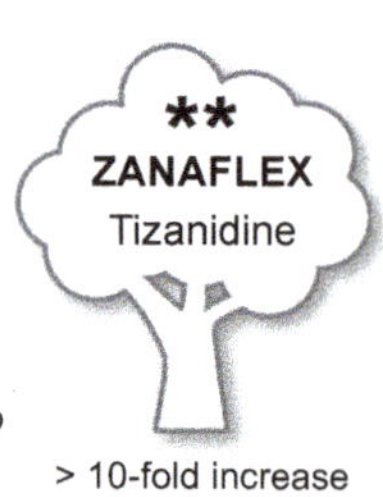

> 10-fold increase by Luvox

* Contraindicated with Luvox
** Contraindicated with Luvox or Cipro

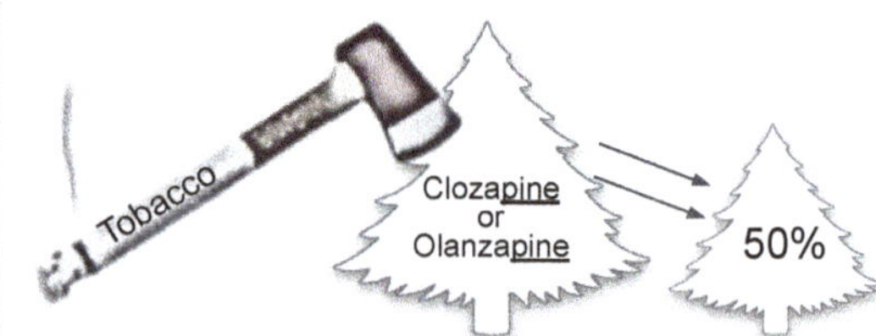

Tobacco Decreases blood levels of these two "pine trees" by about 50%.

Conclusion: Keep in mind that 52% of individuals have a 1A2 ultrarapid metabolizer genotype, and everyone who smokes has a rapid metabolizer phenotype. The effect of smoking on olanzapine and clozapine is worthy of memorization. Memorization of other 1A2 substrates is of lower priority, as long as you remember to refer to this list whenever Luvox is in the mix. Run an interaction check on any medication regimen that includes Luvox. Try to keep Luvox out of the mix entirely—it is nonessential for treatment of OCD because other SSRIs are equally effective at high doses.

Ciprofloxacin, a moderate 1A2 inHibitor, increases clozapine levels about 2-fold.

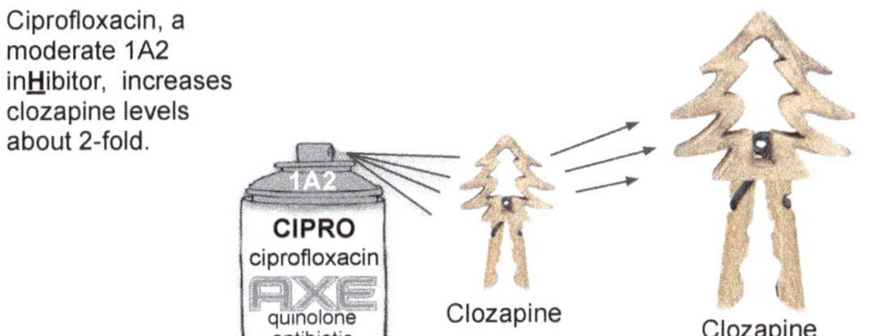

Fluvoxamine, a strong 1A2 inHibitor, increases clozapine levels 3-fold on average, but up to 10-fold in some cases.

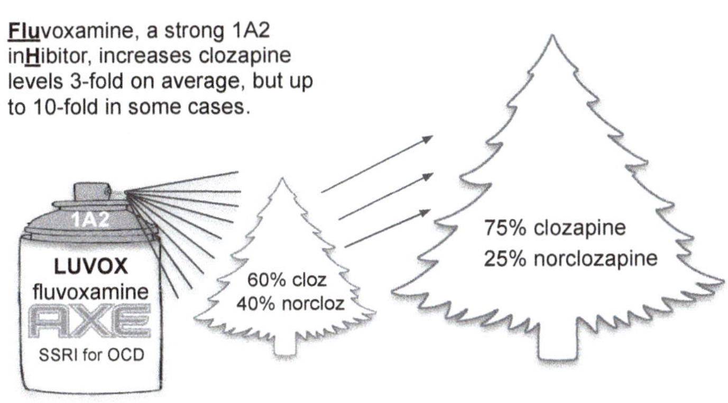

Kinetic interactions can be more complicated than simply increasing/decreasing concentrations of victim substrates.

Combining clozapine and fluvoxamine is hazardous, but can potentially be used for therapeutic advantage. Close monitoring of serum **clozapine levels** would be required.

Norclozapine is the main metabolite of clozapine, formed by 1A2 metabolism. When clozapine blood levels are reported, clozapine and metabolite (norclozapine) levels are provided separately. Through 1A2 inHibition, Luvox increases the **clozapine:norclozapine ratio**. A Higher serum clozapine:norclozapine ratio is generally considered desirable*. Norclozapine provides little antipsychotic benefit and causes weight gain, diabetes, seizures, and neutropenia.

Patients given clozapine 100 mg + Luvox 50 mg daily (compared to clozapine 300 mg monotherapy) demonstrated more improvement with less weight gain. Clozapine levels were similar for both groups with, as expected, lower norclozapine levels for those taking Luvox.
(Lu ML et al, 2018; randomized controlled trial, N=85).

*The negative aspect of a Higher clozapine:norclozapine is greater anticholinergic burden (pages 59-60). Clozapine is anticholinergic, whereas norclozapine is cholinergic. Consequently, clozapine causes constipation, while norclozapine does not. The anticholinergic properties of clozapine may impair cognition, whereas norclozapine may provide cognitive benefits such as enhanced working memory.

Certain physiologic states may increase levels of olanzapine and clozapine up to 2-fold.

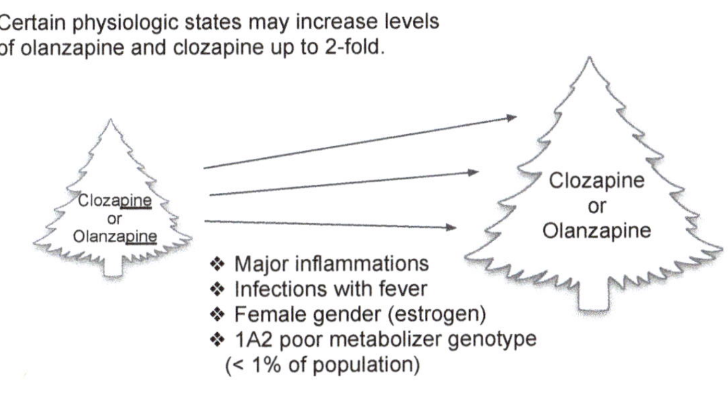

- Major inflammations
- Infections with fever
- Female gender (estrogen)
- 1A2 poor metabolizer genotype (< 1% of population)

For a patient with efficacy or tolerability issues, consider monitoring serum levels of the antipsychotic. The author checks clozapine levels routinely, and olanzapine levels in some cases.

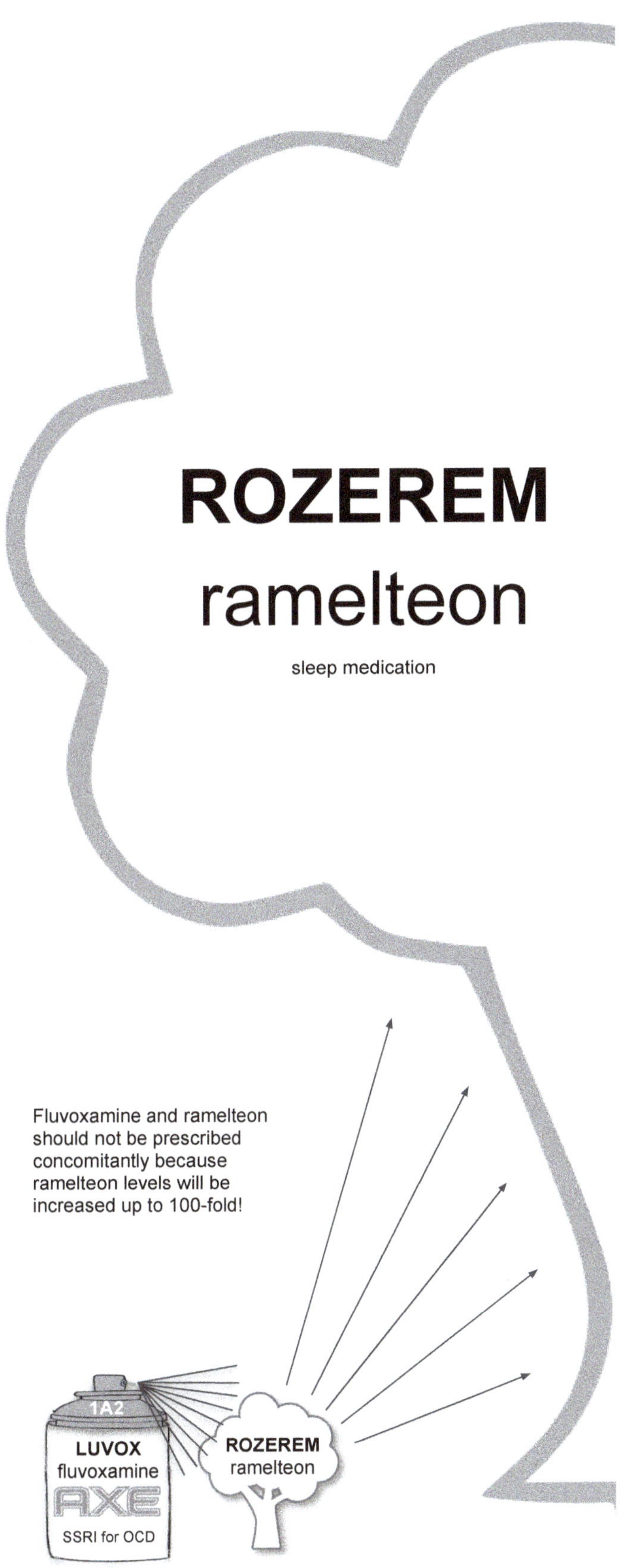

Fluvoxamine and ramelteon should not be prescribed concomitantly because ramelteon levels will be increased up to 100-fold!

No antipsychotics are involved in 2B6 metabolism.

Cytochrome P450 2B6 (CYP2B6)

"Tube Socks"

3% of individuals are 2B6 ultrarapid metabolizers; 7% are poor metabolizers

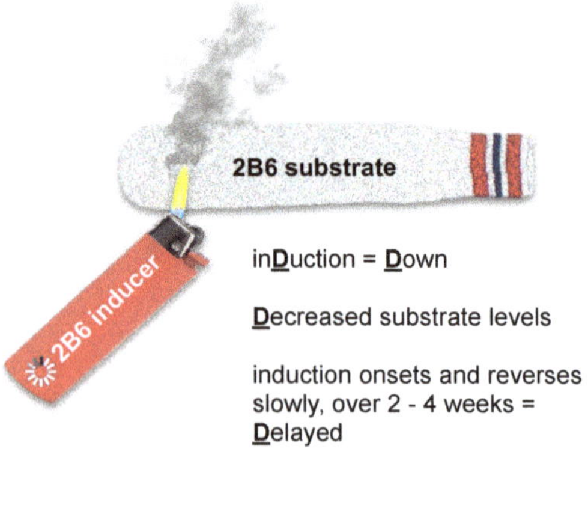

inDuction = Down

Decreased substrate levels

induction onsets and reverses slowly, over 2 - 4 weeks = Delayed

There are no strong 2B6 inducers.

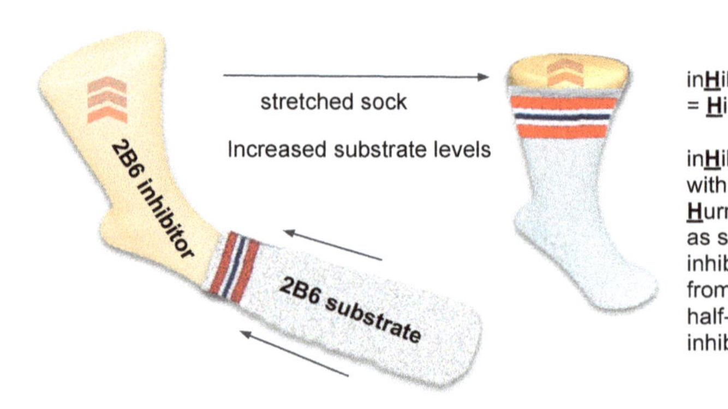

stretched sock

Increased substrate levels

inHibition = High

inHibition happens within Hours = Hurried and reverses as soon as the inhibitor is cleared from the body (five half-lives of the inhibitor)

There are no strong 2B6 inhibitors.

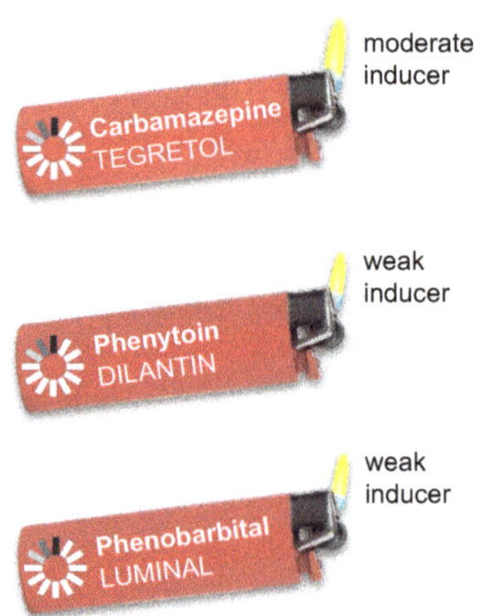

Carbamazepine (TEGRETOL): moderate inducer

Phenytoin (DILANTIN): weak inducer

Phenobarbital (LUMINAL): weak inducer

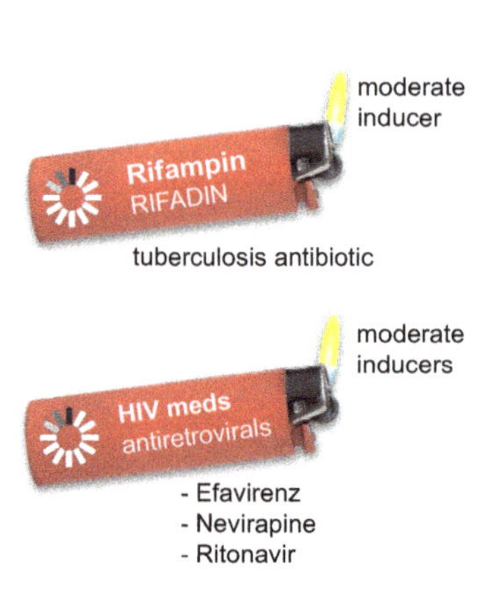

Rifampin (RIFADIN): moderate inducer

tuberculosis antibiotic

HIV meds (antiretrovirals): moderate inducers

- Efavirenz
- Nevirapine
- Ritonavir

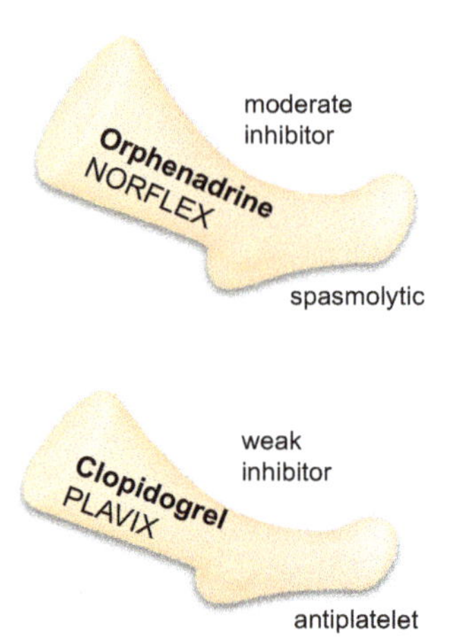

Orphenadrine (NORFLEX): moderate inhibitor

spasmolytic

Clopidogrel (PLAVIX): weak inhibitor

antiplatelet

Antidepressants

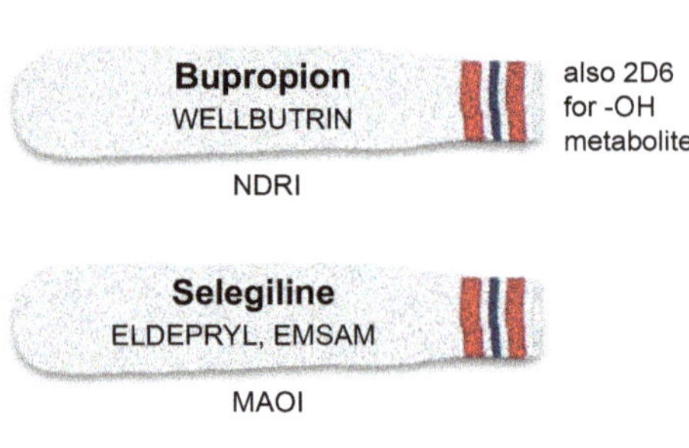

Bupropion (WELLBUTRIN): also 2D6 for -OH metabolite

NDRI

Selegiline (ELDEPRYL, EMSAM)

MAOI

Alkylating Drugs for Cancer

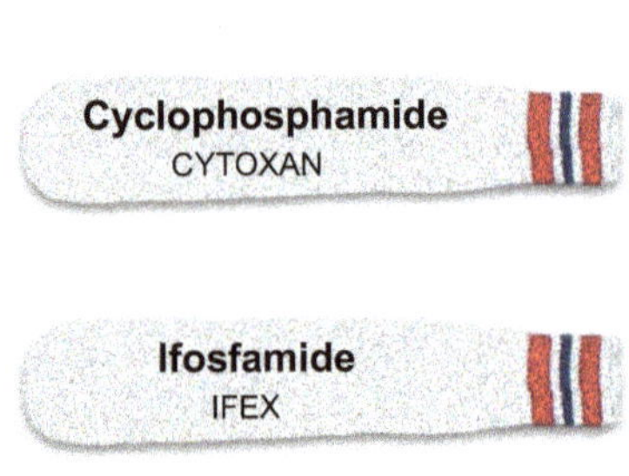

Opioid

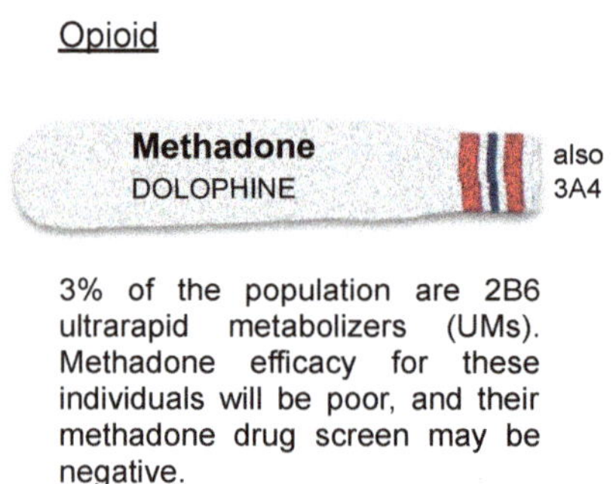

Methadone (DOLOPHINE): also 3A4

3% of the population are 2B6 ultrarapid metabolizers (UMs). Methadone efficacy for these individuals will be poor, and their methadone drug screen may be negative.

Anaesthetics

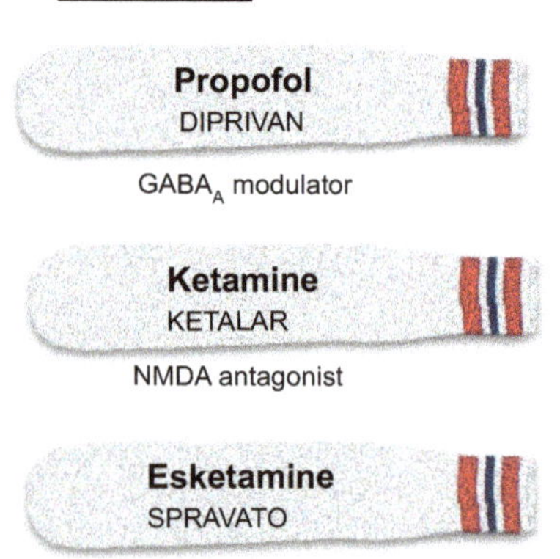

Propofol (DIPRIVAN): $GABA_A$ modulator

Ketamine (KETALAR): NMDA antagonist

Esketamine (SPRAVATO): NMDA antagonist

NNRTIs for HIV

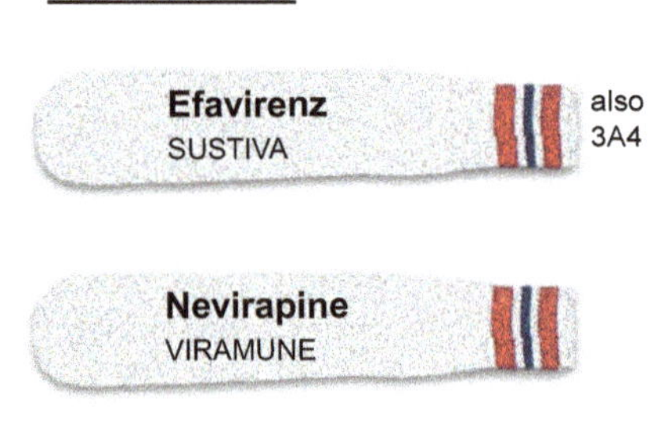

Efavirenz (SUSTIVA): also 3A4

Conclusion: Fortunately, there are no strong inhibitors or inducers of 2B6. For psychiatrists, 2B6 is of minimal significance, unless methadone is being prescribed (see above). You will want to run an interaction check (e.g., ePocrates or Lexicomp) whenever a medication regimen includes a shredder, cancer medication, HIV medication, or systemic antifungal.

For psychiatry, 2C9 interactions are of little clinical significance. No antipsychotics are involved.

Cytochrome P450 2C9 (CYP2C9)

"To See Nice(ly)"

0% of individuals are 2C9 ultrarapid metabolizers; 5% are poor metabolizers

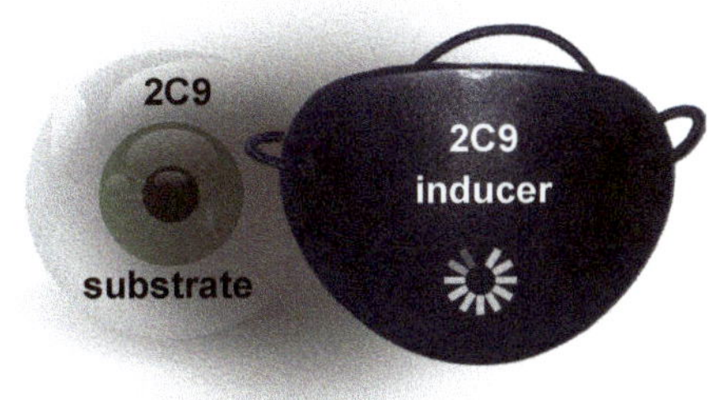

in**D**uction = **D**own

Decreased substrate levels

induction onsets and reverses slowly, over 2 - 4 weeks = **D**elayed

There are no strong 2C9 inducers.

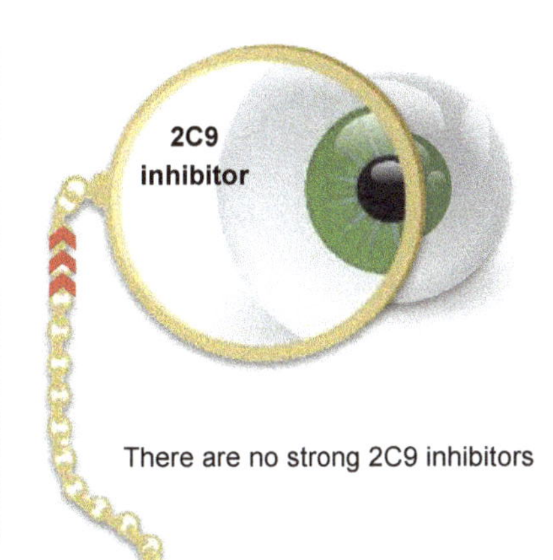

in**H**ibition = **H**igh

Increased substrate levels

in**H**ibition happens within **H**ours = **H**urried

Inhibition reverses as soon as the inhibitor is cleared from the body (five half-lives of the inhibitor)

There are no strong 2C9 inhibitors

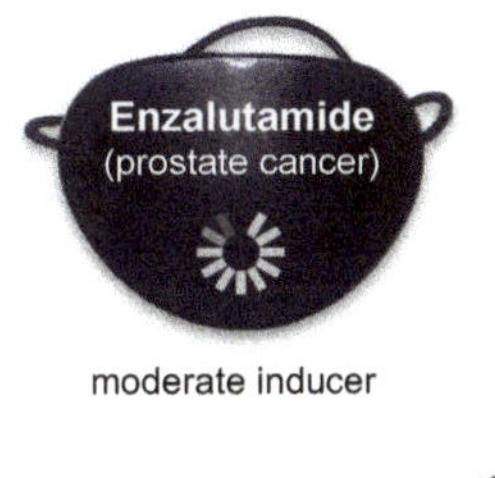

moderate inducer

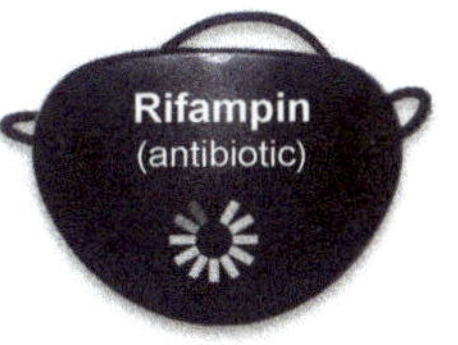

moderate inducer

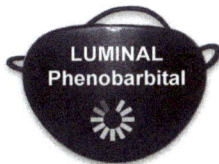

LUMINAL
Phenobarbital

weak inducer

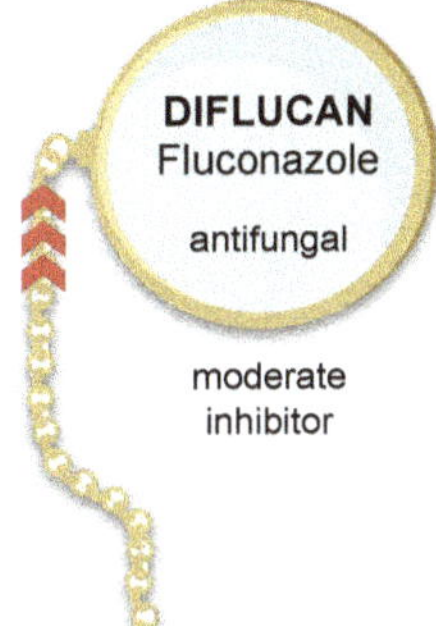

moderate inhibitor

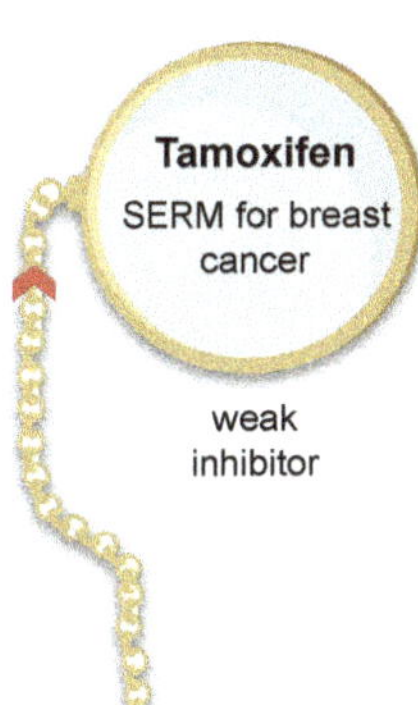

weak inhibitor

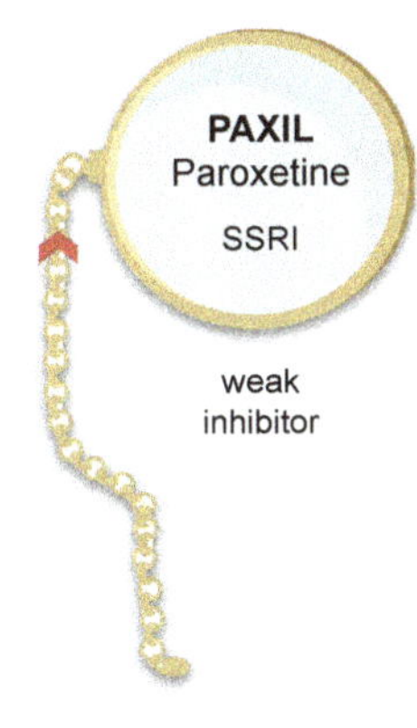

weak inhibitor

Antiepileptics

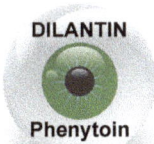

DILANTIN
Phenytoin

"d-EYE-lantin; phen-EYE-toin"

Also 2C19

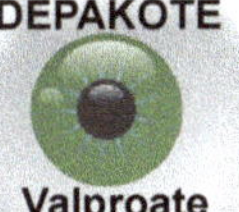

"Dep-EYE-kote"

2C9 contributes only 25% to the metabolism of VPA

Anticoagulant

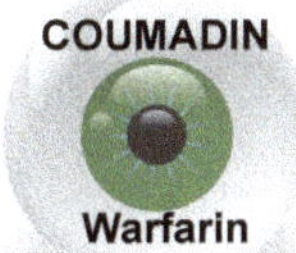

"coum-EYE-din"

Also 2C19

Sulfonylureas for DM

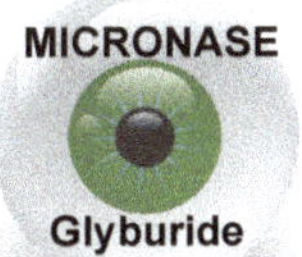

"glybur-EYED"

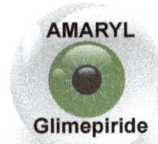

AMARYL
Glimepiride

"glimepir-EYED"

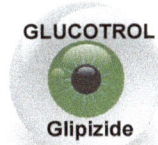

GLUCOTROL
Glipizide

"Glipiz-EYED"

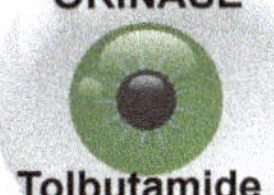

"tolbutam-EYED"

ARB for HTN

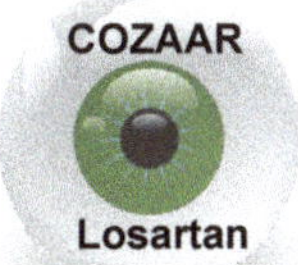

"Coz-EYEr"

Also 3A4

Lipid lowering

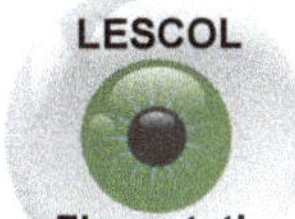

"fluv-EYE-statin"

Libido enhancer

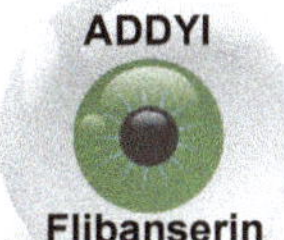

"Add-EYE"

NSAID

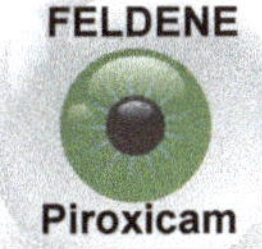

"p-EYE-roxicam"

COX-2 inhibitor

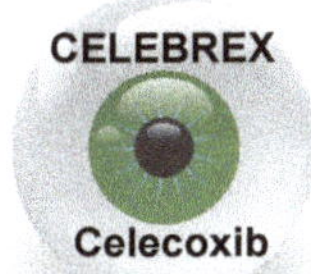

"cel-EYE-brex"

Conclusion: Consider checking valproic acid (VPA) levels more often if the patient is taking enzalutamide, rifampin or diflucan; but don't expect much variance from baseline. Avoid prescribing paroxetine (Paxil) entirely.

No antipsychotics are involved in 2C19 metabolism, unless you count CBD oil.

Cytochrome P450 2C19 (CYP2C19)

"To See Nice Things (grow)"

10% of individuals are 2C19 ultrarapid metabolizers; 5% are poor metabolizers

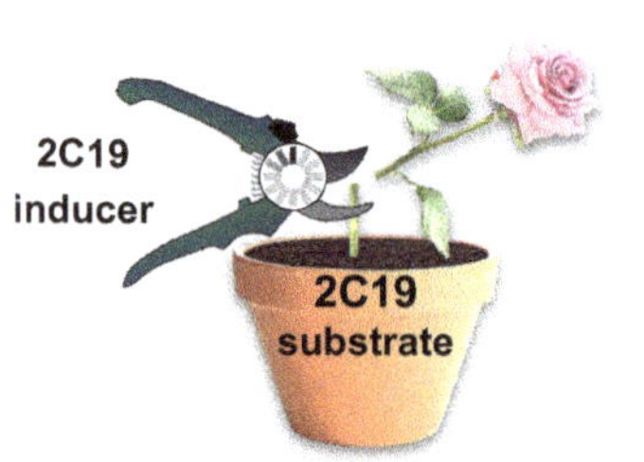

in**D**uction = **D**own

Decreased substrate levels

induction onsets and reverses slowly, over 2 - 4 weeks = **D**elayed

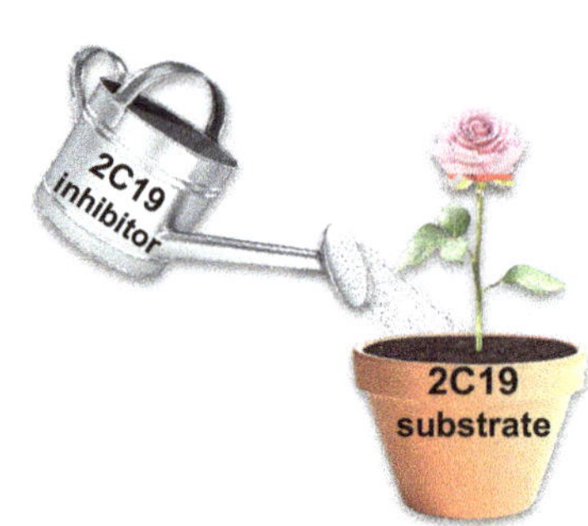

2C19
Inhibitor
2C19
substrate

in**H**ibition = **H**igh

Increased substrate levels

in**H**ibition happens within **H**ours = **H**urried

Inhibition reverses as soon as the inhibitor is cleared from the body (five half-lives of the inhibitor)

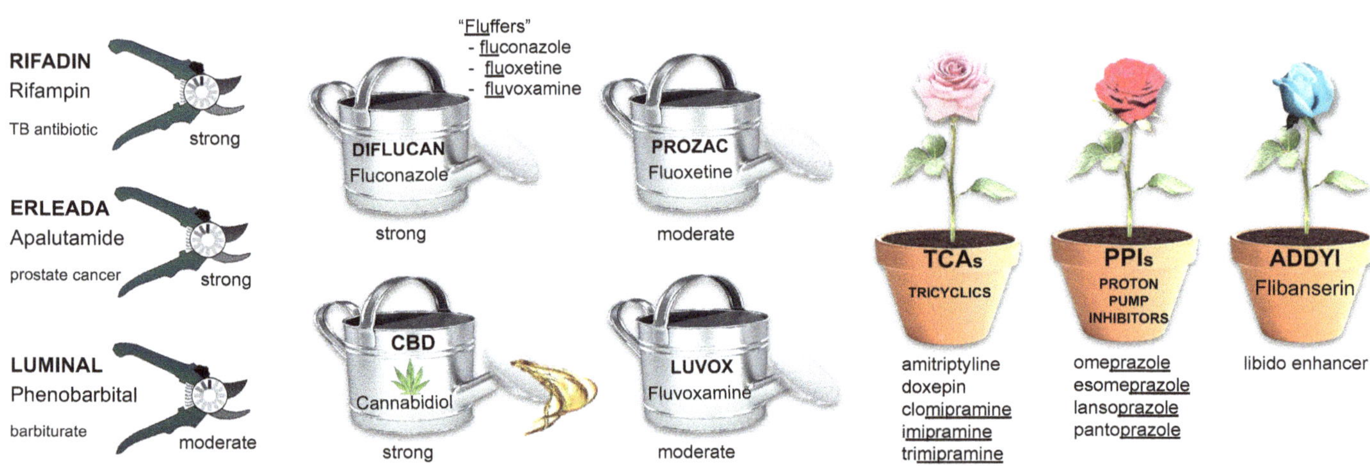

RIFADIN
Rifampin
TB antibiotic
strong
ERLEADA
Apalutamide
prostate cancer
strong
LUMINAL
Phenobarbital
barbiturate
moderate
"Fluffers"
- fluconazole
- fluoxetine
- fluvoxamine
DIFLUCAN
Fluconazole
strong
PROZAC
Fluoxetine
moderate
CBD
Cannabidiol
strong
LUVOX
Fluvoxamine
moderate
TCAs
TRICYCLICS
PPIs
PROTON PUMP INHIBITORS
ADDYI
Flibanserin

amitriptyline
doxepin
clomipramine
imipramine
trimipramine

omeprazole
esomeprazole
lansoprazole
pantoprazole

libido enhancer

SSRI antidepressants

Sedative/Antiepileptic

Anticoagulant

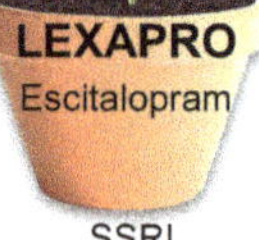

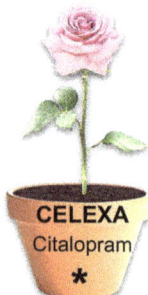

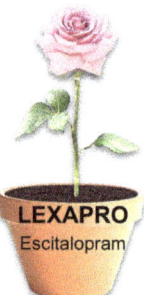

- CELEXA Citalopram * — SSRI
- LEXAPRO Escitalopram — SSRI
- ZOLOFT Sertraline — SSRI
- SOMA Carisoprodol — spasmolytic
- LUMINAL Phenobarbital — barbiturate
- DILANTIN Phenytoin — antiepileptic
- VALIUM Diazepam — BZD
- ONFI Clobazam — BZD
- COUMADIN Warfarin — Vitamin K "antagonist"

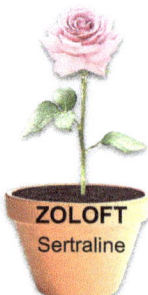

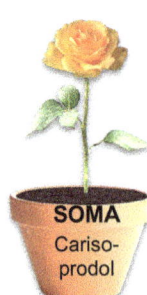

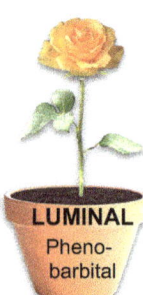

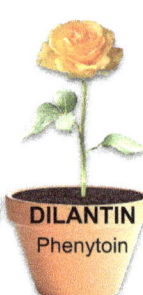

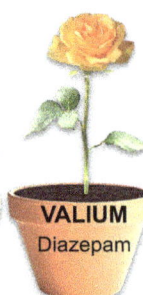

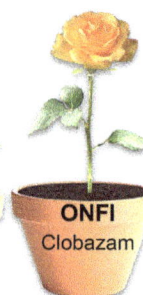

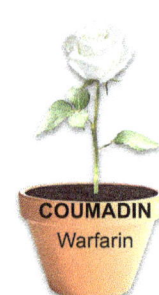

2C19 poor metabolizers (PM)

Individuals with a 2C19 PM genotype clear 2C19 substrates slowly, leading to **H**igher blood levels (as if they were taking a 2C19 in**H**ibitor). Standard doses of 2C19 substrates may be too strong.

* 2C19 poor metabolizers should not exceed 20 mg of citalopram (QT prolongation).

5% of population (20% of Asians)

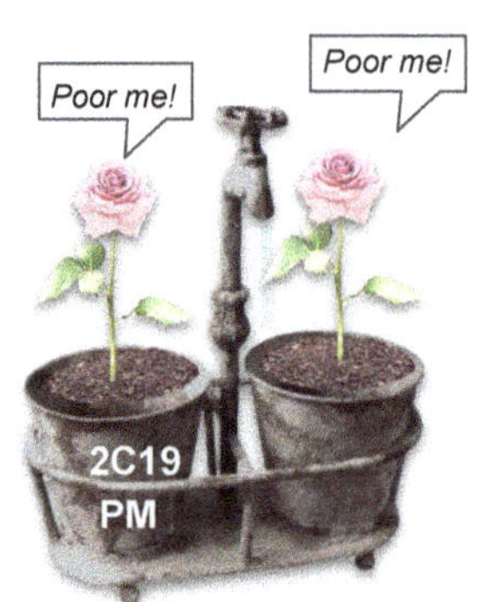

Poor me!
Poor me!
2C19
PM

2C19 ultrarapid metabolizers (UM)

2C19 UM individuals clear 2C19 substrates quickly, leading to low blood levels. These individuals are more likely to be non-responders to 2C19 substrates.

10% of population

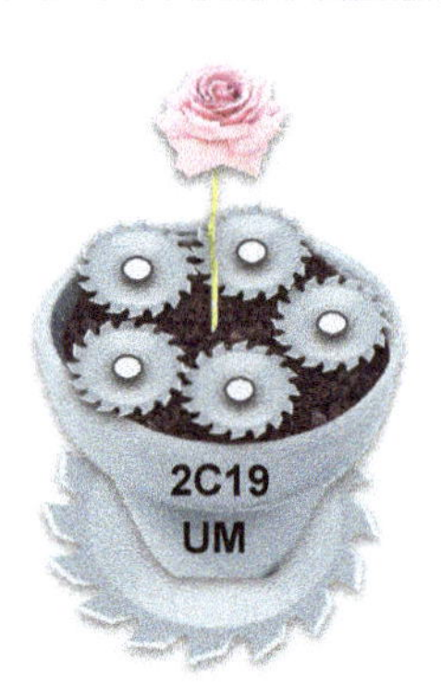

2C19
UM

Conclusion: 2C19 genotyping is not typically ordered as a standalone test, but if 2C19 metabolizer genotype is known (e.g., from GeneSight or Genecept), the information can be put to good use when dosing (es)citalopram and sertraline. Knowledge of metabolizer status is not essential because these SSRIs can be titrated the old-fashioned way, according to response and side effects. In any event, avoid prescribing Soma, Valium, or phenobarbital for anxiety due to their particularly high risk of abuse and dependence. Avoid St. John's Wort due to interactions, and because it only works for mild depression.

2D6 metabolizes ~ 12% of prescription drugs. Notice how all of the -oxetine's are 2D6 inhibitors and/or substrates.

Cytochrome P450 2D6 (CYP2D6)

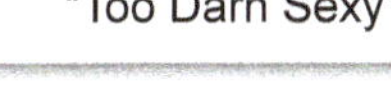

5% of individuals are 2D6 ultrarapid metabolizers (UM).
10% are poor metabolizers (PM).

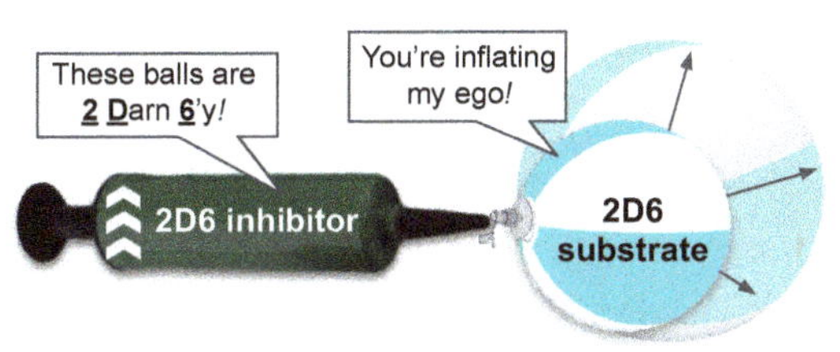

2D6 enzymes cannot be induced.

inHibition = High

Increased substrate levels

inHibition happens within Hours = Hurried

Inhibition reverses as soon as the inhibitor is cleared from the body (five half-lives of the inhibitor)

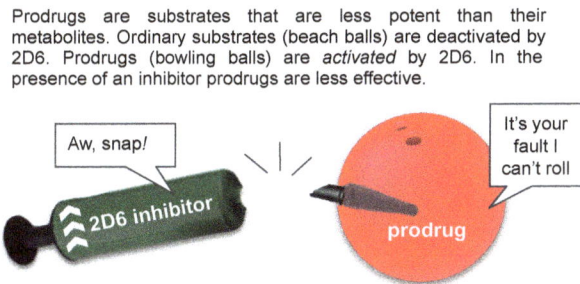

Prodrugs are substrates that are less potent than their metabolites. Ordinary substrates (beach balls) are deactivated by 2D6. Prodrugs (bowling balls) are *activated* by 2D6. In the presence of an inhibitor prodrugs are less effective.

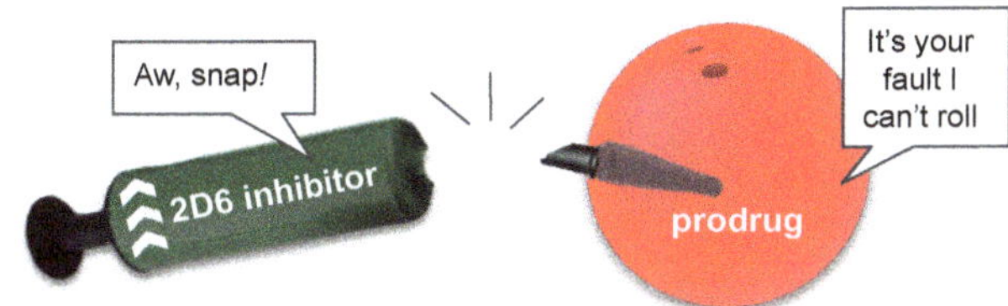

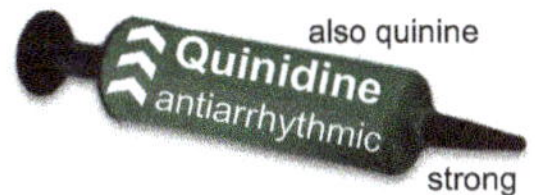

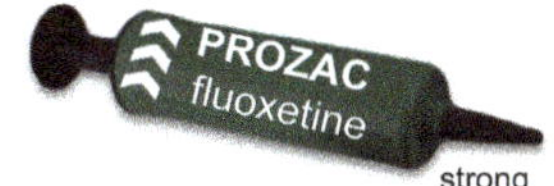

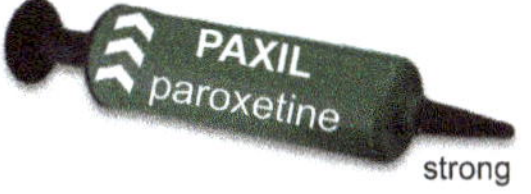

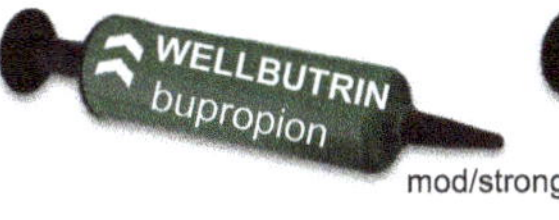

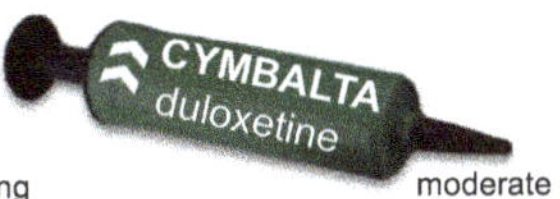

Antidepressants

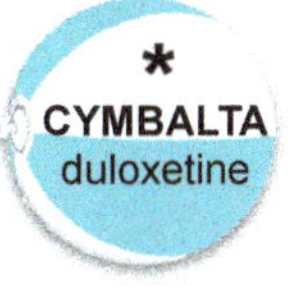

SNRI

SNRI for ADHD

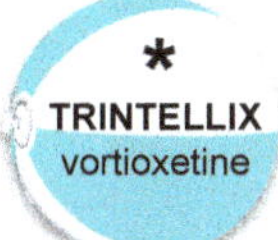

SPARI

active metabolite of bupropion (Wellbutrin)

especially:
amoxapine
protriptyline
(nortriptyline)
(desipramine)

VMAT inhibitors

tetrabenazine
deutetrabenazine
valbenazine

Antitussive

Anti-HTN

beta blocker

1st Gen Antipsychotics (FGA)

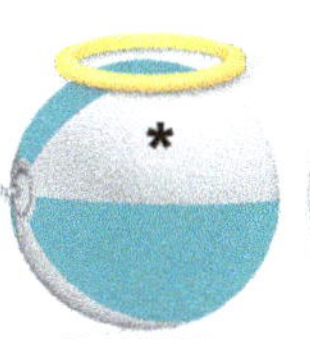

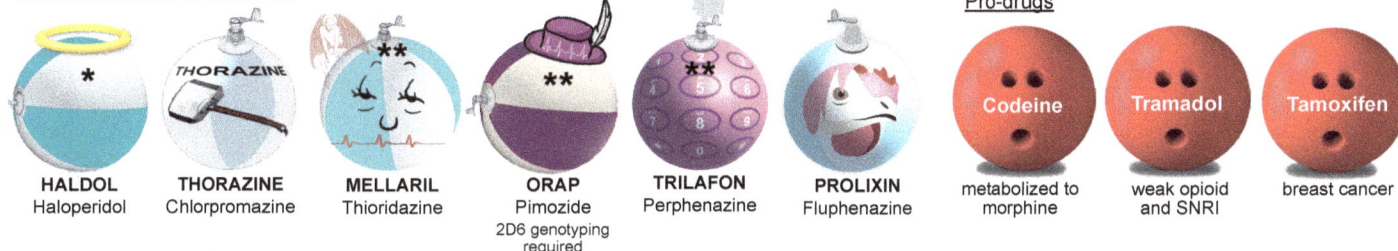

HALDOL
Haloperidol

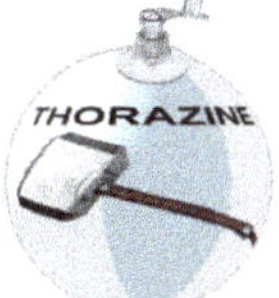

THORAZINE
Chlorpromazine

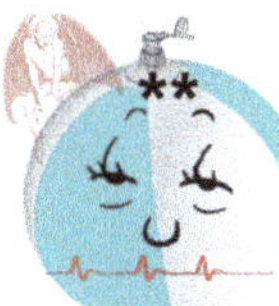

MELLARIL
Thioridazine

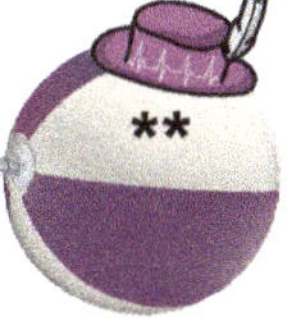

ORAP
Pimozide
2D6 genotyping required

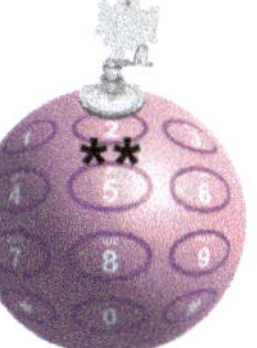

TRILAFON
Perphenazine

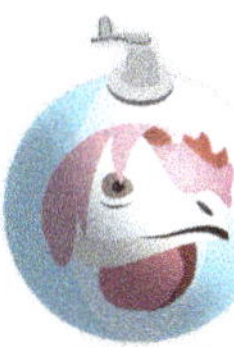

PROLIXIN
Fluphenazine

Pro-drugs

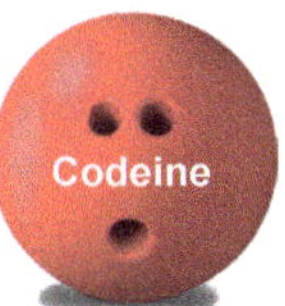
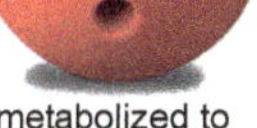

metabolized to morphine

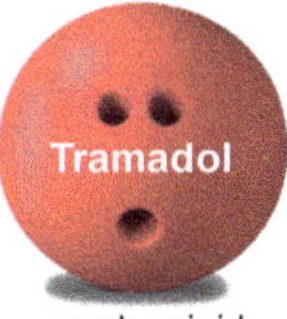

weak opioid and SNRI

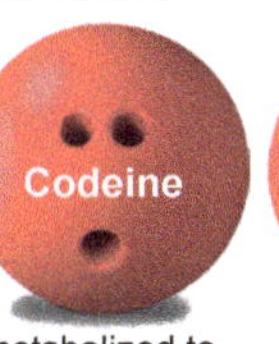
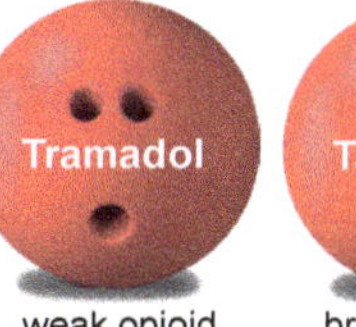

breast cancer

2nd Gen Antipsychotics (SGA)

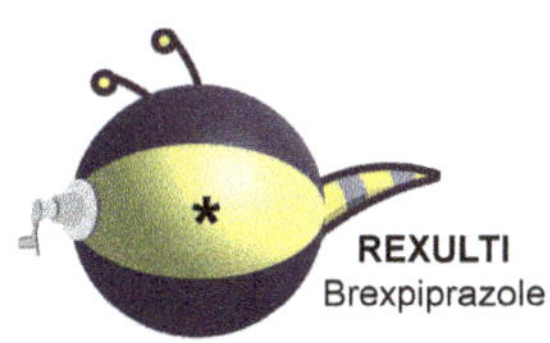

REXULTI
Brexpiprazole

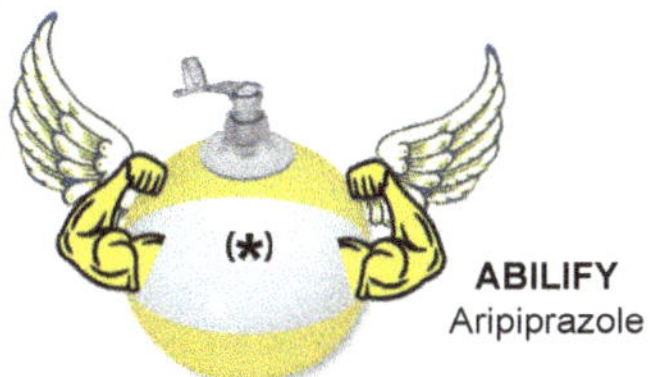

ABILIFY
Aripiprazole

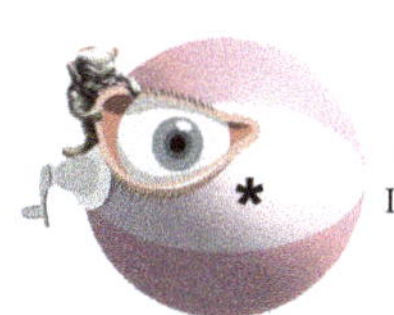

FANAPT
Iloperidone

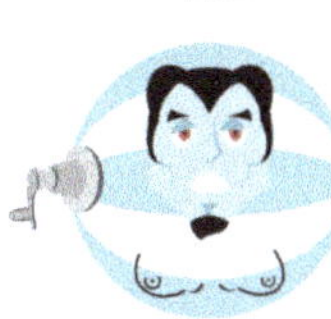

RISPERDAL
Risperidone

2D6 <u>poor</u> <u>metabolizers</u>

2D6 **poor metabolizers** have defective 2D6 enzymes. Substrates are cleared slowly (by other pathways) or are unmetabolized leading to Higher blood levels, **as if** the patient were taking an inHibitor.

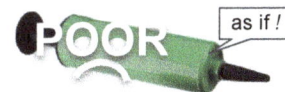

****** 2D6 genotyping is recommended prior to starting these medications, which are increased 3--4-fold with 2D6 PMs. Mellaril is contraindicated for 2D6 PMs.

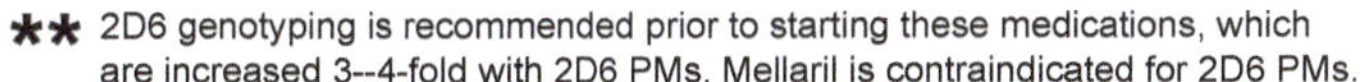

***** 50% dose reduction is recommended for 2D6 poor metabolizers

(*) According to the label, use 75% of Abilify dose if the individual is a 2D6 PM. Use 50% Abilify dose if 2D6 PM and taking a 3A4 inhibitor.

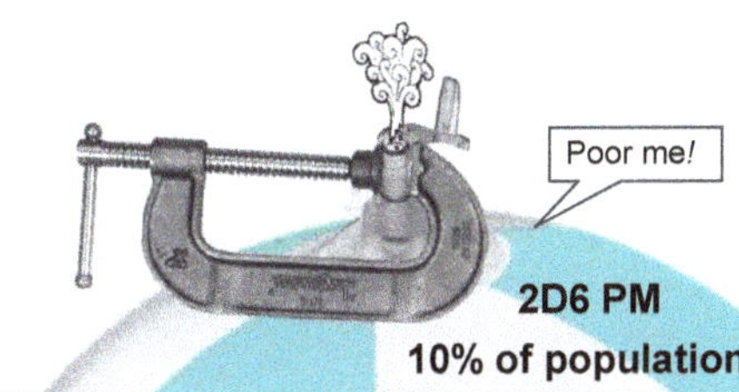

2D6 extensive metabolizers

have the typical genotype and process 2D6 substrates as expected

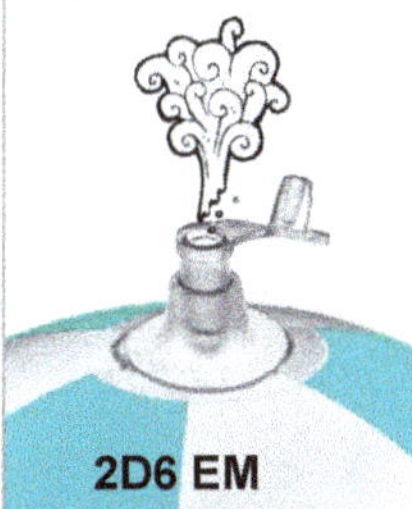

2D6 ultrarapid metabolizers

clear 2D6 substrates quickly. These individuals are more likely to be non-responders to 2D6 substrates (excluding 2D6 prodrugs, which may be too strong). This genotype is relatively common among those with Middle Eastern or North African heritage.

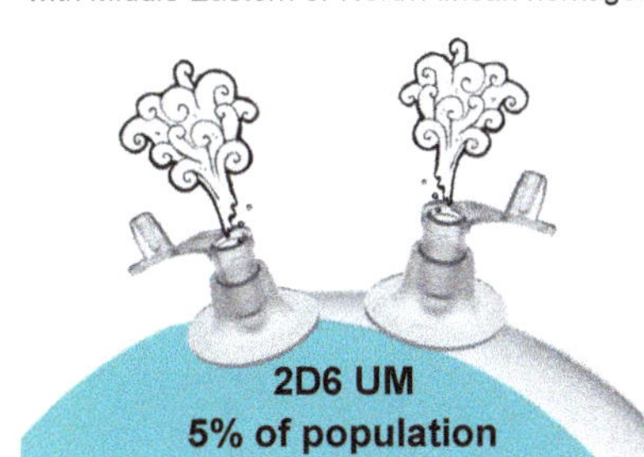

Conclusion: 2D6 interactions need to be understood by prescribers of antidepressants and antipsychotics. To avoid 2D6 interactions, use Lexapro or Zoloft instead of Prozac/Paxil. Consider Invega ($330) instead of Risperdal ($12), although cost is an issue.

Among the CYP genetic assays, 2D6 is the most useful. The test is about $200 as a standalone, and is recommended prior to starting Trilafon, Mellaril, or Orap—three antipsychotics that psychiatrists rarely prescribe. For the other 2D6 substrates, serum drug levels may be more useful than genotyping. The author checks blood levels of haloperidol, risperidone and aripiprazole when there are issues with efficacy or tolerability.

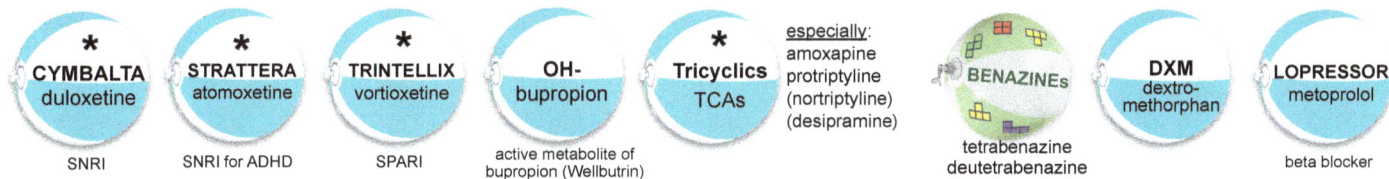

Cytochrome P450 3A4 (CYP3A4)

"3 A's For (fishing)"

> 50% of prescription drugs are 3A4 substrates – plenty of fish!

0% of individuals are 3A4 ultrarapid metabolizers; <1% are poor metabolizers

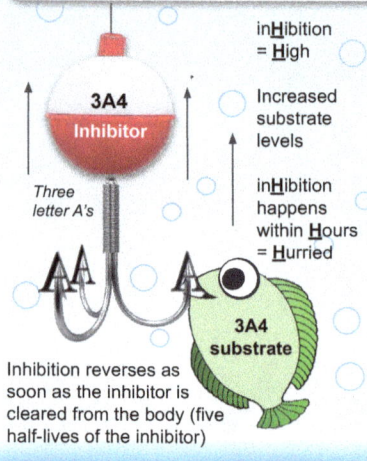

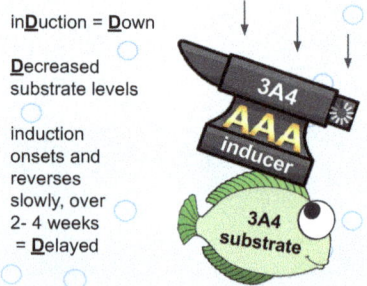

3A4 Inhibitor

Three letter A's

inHibition = High

Increased substrate levels

inHibition happens within Hours = Hurried

3A4 substrate

Inhibition reverses as soon as the inhibitor is cleared from the body (five half-lives of the inhibitor)

inDuction = Down

Decreased substrate levels

induction onsets and reverses slowly, over 2- 4 weeks = Delayed

3A4 AAA inducer

3A4 substrate

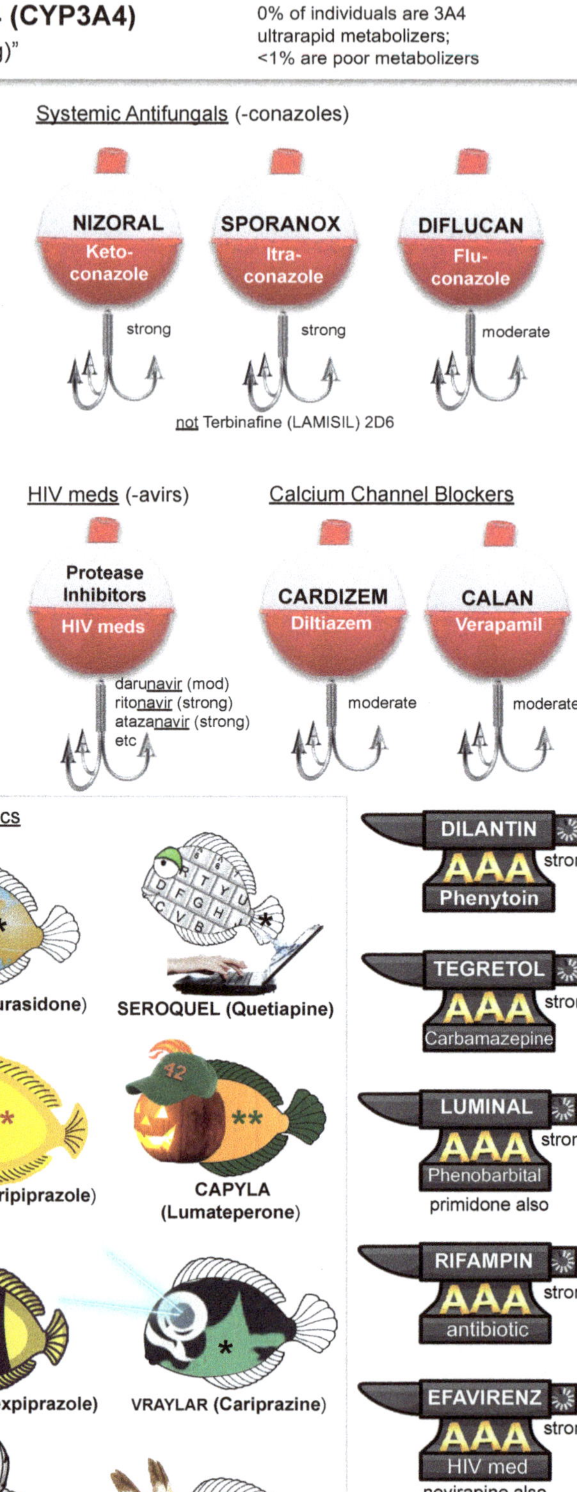

Macrolide Antibiotics (-mycins)

- BIAXIN Clarithromycin — strong
- E-MYCIN Erythromycin — moderate

not Azithromycin (ZITHROMAX)

Systemic Antifungals (-conazoles)

- NIZORAL Ketoconazole — strong
- SPORANOX Itraconazole — strong
- DIFLUCAN Fluconazole — moderate

not Terbinafine (LAMISIL) 2D6

Grapefruit Juice — moderate

Antidepressant

- SERZONE Nefazodone SARI — strong

HIV meds (-avirs)

- Protease Inhibitors HIV meds — darunavir (mod), ritonavir (strong), atazanavir (strong), etc

Calcium Channel Blockers

- CARDIZEM Diltiazem — moderate
- CALAN Verapamil — moderate

PDE-5 inhibitors * — Viagra, etc

ADDYI Flibanserin **

Contraceptives — estrogens, progestins

VIIBRYD Vilazodone *

BUSPAR Buspirone *

SUBOXONE Buprenorphine

BELSOMRA Suvorexant — also lemborexant (Dayvigo)

INGREZZA (Valbenazine) *

Benzodiazepines

- XANAX Alprazolam **
- LIBRIUM Chlordiazepoxide
- KLONOPIN Clonazepam

also:
Diazepam (Valium)
Estazolam (Prosom) **
Midazolam (Versed) **
Triazolam (Halcion) **
Clorazepate(Tranxene)

not:
Lorazepam (Ativan)
Oxazepam (Serax))
Temazepam (Restoril)
Clobazam (Onfi) 2C19

Antipsychotics

- LATUDA (Lurasidone) **
- SEROQUEL (Quetiapine) *
- ABILIFY (Aripiprazole) * — also 2D6
- CAPYLA (Lumateperone) **
- REXULTI (Brexpiprazole) *
- VRAYLAR (Cariprazine) *
- ORAP (Pimozide) ** — also 2D6
- Pimavanserin (NUPLAZID) *

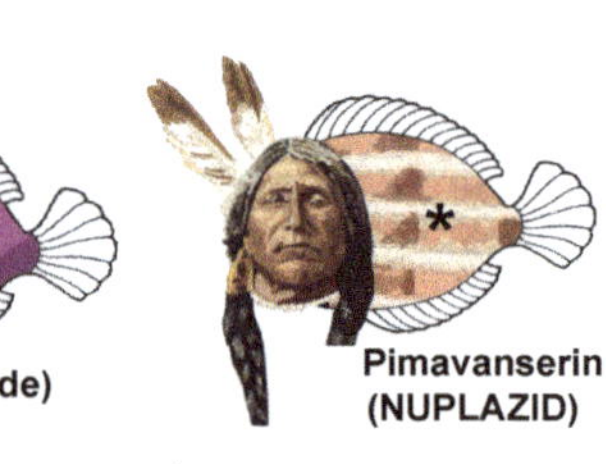

minor 3A4 substrates:
Chlorpromazine (Thorazine)
Clozapine (Clozaril)
Haloperidol (Haldol)
Iloperidone (Fanapt)
Loxapine (Loxitane)
Perphenazine (Trilafon)
Risperidone (Risperdal)
Ziprasidone (Geodon)

not:
Asenapine (Saphris) 1A2
Fluphenazine (Prolixin) 2D6
Molindone (Moban)
Olanzapine (Zyprexa) 1A2
Paliperidone (Invega)
Promethazine (Phenergan)
Thiothixene (Navane) 1A2
Trifluoperazine (Stelazine) 1A2

Inducers (AAA):

- DILANTIN Phenytoin — strong
- TEGRETOL Carbamazepine — strong
- LUMINAL Phenobarbital — strong; primidone also
- RIFAMPIN antibiotic — strong
- EFAVIRENZ HIV med — strong; nevirapine also
- St John's Wort (SJW) — mod

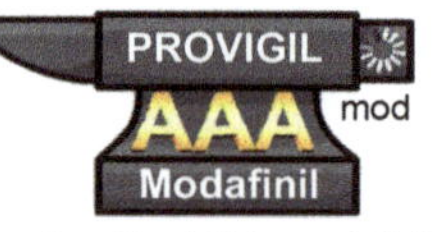

- PROVIGIL Modafinil — mod

weaker: Nuvigil (armodafinil)

There is risk of rhabdomyolysis when HMG-CoA reductase inhibitors (statins) are combined with 3A4 inHibitors.

STATINS ** — simvastatin, atorvastatin

not:
Pravastatin (Pravachol)
Rosuvastatin (Crestor)
Fluvastatin (Lescol)

* Dosing adjustments defined

** Has contraindications related to kinetic interactions

Conclusion: 3A4 is the workhorse of CYP metabolism, accounting for 30% of hepatic CYP activity and 70% of CYP activity in the gut. Since >50% of drugs are 3A4 substrates, think twice before prescribing strong 3A4 inhibitors or inducers.

UGT interactions

Phase II metabolism

18% of individuals are UGT1A4 ultrarapid metabolizers; 0% are poor metabolizers

There are two phases of drug metabolism. CYP enzymes are responsible for most phase I reactions, which make chemicals less fat soluble (i.e., more water-soluble), usually by oxidation. Phase II reactions are usually by conjugation with glucuronic acid to render the chemical even more water-soluble. Chemicals conjugated with glucuronic acid are ready to be excreted in the urine or feces. The main phase II enzyme is UDP- glucuronosyltransferase (UGT), as in "U Got Tagged!" with glucuronic acid. The most relevant specific UGT enzyme for metabolism of lamotrigine and lumateperone is UGT1A4.

Psychiatric drugs metabolized by Phase II conjugation include valproic acid (VPA) and lamotrigine (Lamictal). UGT enzymes attach more strongly to VPA than to lamotrigine.

The presence of VPA slows the rate of Phase II metabolism of lamotrigine, causing lamotrigine blood levels to double.

There are several glucuronidation pathways involving several specific UGT enzymes. In this book, UGT activity and phase II metabolism are only visualized in the context of lamotrigine and the antipsychotic lumateperone (Caplyta)—both substrates of UGT1A4. Other UGT1A4 substrates (that could be depicted as sheep) include amitriptyline, doxepin, valproate, haloperidol, clozapine, olanzapine, and asenapine. GeneSight reports UGT**1A**4 and UGT**2B**15 (easy-to-recall sequence) metabolizer genotypes.

UGT2B15 is not visualized in this book. UGT2**B**15 substrates include the "LOT" **B**enzos—lorazepam, oxazepam and temazepam. The major UGT2B15 inHibitor is VPA. Nobody is a UGT2B15 ultrarapid or poor metabolizer, although some individuals are intermediate metabolizers.

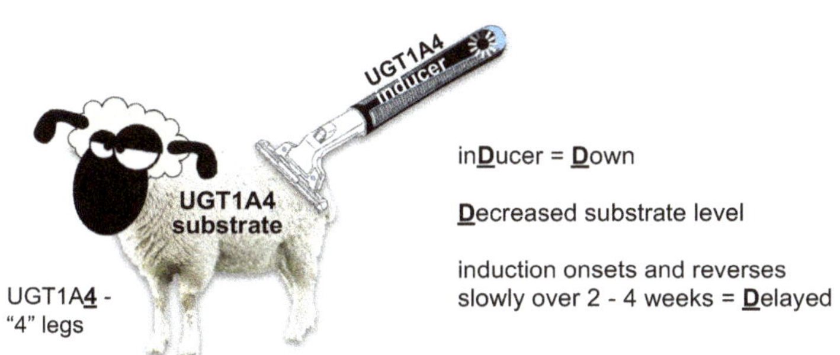

in**D**ucer = **D**own

Decreased substrate level

induction onsets and reverses slowly over 2 - 4 weeks = **D**elayed

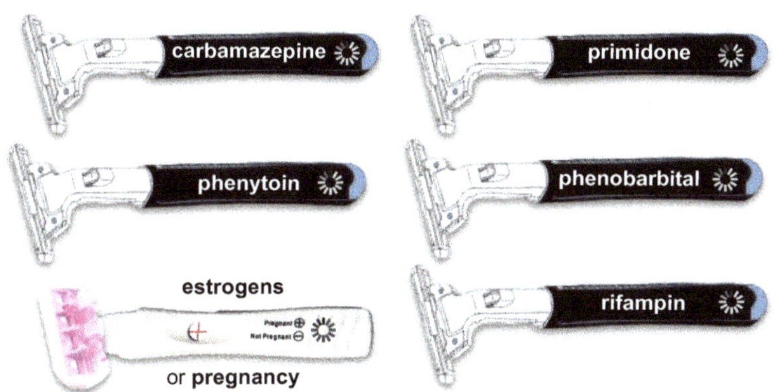

in**H**ibitor = **H**igh

Increased substrate level

in**H**ibition happens within **H**ours = **H**urried

Inhibition reverses as soon as the inhibitor is cleared from the body (five half-lives of the inhibitor). In the case of VPA, 5 x 14 hours = about 3 days.

VPA doubles lamotrigine levels.

UGT1A4 substrates

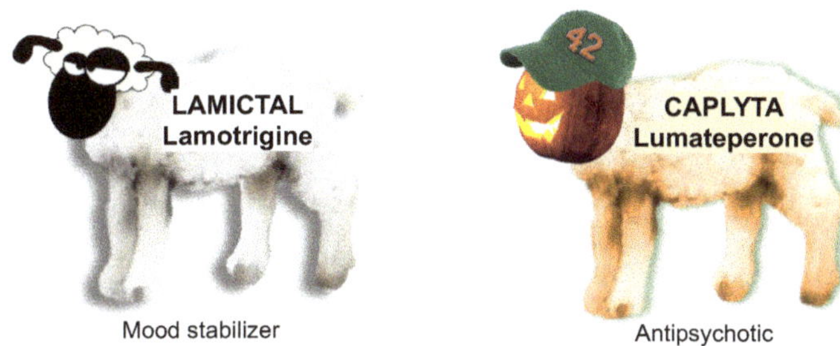

Mood stabilizer

Antipsychotic

Conclusion: In management of bipolar disorder, lamotrigine can be combined with any mood stabilizer or antipsychotic. Lamictal plus lithium is a favorable pairing, as long as renal function is normal. The combination of lamotrigine and VPA may increase the risk of Stevens-Johnson syndrome. For patients on lamotrigine plus VPA or carbamazepine (CMZ), consider checking lamotrigine blood levels before discontinuation of VPA/CMZ and after lamotrigine dose is adjusted to account for reversal of inhibition/induction (page 7). Do not combine lumateperone with VPA.

UGT1A4 ultrarapid metabolizers (UM)

Represented by a fast-shedding sheep, individuals who have a UGT1A4 ultrarapid metabolizer genotype clear UGT1A4 substrates quickly. These individuals are more likely to be non-responders to lamotrigine and lumateperone.

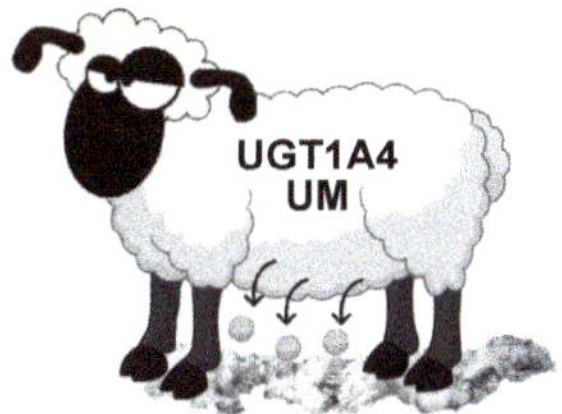

18% of population

Non-participants

Medications that do not become significantly involved in <u>kinetic</u> interactions are depicted **"in a bubble"**.

Some of these medications are **"in a box"** (with a hole in it) to indicate that kinetic interactions exist, but usually do not need be taken into consideration when prescribing the medication.

<u>Dynamic</u> interactions still apply to bubbled/boxed medications.

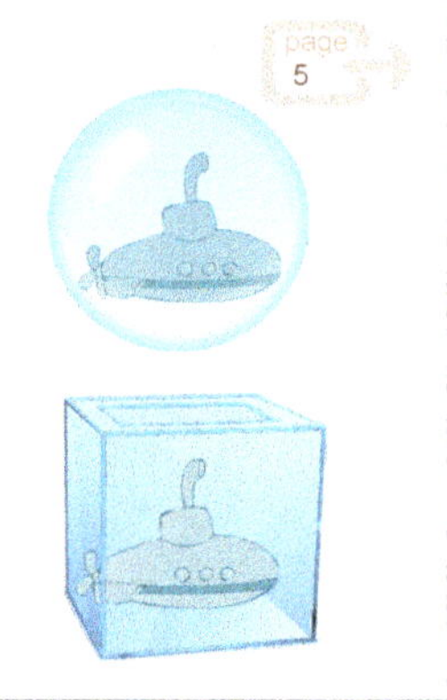

We will display medications "in a bubble" or "in a box" if they are not expected to serve as *clinically significant* substrates, inducers or inhibitors. There is a hole at the top of the boxes to indicate some degree of vulnerability to relevant kinetic interactions, but not to an extent prescribers need to worry about. In general, medications that are renally cleared have relatively few drug–drug interactions because their metabolism does not rely on hepatic enzymes.

For a substrate metabolized through multiple pathways, serum levels are not significantly affected by in**<u>Hi</u>**bition of a single CYP. For instance, over half of prescription drugs are 3A4 substrates, but will not be depicted as fish (page 16) if they are multi-CYP substrates. Multi-CYP substrates are depicted in a box (not a bubble) because interactions do occur but are unlikely to matter much.

A multi-CYP substrate is more likely to be victimized by an in**<u>D</u>**ucer than by an in**<u>H</u>**ibitor. It is worthwhile to run an interaction check on a patient's medication list if they are taking a "shredder" in**<u>D</u>**ucer (page 7), even for the boxed medications.

A bubble/box certifies the medication is:

- ❖ No worse than a mild CYP inducer or inducer, and...
- ❖ Either a multi-CYP substrate or a substrate not metabolized by any CYP

A bubble does **not** imply that a medication does not participate in <u>dynamic</u> interactions, because almost all drugs do. Acamprosate (Campral) and N-acetylcysteine (NAC) are rare exceptions, depicted in a double bubble.

Cafer's Psychopharmacology contains over 270 monographs of medications with mascots designed to help you pair trade names with generic names, and to remember kinetic interactions. The mascots inside the bubbles/boxes are introduced in other books in this series.

Dynamic interactions:
Not applicable to every drug in class

"Bubbled" or "boxed" medications are unlikely to be involved in clinically significant <u>kinetic</u> interactions:

<u>Antipsychotics</u>

- ❖ EPS (page 25)
- ❖ Sedation
- ❖ Weight gain (page 47)
- ❖ Hyperglycemia
- ❖ QT prolongation (page 23)
- ❖ Myelosuppression
- ❖ Anticholinergic (page 59)
- ❖ Proconvulsant (page 47)

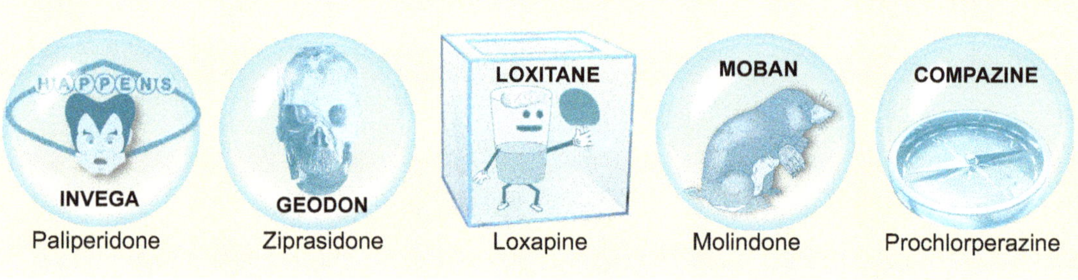

Paliperidone | Ziprasidone | Loxapine | Molindone | Prochlorperazine

<u>Antidepressants</u>

- ❖ Serotonergic
- ❖ QT prolongation
- ❖ Sedation (some)
- ❖ Weight gain
- ❖ Hyponatremia
- ❖ Antiplatelet
- ❖ Hypotensive (some)
- ❖ Hypertensive (others)

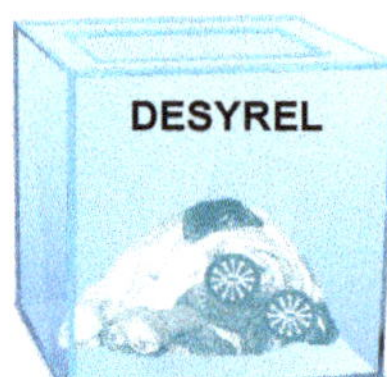

Trazodone

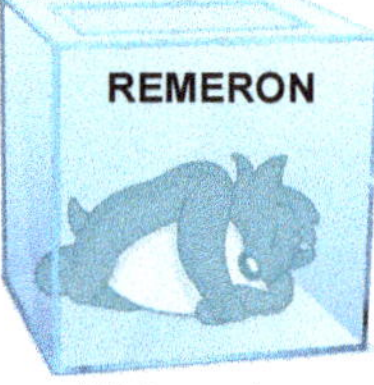

Mirtazapine

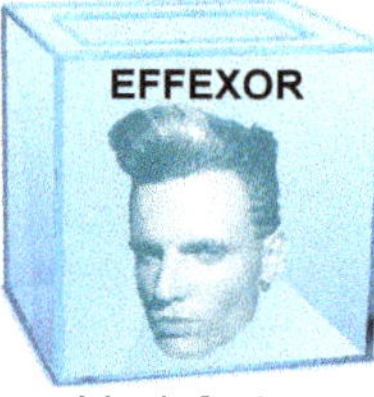

Venlafaxine

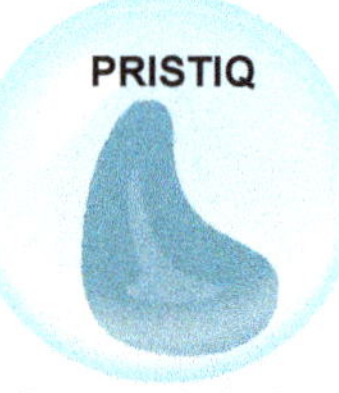

Desvenlafaxine

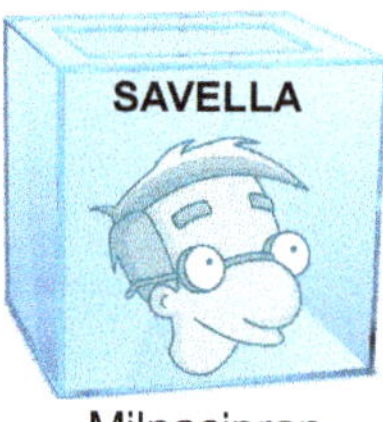

Milnacipran

<u>Antiepileptics</u>

- ❖ Sedation
- ❖ Stevens-Johnson Syndrome
- ❖ Hyponatremia
- ❖ Acidosis
- ❖ Myelosuppression

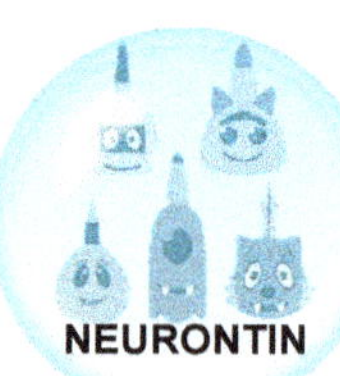

Gabapentin

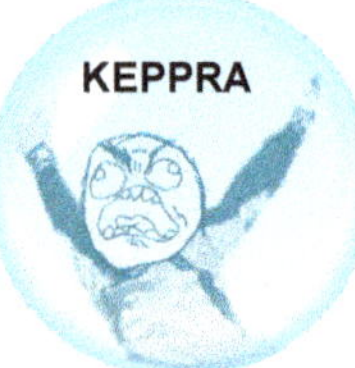

Levetiracetam

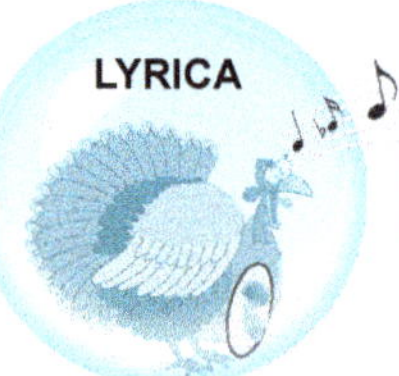

Pregabalin

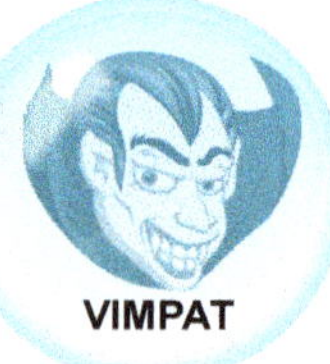

Lacosamide

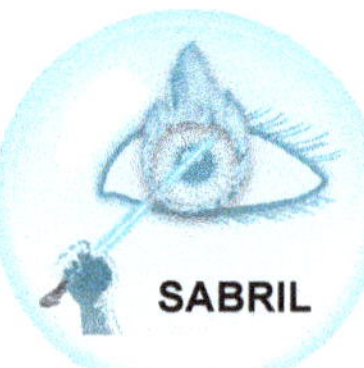

Vigabatrin

<u>Sedatives</u>

- ❖ Sedation
- ❖ Respiratory depression

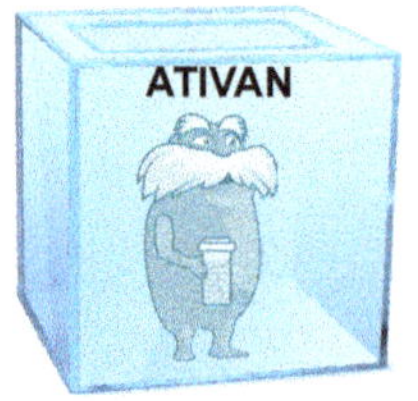

<u>L</u>orazepam

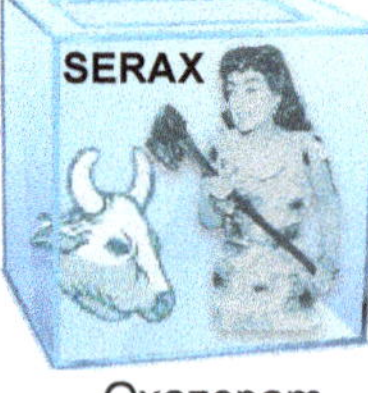

<u>O</u>xazepam

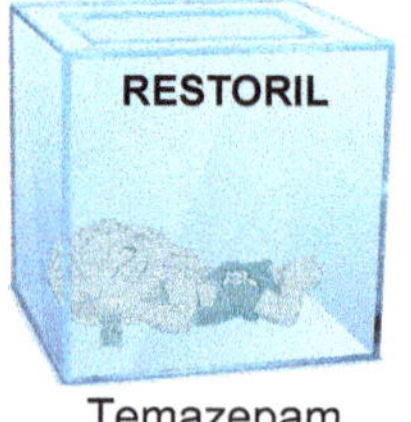

<u>T</u>emazepam

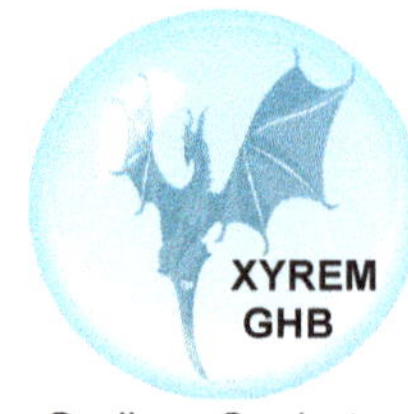

Sodium Oxybate

The 3 "<u>LOT</u>" benzos—No CYP interactions but levels may double due to UGT2B15 inHibition with VPA (Depakote)

Dynamic interactions:
Not applicable to every drug in class

"Bubbled" or "boxed" medications are unlikely to be involved in clinically significant kinetic interactions:

Antihistamines

- ❖ Anticholinergic
  - constipation
  - urinary retention
  - cognitive impairment
- ❖ Sedation

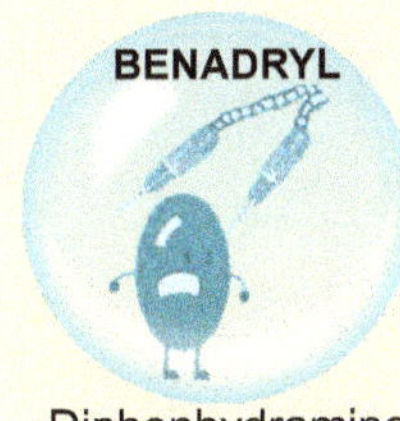

Diphenhydramine

UNISOM
Doxylamine

VISTARIL
Hydroxyzine

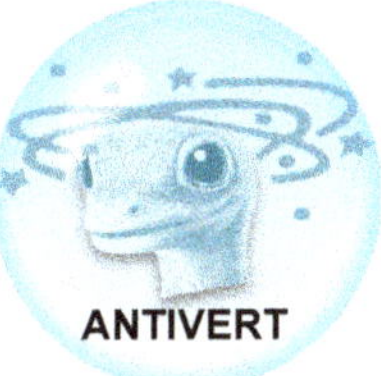

Meclizine

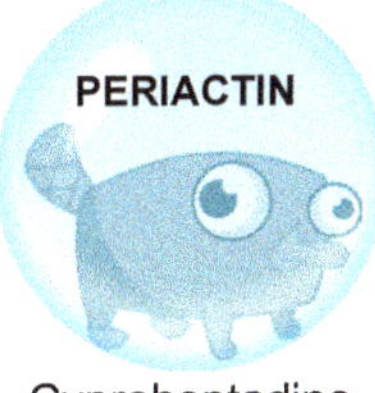

Cyproheptadine

Anticholinergics

- ❖ Anticholinergic
  - constipation
  - urinary retention
  - cognitive impairment
- ❖ Sedation

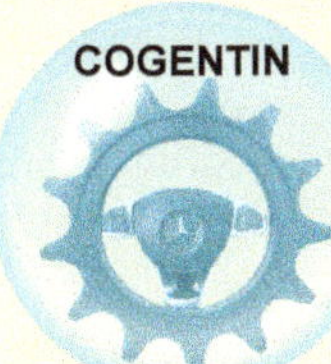

Benztropine

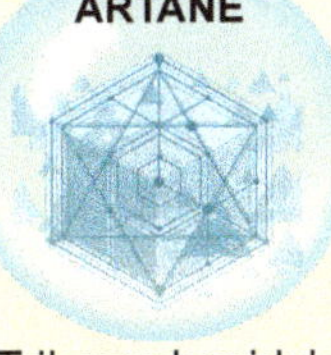

Trihexyphenidyl

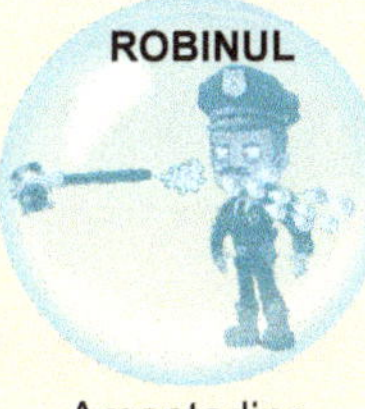

Amantadine

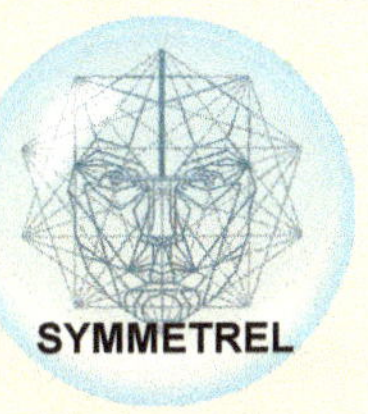

Glycopyrrolate

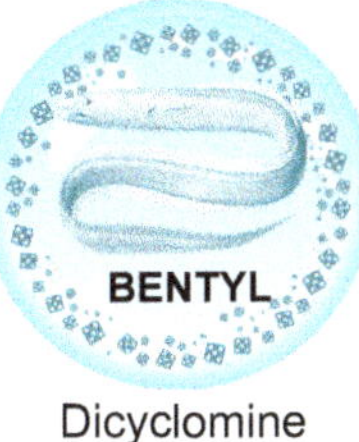

Dicyclomine

Cognitive Enhancers

- ❖ Cholinergic
- ❖ Proconvulsant

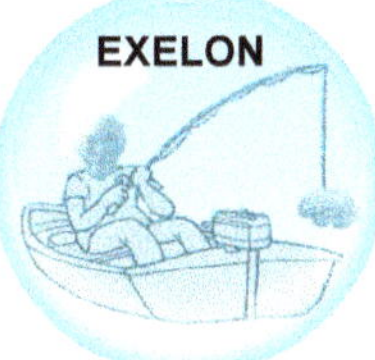

Rivastigmine

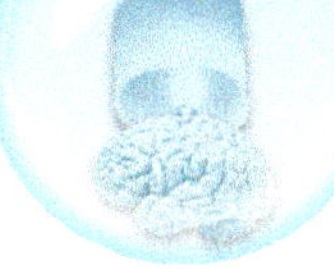

Galantamine

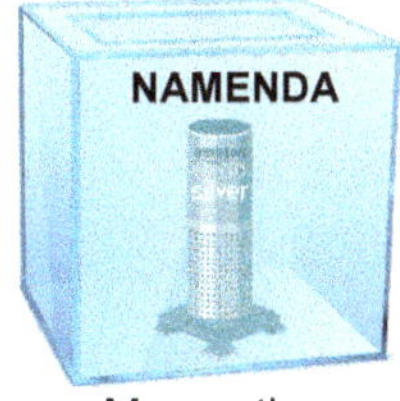

Memantine

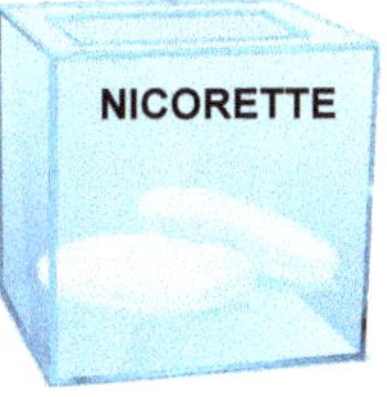

Nicotine

The hydrocarbons in smoked tobacco in**D**uce 1A2. Nicotine itself does not.

Addiction Medicine

For some, dynamic interactions are part of their mechanism of action, e.g., opioid antagonism by naltrexone and naloxone.

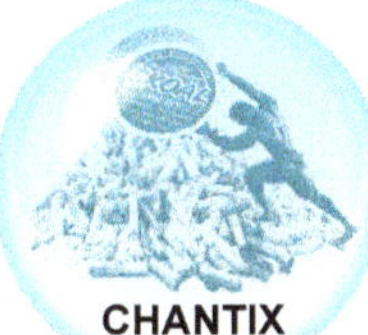

Varenicline

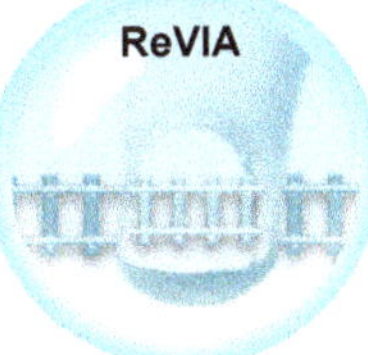

Naltrexone

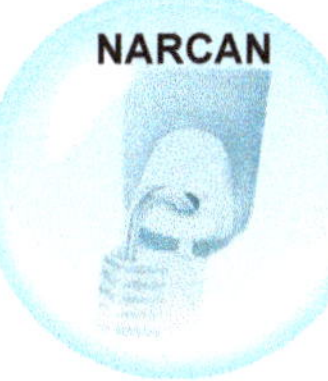

Naloxone

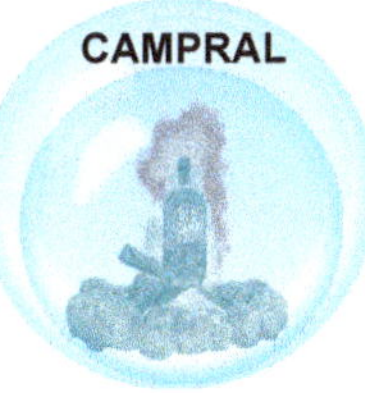

Acamprosate

Double bubble: Campral has no known kinetic or dynamic interactions.

Antihypertensives

- ❖ Hypotension
- ❖ Bradycardia
- ❖ Sedation
- ❖ Depression (some)

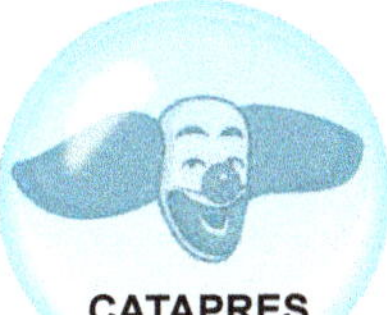

Clonidine

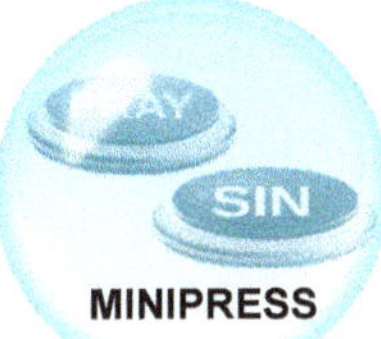

Prazosin

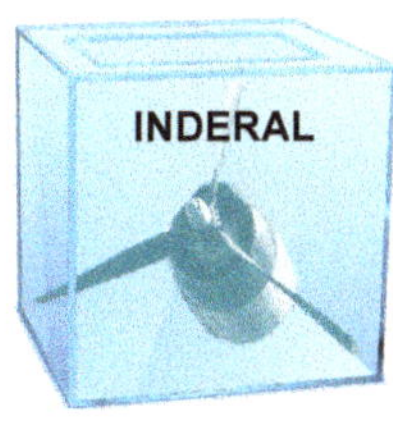

Propranolol

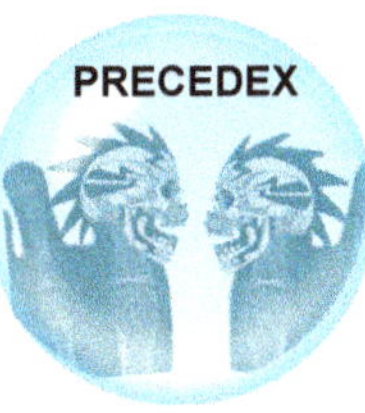

Dexmedetomidine

Spasmolytics

- ❖ Sedation
- ❖ Hypotensive
- ❖ Proconvulsant (some)

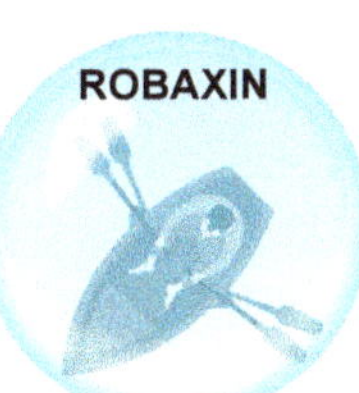

Methocarbamol

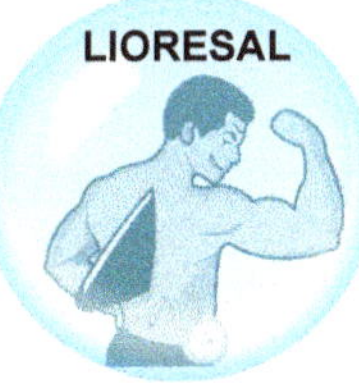

Baclofen

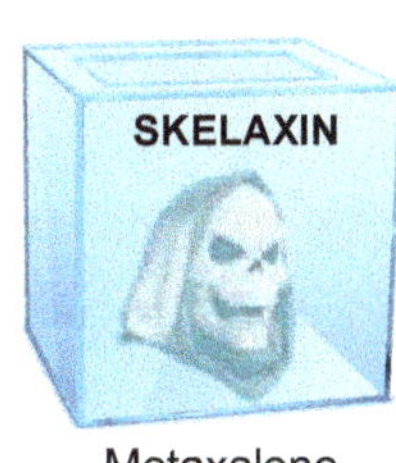

Metaxalone

Stimulants

- ❖ Proconvulsant
- ❖ Hypertensive
- ❖ Dopaminergic
- ❖ Noradrenergic

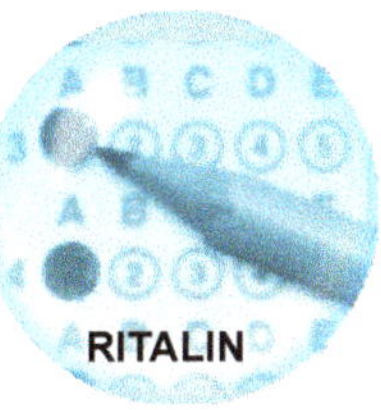

Methylphenidate

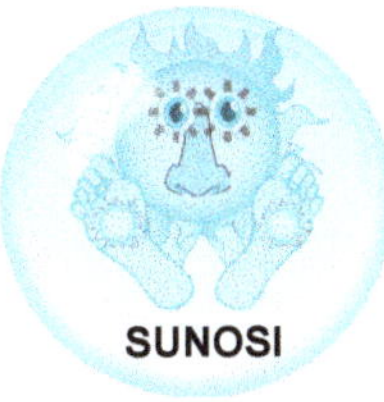

Solriamfetol

Supplements

Double bubble: NAC has no known kinetic or dynamic interactions.

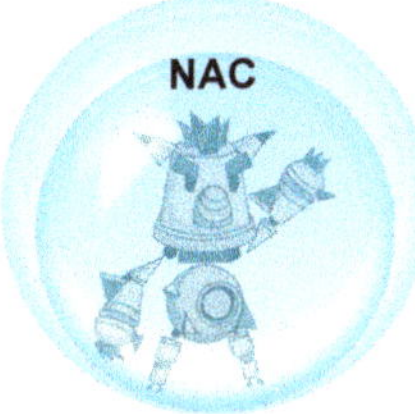

N-acetylcysteine

RELEVANT PHARMACOKINETIC INTERACTIONS, general overview with included medications highlighted

INDUCERS	INHIBITORS	SUBSTRATES
InDuction Decreases substrates slowly, over 2 to 4 weeks (Delayed). With smoked tobacco, induction (1A2) starts in 3 days and reverses in about 1 week	InHibition increases substrate levels (High), happening within Hours (Hurried). Inhibition reverses as soon as the inhibitor is cleared from the body (five half-lives of the inhibitor)	"Victims" of inducers and inhibitors
1A2 inducers Ψ Tobacco/Cannabis (faster on/off) Ψ Carbamazepine Ψ Phenytoin	1A2 inhibitors Ψ **Fluvoxamine** Ciprofloxacin	1A2 substrates Ψ Asenapine Ψ **Clozapine** Ψ Duloxetine Ψ Olanzapine Ψ **Ramelteon** Ψ Thiothixene
2B6 inducers Ψ Carbamazepine Rifampin HIV MEDS	2B6 inhibitors Ψ Orphenadrine (Norflex)	2B6 substrates HIV MEDS CANCER MEDS Ψ Bupropion Ψ Ketamine Ψ Methadone Ψ Selegiline
2C9 inducers **Rifampin** Ψ St John's Wort	2C9 inhibitors **Fluconazole**	2C9 substrates Ψ Valproate (VPA)
2C19 inducers Ψ Phenobarbital Rifampin Apalutamide ***Ultrarapid metabolizers (10%)***	2C19 inhibitors Ψ **Cannabidiol** (CBD) **Fluconazole** Ψ Fluoxetine Ψ Fluvoxamine ***Poor metabolizers (5%)***	2C19 substrates Ψ Citalopram Ψ Diazepam Ψ Escitalopram Ψ Phenobarbital Ψ Phenytoin Ψ Sertraline Ψ Methadone Warfarin
2D6 inducers None ***Ultrarapid metabolizers (5%)***	2D6 inhibitors Ψ **Bupropion** Ψ Duloxetine Ψ **Fluoxetine** Ψ **Paroxetine** **Quinidine** ***Poor metabolizers (10%)***	2D6 substrates Ψ Tricyclics (TCAs) Ψ Aripiprazole Ψ Atomoxetine Ψ Brexpiprazole Ψ Bupropion-OH Ψ Codeine *PRODRUG* Ψ Deutetrabenazine Ψ Dextromethorphan Ψ Duloxetine Ψ Haloperidol Ψ Iloperidone Ψ **Perphenazine** Ψ **Pimozide** Ψ Risperidone Tamoxifen *PRODRUG* Ψ Tetrabenazine Ψ **Thioridazine** Ψ Tramadol *PRODRUG* Ψ Vortioxetine
3A4 inducers Ψ **Carbamazepine** Ψ Modafinil Ψ **Phenobarbital** Ψ **Phenytoin** **Rifampin** Ψ St John's Wort	3A4 inhibitors Protease Inhibitors (HIV) Clarithromycin Diltiazem Grapefruit juice **Ketoconazole** **Itraconazole** Ψ **Nefazodone** Verapamil	3A4 substrates Immunosuppressants Progestins Ψ Alprazolam Ψ Aripiprazole Ψ Brexpiprazole Ψ Buprenorphine Ψ **Buspirone** Ψ Carbamazepine Ψ Cariprazine Ψ Chlordiazepoxide Ψ Clonazepam Ψ **Flibanserin** Ψ Lemborexant Ψ **Lumateperone** Ψ **Lurasidone** Ψ Pimavanserin Ψ Pimozide Ψ **Quetiapine** Sildenafil **Simvastatin** Ψ Suvorexant Tadalafil Ψ Valbenazine Ψ **Vilazodone**
UGT inducers Ψ Carbamazepine Estrogens Ψ Phenobarbital Ψ Phenytoin Rifampin	UGT inhibitors Ψ Valproate (VPA)	UGT substrates Ψ **Lamotrigine** Ψ **Lumateperone**

Lithium levels	Decreased by:	Increased by:
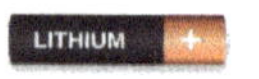	Acetazolamide Ψ Caffeine Mannitol Theophylline Ψ Topiramate Ψ Zonisamide 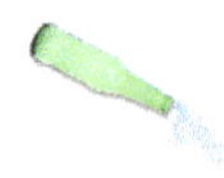	**Thiazides:** - HCTZ - Chlorthalidone **NSAIDS:** - Celebrex - Ibuprofen - Indomethacin - Naproxen - Diclofenac **ACE Inhibitors** "-prils" **ARBs** "-sartans" **Antimicrobials:** - Tetracyclines - Metronidazole 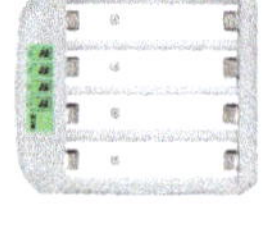

Ψ = CNS meds (psychoactive)

Pharmacokinetic Drug-Drug Interactions with included medications highlighted

INDUCERS

In**D**uction decreases (**D**own) substrates slowly, over 2 to 4 weeks* (**D**elayed).

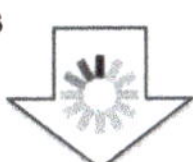

Inducer	CYP
Ψ Armodafinil	(3A4)
Apalutamide (prostate cancer)	2C19, 3A4 & (2C9)
Ψ Cannabis	1A2 fast
Chargrilled meat	1A2
Ψ Carbamazepine (Tegretol)	3A4, 2B6 & (1A2)
Efavirenz (HIV)	3A4, 2B6
Enzalutamide (prostate cancer)	3A4, 2C9 & 2C19
Estradiol	UGT
Ψ Modafinil	3A4
Nevirapine	2B6 (3A4)
Ψ Phenobarbital (Luminal)	3A4 (1A2), (2B6, 2C9) & UGT
Ψ Phenytoin (Dilantin)	3A4 (1A2), (2B6), UGT
Ψ Primidone (Mysoline) metab to phenobarb	3A4 (1A2), (2B6, 2C9) & UGT
Rifampin (Rifadin)	2C19, 3A4, 2B6, 2C9 (1A2) & UGT
Ritonavir (HIV)	2B6 (2C19) (1A2, 2C9)
Ψ St John's Wort	1A2, 2C9 & 3A4
Ψ Tobacco	1A2 fast
Ψ Topiramate ≥200 mg	(3A4)

in**D**uction reverses gradually over a few weeks* after the inducer is discontinued.

*With smoking (tobacco or cannabis), induction is faster (a few days).

INHIBITORS

In**H**ibition increases substrate levels (**H**igh). Inhibition happens within **H**ours (**H**urried).

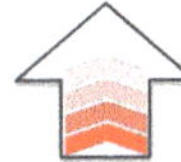

Inhibitor	CYP
Amiodarone	(2C9, 2D6, 3A4)
Ψ Asenapine	(2D6) weak
Ψ Bupropion	2D6
Ψ Cannabidiol	2C19, UGT
Cimetidine	(multi) weak
Ciprofloxacin	1A2, (3A4)
Clarithromycin	3A4
Clopidogrel	(2B6)
Darunavir (HIV)	3A4, (2D6)
Diltiazem	3A4, (2D6)
Ψ Duloxetine	2D6
Efavirenz (HIV)	2C9, 2C19
Erythromycin	3A4
Esomeprazole	(2C19) weak
Fluconazole	2C9, 2C19, 3A4
Ψ Fluoxetine	2D6, 2C19
Ψ Fluvoxamine (Luvox)	1A2, 2C19, & (3A4, 2C9)
Grapefruit juice	3A4
Isoniazid	(3A4) weak
Indinavir	3A4
Itraconazole	3A4
Ketoconazole	3A4, (2C19)
Ψ Methadone	(2D6) weak
Ψ Modafinil	(2C19) weak
Nelfinavir	3A4
Omeprazole	2C19
Ψ Nefazodone	3A4
Ψ Orphenadrine	2B6
Ψ Paroxetine	2D6
Quinidine	2D6, (3A4)
Ritonavir	3A4 Black Box
Ψ Sertraline ≥150mg	(2D6)
Terbinafine	2D6
Ψ Thioridazine	2D6
Ψ Valproate (VPA)	UGT
Voriconazole	3A4,2C19,(2C9)
Verapamil	3A4, (1A2)

In**H**ibition is reversed as soon as the inhibitor is cleared, which will be about 5 half-lives after it is discontinued.

UGT refers to UGT1A4.

( ) = weak inducer/inhibitor; less susceptible substrate

Ψ = CNS medication (psychoactive)

SUBSTRATES

"Victims" of inducers and inhibitors

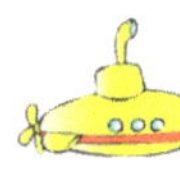

In general, substrates that are metabolized through only one pathway are more vulnerable to drug interactions. For drugs metabolized by multiple CYPs, strong in**D**uction of a single CYP is likely to reduce substrate levels, but in**H**ibition of one CYP is unlikely to significantly increase substrate levels.

Substrate	CYP
Atazanavir (HIV)	3A4
Ψ Alprazolam	3A4
Ψ Amitriptyline	2D6, 2C19
Amlodipine	3A4
Ψ Amoxapine	2D6
Ψ Amphetamine salts	(2D6)
Ψ Aripiprazole	2D6, 3A4
Ψ Armodafinil	3A4
Ψ Asenapine	(1A2)
Ψ Atomoxetine	2D6, (2C19)
Atorvastatin	3A4
Avanafil	3A4
Ψ Brexpiprazole	2D6, 3A4
Ψ Buprenorphine	3A4
Ψ Bupropion	2B6; 2D6 (OH-)
Ψ Buspirone	3A4, (2D6)
Ψ Caffeine	1A2 (etc)
Ψ Carbamazepine	3A4
Ψ Cariprazine	3A4, (2D6)
Ψ Carisoprodol	2C19
Carvedilol	2D6 (etc)
Celecoxib	2C9, (3A4)
Ψ Chlordiazepoxide	3A4
Ψ Chlorpromazine	2D6, (1A2,3A4)
Ψ Citalopram	2C19,3A4(2D6)
Clarithromycin	3A4
Ψ Clomipramine	2D6, 2C19, 1A2
Ψ Clonazepam	3A4
Clopidogrel	2C19, (3A4)
Ψ Clozapine	1A2 (2D6, etc)
Ψ Codeine *2D6 prodrug	*2D6, (3A4)
Ψ Cyclobenzaprine	1A2, (2D6, 3A4)
Cyclophosphamide	2B6, 2C19
Cyclosporine	3A4 (etc)
Ψ Desipramine	2D6, (1A2)
Ψ Deutetrabenazine	2D6
Ψ Dextromethorphan	2D6 (etc)
Ψ Diazepam	2C19, 3A4
Diclofenac	multi
Diltiazem	3A4 (2C19,3A4)
Ψ Doxepin	2D6, 2C19 (etc)
Ψ Donepezil	(2D6, 3A4)
Ψ Duloxetine	2D6, 1A2
Efavirenz (HIV)	2B6, 3A4
Ψ Escitalopram	2C19,3A4(2D6)
Esomeprazole	2C19, (3A4)
Estradiol	1A2, 2C9, 3A4
Ψ Eszopiclone	3A4
Ψ Fentanyl 3A4 Black Box	3A4 (etc)
Flecainide	2D6, 1A2
Ψ Flibanserin 3A4 Black Box	3A4, 2C9, 2C19
Ψ Fluoxetine	2D6, 2C9 (etc)
Ψ Fluphenazine	2D6
Ψ Flurazepam	3A4
Fluvastatin	2C9 (2B6, 3A4)
Ψ Fluvoxamine	2D6, 1A2
Ψ Galantamine	(2D6, 3A4)
Glimepiride	2C9
Glipizide	2C9
Glyburide	2C9
Ψ Guanfacine	3A4
Ψ Haloperidol	2D6, 3A4, (1A2)
Ψ Hydrocodone Black Box	3A4
Ifosfamide	2B6 (& others)
Ψ Iloperidone	2D6, (3A4)
Ψ Imipramine	2D6, 2C19 (etc)
Ψ Ketamine	2B6, 2C9, 3A4
Ψ Lamotrigine	UGT
Lansoprazole	2C19, 3A4
Ψ Lemborexant	3A4
Ψ Levomilnacipran	3A4, (2D6)
Losartan	2C9, 3A4
Ψ Loxapine	(1A2, 2D6,3A4)
Ψ Lumateperone	3A4, UGT
Ψ Lurasidone *contraind*	3A4
Medroxyprogesterone	3A4
Meloxicam	2C9, (3A4)
Ψ Meperidine Black Box	3A4
Ψ Methadone	3A4, 2B6, (etc)
Ψ Methamphetamine	2D6
Metoprolol	2D6, (2C19)
Mexiletine	1A2, 2D6
Ψ Midazolam	3A4, (2B6)
Ψ Mirtazapine	2D6, 3A4, 1A2
Ψ Modafinil	3A4 (2D6)
Nevirapine	3A4 (2B6, 2D6)
Ψ Nefazodone	3A4; 2D6 mCPP
Nifedipine	3A4, (2D6)
Norethindrone	3A4
Ψ Nortriptyline	2D6 (etc)
Ψ Olanzapine	1A2; (2D6)
Omeprazole	2C19 (etc)
Ψ Oxycodone	3A4, (2D6)
Pantoprazole	2C19,(2D6, 3A4)
Ψ Paroxetine	2D6
Ψ Perphenazine	2D6 (etc)
Ψ Phenobarbital	2C19,(2C9)
Ψ Phenytoin	2C9, 2C19,(3A4)
Ψ Pimavanserin	3A4
Ψ Pimozide	2D6, 3A4 (1A2)
Piroxicam	2C9
Ψ Promethazine	(2B6, 2D6)
Propafenone	2D6, (1A2, 3A4)
Ψ Propofol	2B6 (etc)
Ψ Propranolol	2D6, 1A2,(2C19)
Ψ Protriptyline	2D6
Ψ Quetiapine	3A4, (2D6)
Ψ Ramelteon	1A2 (3A4,2C19)
Ψ Risperidone	2D6, (3A4)
Ψ Selegiline	2B6 (etc)
Ψ Sertraline	2C19 (2B6,2D6)
Sildenafil	3A4, (etc)
Simvastatin	3A4
Ψ Suvorexant	3A4
Tacrolimus	3A4
Tadalafil	3A4
Tamoxifen *2D6 prodrug	*2D6, 3A4, 2C9
Ψ Tasimelteon	1A2, 3A4
Ψ Tetrabenazine	2D6
Theophylline	1A2, (3A4)
Ψ Thioridazine	2D6, (2C19)
Ψ Thiothixene	1A2
Ψ Tiagabine	3A4
Ψ Tizanidine	1A2
Tolbutamide	2C9, (2C19)
Ψ Tramadol *2D6 prodrug*	3A4,(2D6*; 2B6)
Ψ Trazodone	3A4 (2D6 mCPP)
Ψ Triazolam	3A4
Ψ Trifluoperazine	1A2
Ψ Trimipramine	2D6, 2C19, 3A4
Ψ Valproate (VPA)	(multi); Aspirin*
Ψ Valbenazine	3A4 (2D6)
Vardenafil	3A4
Ψ Venlafaxine	2D6, 3A4,(2C19)
Ψ Vilazodone	3A4,(2C19,2D6)
Vincristine	3A4
Voriconazole	2C9, 2C19, 3A4
Ψ Vortioxetine	2D6, 3A4, etc
Warfarin	2C9, 2C19,(3A4)
Ψ Zaleplon	(3A4)
Ψ Zolpidem	3A4 (etc)

Lithium levels

LITHIUM +

Decreased by:

- Acetazolamide
- Ψ Caffeine
- Mannitol
- Theophylline
- Ψ Topiramate
- Ψ Zonisamide (weak)

Increased by:

- Benazepril
- Celecoxib
- Chlorthalidone
- Diclofenac
- Doxycycline
- Enalapril
- Etodolac
- HCTZ
- Ibuprofen
- Indomethacin
- Irbesartan Lisinopril
- Tetracycline
- Losartan
- Metronidazole
- Minocycline
- Naproxen
- Olmesartan
- Ramipril
- Valsartan

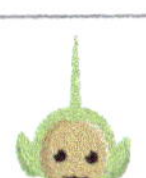

With high-dose aspirin, Depakote (VPA) will be stronger than suggested by total VPA level because aspirin (highly protein-bound) bumps VPA off of albumin.

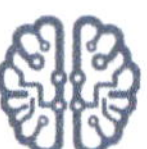

Neurotransmitters

Here is a simplified overview of important neurotransmitters in the brain. Serotonin, norepinephrine, epinephrine and histamine are referred to as monoamine neurotransmitters because they contain a single amine group (--NH_2). The monoamine neurotransmitter dopamine is heavily implicated in psychotic disorders, and is the target of nearly all available antipsychotic medications.

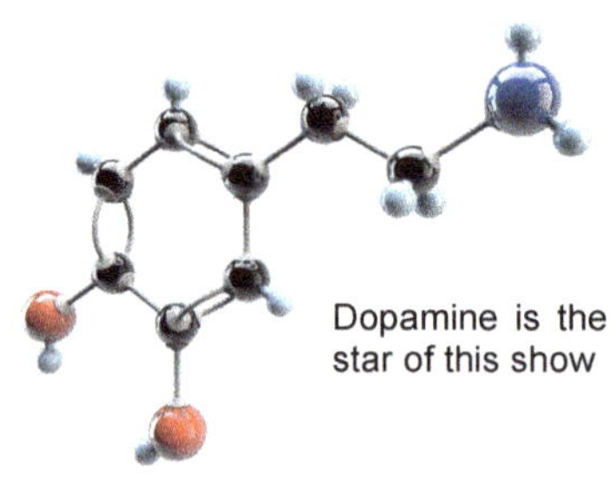

Dopamine is the star of this show

Neurotransmitter	Abbrev	Normal activity	Low activity	High activity	Comments
Serotonin (5-hydroxytryptamine)	5-HT	"Serenity" Calmness Satisfaction Euthymic mood Sleep	Depression Anxiety OCD	Sexual dysfunction, Muscle twitching, Hyperreflexia, Dilated pupils, Restlessness, GI distress/nausea, Serotonin syndrome, Hallucinations (LSD)	Most antidepressants are serotonergic, i.e., enhance 5-HT activity.
Norepinephrine	NE	Energy, Motivation, Ability to focus and respond to stress	Fatigue Inattention Sexual dysfunction Hypotension	Insomnia Anxiety Loss of appetite Hypertension Seizure	NE is also known as noradrenaline. Stimulants increase noradrenergic (NE) activity.
Dopamine	DA	Ability to experience pleasure and strong emotions	Anhedonia, Inattention, Sexual dysfunction, Parkinsonism, Akathisia, Dystonia, Neuroleptic malignant syndrome (NMS), Restless legs syndrome, Antiemetic	Mania, Euphoria, Agitation, Anger, Aggression, Chemical "high", Paranoia, Auditory hallucinations, Compulsive behaviors, Hypersexuality, Insomnia, Nausea	Think pleasure, passion, paranoia. Drugs of abuse, colloquially known as "dope", cause euphoria by spiking DA in the nucleus accumbens.
Acetylcholine	ACh	"Rest and digest" parasympathetic activity; Normal cognitive function	"Dry as a bone" - Constipation, urinary retention, dry mouth; "Mad as a hatter" - confusion, delirium with visual hallucinations; dilated pupils, tachycardia	"SLUDGE" - Salivation, lacrimation, urination, diaphoresis, GI upset (including diarrhea), emesis; constricted pupils	Acts on muscarinic and nicotinic receptors. What are commonly described as "anticholinergic" effects would be more accurately termed "antimuscarinic".
Histamine	H	Not sedated; Not having an allergic reaction	Sedation Weight gain	Allergic reaction Pruritus	Antihistamines are used for sleep and allergies; H2 blockers (ranitidine, etc) reduce stomach acid.

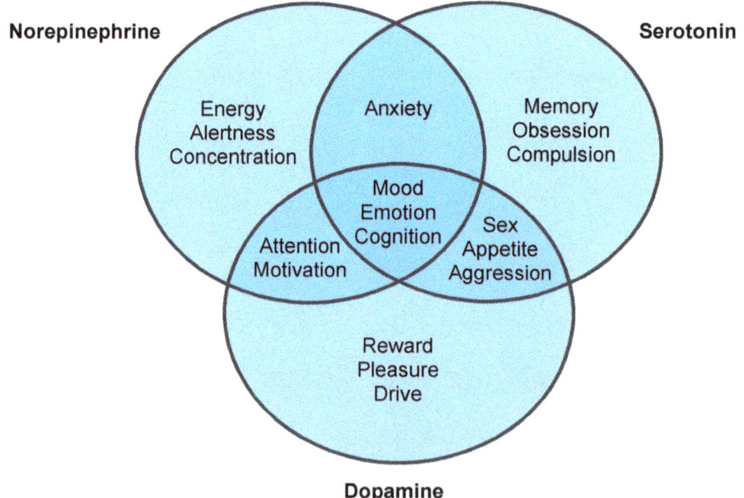

QT prolongation

"Cutie heart"

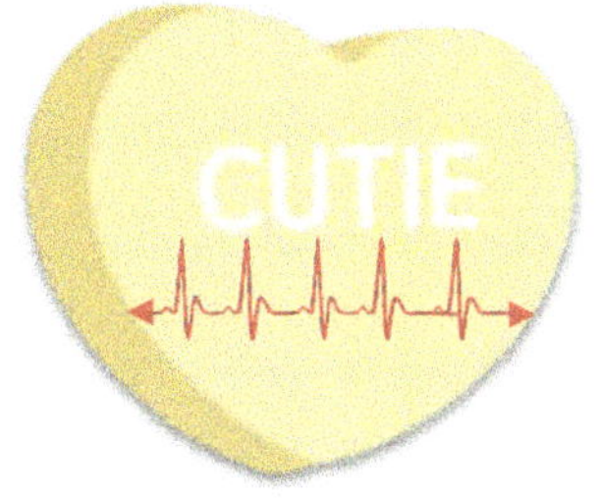

In this book, an ECG tracing like the one on this candy heart means that the medication prolongs QT interval.

On electrocardiogram (ECG), the QT interval, measured from the beginning of the QRS complex to the end of the T-wave, reflects the rate of electrical conduction of the heart. The useful number for our purposes is the QTc interval, which is QT corrected for heart rate.

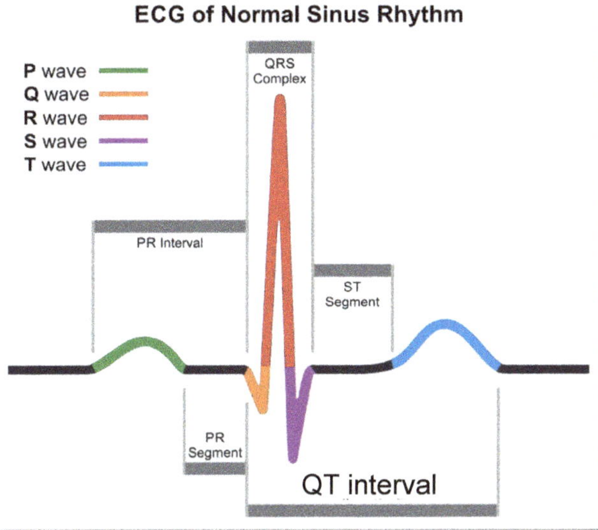

QT prolongation is a delay in cardiac conduction that can trigger ***Torsades de pointes*** (French "twisting of points"). This may precede sudden death.

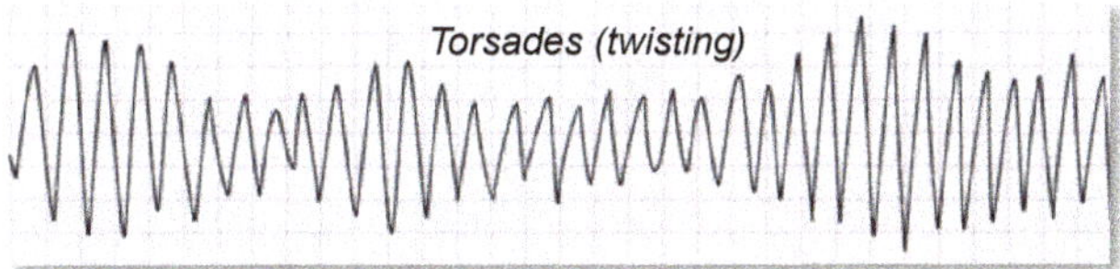

Many psychotropic medications prolong QT interval, including most antidepressants and antipsychotics. In overdose scenarios involving antidepressants or antipsychotics, QT interval is usually long, necessitating a trip to the ICU. Tricyclic antidepressants (TCAs) are particularly deadly in overdose due to disruption of cardiac conduction manifested by, among other measures, prolonged QT.

Roughly speaking, QTc > 460 milliseconds is long and QTc > 500 msec is dangerous. An increase in QTc > 60 msec caused by a medication would be of concern.

The risk of torsades is the highest within the first few days of initiating treatment with a QT prolonger. For most drugs that prolong QT, the risk of torsades is so low that routine ECG screening is unnecessary. Although combining QT prolonging medications does prolong QT interval, the magnitude of the effect is likely to be tiny, with a very low probability of clinical consequences (Carlat Report, March 2018). However, it is prudent to check an ECG for patients taking high doses of multiple QT prolonging medications, or individuals with these risk factors:

Risk factors for QT prolongation
- Hypokalemia (low K+)
- Hypomagnesemia (low Mg+)
- Bradycardia
- Left ventricular hypertrophy

Patients with congenital long QT syndrome should not be given QT prolonging medications. Do not add a QT prolonging medication when QTc is near 500 msec.

QT prolongation by psychotropic medications:

Risk	Medication	Class
Highest	Thioridazine (Mellaril)	Antipsychotic
High	Pimozide (Orap) Ziprasidone (Geodon)	Antipsychotic Antipsychotic
Moderate	Iloperidone (Fanapt) Chlorpromazine (Thorazine) Haloperidol (Haldol)* Amitriptyline (Elavil) Desipramine (Norpramin) Imipramine (Tofranil) Maprotiline (Ludiomil) Citalopram (Celexa) Methadone (Dolophine)	Antipsychotic Antipsychotic Antipsychotic TCA TCA TCA TCA SSRI Opioid
Low risk except in combination or overdose	Most antidepressants Most antipsychotics	

*Intravenous haloperidol poses high risk of QT prolongation.

Due to the extent of QT prolongation caused by thioridazine (Mellaril), most psychiatrists avoid prescribing it. For healthy patients taking ziprasidone (Geodon), the author checks an ECG before exceeding the FDA maximum dose of ziprasidone (80 mg BID) or when combining 3 or more medications known to prolong QT interval. Check an ECG if a patient taking QT prolonging medications experiences palpitations or syncope/presyncope.

Other medications that prolong QT interval:

Class	Medication
Antiarrhythmic	Amiodarone (Cordarone) Flecainide (Tambocor) Quinidine Sotalol (Betapace)
Antimicrobial	Azithromycin (Zithromax) Ciprofloxacin (Cipro) Clarithromycin (Biaxin) Erythromycin (Erythrocin) Fluconazole (Diflucan) Hydroxychloroquine (Plaquenil) Levofloxacin (Levaquin)
Other	Cocaine Opioids (most) - generally mild except methadone Ondansetron (Zofran) - antiemetic (IV route) Propofol (Diprivan) - anesthetic

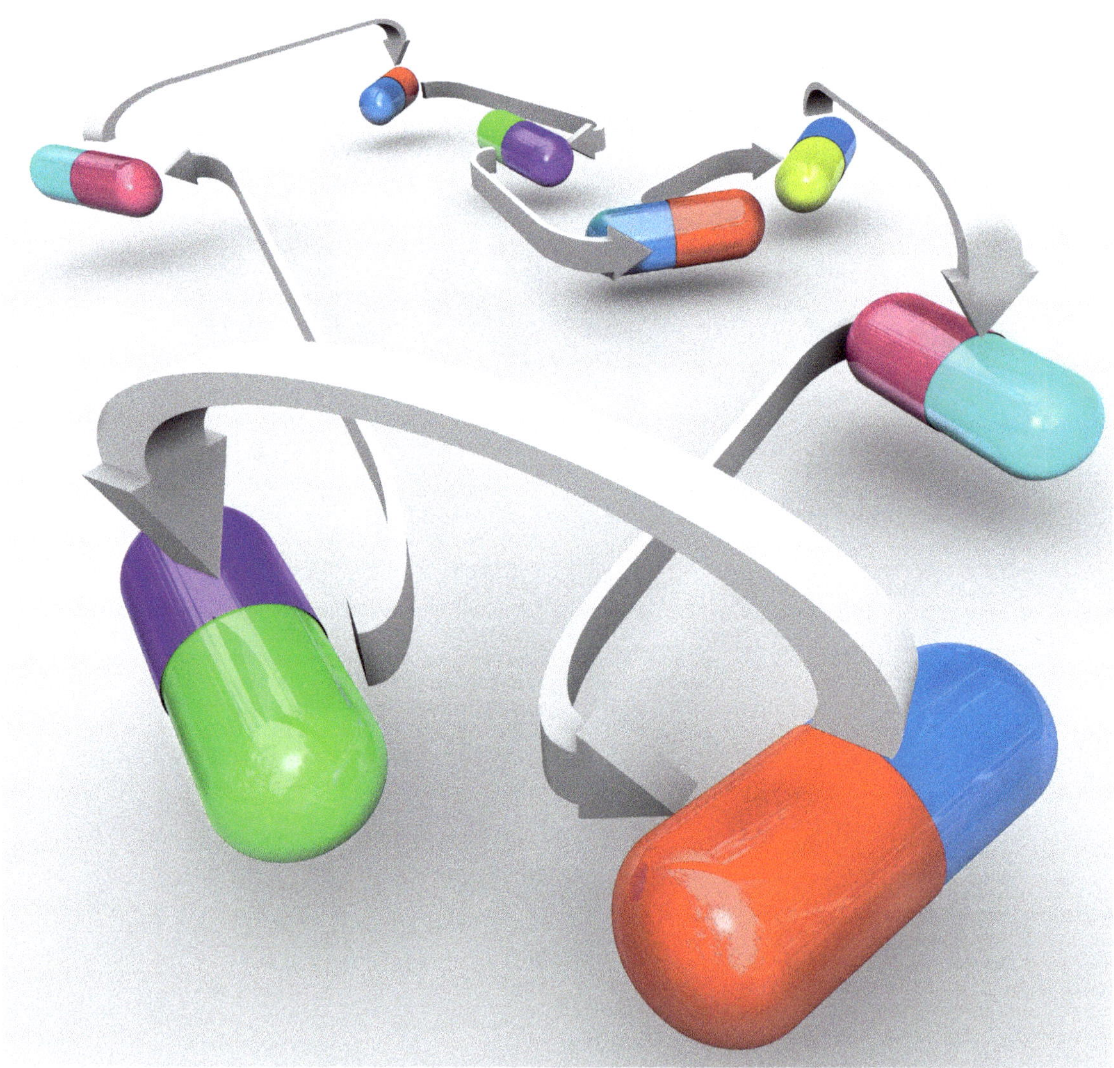

D2

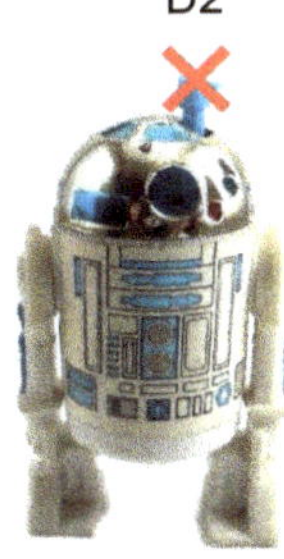

Antipsychotics work by blocking D2 dopamine receptors. Think Star Wars droid R2**D2**.

In the book *Memorable Psychopharmacology*, Dr. Heldt provides the mnemonic for antipsychotics as D2 receptor (D_2R) blockers for psychotic patients taking a "D_2R (detour) from reality".

Antipsychotics slow down thoughts. This effect is useful for treatment of mania, but can be detrimental for schizophrenia patients—manifested by worsening of negative symptoms (amotivation, anhedonia, blunting of affect).

When it comes to treatment of schizophrenia, the patient is generally started on the minimum effective dose for a given antipsychotic and considered for dose increase at two weeks. For aggressive patients, or for those hospitalized with acute psychosis, the dose can be titrated much faster. For first episode psychosis, it is a good idea to decrease dose of the antipsychotic after 6 months of remission. When the antipsychotic dose is reduced by 50% at 6 months, patients had better overall functioning 7 years later (Wunderlink et al, 2013).

It is considered best practice to stick with a single antipsychotic rather than combining two antipsychotics. For a psychiatric hospital to maintain accreditation, the psychiatrist must document the justification for multiple antipsychotics. The Joint Commission has identified three appropriate reasons for discharging a patient from the hospital on more than one antipsychotic:

- three failed trials of monotherapy
- cross-taper to monotherapy
- augmentation of clozapine (Clozaril)

In other words, the concurrent use of two or more antipsychotic medications should generally be avoided except in cases of three failed trials of monotherapy, preferably including clozapine—the most effective medication for refractory psychosis.

Antipsychotics commonly cause extrapyramidal symptoms (EPS). The extrapyramidal system ("outside of the pyramids") is an imprecise anatomic term referring to motor tracts other than those projecting through the pyramids of the medulla oblongata. The pyramidal system allows voluntary movements, while the extrapyramidal system coordinates motor activity without directly innervating motor neurons. Dysfunction of the extrapyramidal system leads to involuntary movements. Short term exposure to antipsychotic drugs may cause EPS resembling Parkinson's disease, while long term exposure can cause tardive dyskinesia, which resembles the choreiform movements of Huntington's disease.

The likelihood that an antipsychotic will cause EPS is proportional to its efficacy in blocking D2 receptors. Haloperidol (Haldol) is a high potency D2 blocker that commonly causes EPS. Since the likelihood of EPS is dose-related, haloperidol should be dosed at low strength. EPS is caused by a relative deficiency of dopamine and an excess of acetylcholine in the nigrostriatal pathway. This explains why anticholinergic medications such as benztropine (Cogentin) can quickly alleviate dystonia. Some of the newer antipsychotics are likely to cause akathisia (restlessness) but are relatively unlikely to cause the other kinds of EPS shown below. Note that "tardive" refers to delayed onset. Management would include dose reduction or discontinuation of the offending medication, or switching to a medication with minimal EPS such as quetiapine (Seroquel), clozapine (Clozaril), or possibly pimavanserin (Nuplazid).

All antipsychotics now have a black box warning: "Not approved for dementia-related psychosis; increased mortality risk in elderly dementia patients."

Antipsychotics may cause an elevation in core body temperature that can be exacerbated by strenuous exercise and anticholinergic medications ("hot as a hare").

To maintain effectiveness, multiple daily dosing may not be needed. A continuous dopamine D2 receptor blockade is generally not necessary to sustain antipsychotic response. For instance, perphenazine (Trilafon) has a 10-hour half-life and, although the label instructs BID-TID dosing, once-daily dosing was found to be equally effective for maintenance treatment (Takeuchi et al, 2014).

Types of Extrapyramidal Symptoms (EPS)

Type of EPS	Usual onset	Description	Reversible?	Treatment
Dystonia	Quickly	Muscle contraction in the face, neck, trunk or extremities, and even the larynx. "Oculogyric crisis" is a dystonic reaction with prolonged upward deviation of the eyes.	Yes	Anticholinergics: - Benztropine (Cogentin) - Diphenhydramine (Benadryl)
Akathisia	Acute akathisia - quickly; Tardive akathisia - after several months	*Akathemi* is Greek for "never sit down". Akathisia is an uncomfortable feeling of internal motor restlessness with difficulty sitting still. The patient may fidget, pace, or rock back and forth.	Yes	Propranolol (Inderal) Benzodiazepines Anticholinergics (less effective)
Pseudo-parkinsonism	Months–years	Pill-rolling Parkinsonian tremor; Bradykinesia (e.g., "Thorazine shuffle" gait); Does not progress to Parkinson's disease	Usually	Amantadine (Symmetrel) Benzodiazepines
Tardive Dyskinesia	6 months - year(s)	Movement disorder that is often irreversible, characterized by tongue movements, lip smacking, excessive blinking, grimacing or raising of eyebrows; irregular finger movements as if playing an invisible piano or air guitar; chorea of extremities in severe cases. Often the patient is unaware of the movements. Older adults are at higher risk.	Usually not	Valbenazine (Ingrezza) Deutetrabenazine (Austedo) Benzodiazepines Amantadine (Symmetrel)

Antipsychotics are not always to blame for the involuntary movements presumed to be tardive dyskinesia. In the pre-antipsychotic era, there was a 4% incidence of dyskinesia with the first psychotic episode. 40% of those over age 60 with chronic schizophrenia demonstrated dyskinesia despite never taking an antipsychotic (Fenton, 2013). Spontaneous dyskinesia (unrelated to antipsychotic use) is also more prevalent in nonpsychotic first-degree relatives of schizophrenic individuals, likely due to genetically-based dopamine dysfunction (Koning et al, 2010).

All antipsychotics are labeled with a black box warning of increased mortality in elderly patients with dementia-related psychosis. However, antipsychotics are commonly prescribed for this population, not only for psychosis but also for aggression and agitation associated with dementia. These symptoms are referred to as "behavioral and psychological symptoms of dementia" (BPSD). After BPSD symptoms are controlled with an antipsychotic for at least 3 months, it is recommended to gradually taper off of the medication (Bjerre et al, 2018).

Serotonin Syndrome -vs- Neuroleptic Malignant Syndrome (NMS)

Serotonin (5-HT) Syndrome and Neuroleptic Malignant Syndrome are rare psychiatric emergencies. These syndromes should be considered when an individual taking several psychotropic medications becomes acutely ill. Since some symptoms overlap, here is a head-to-head comparison.

5-HT "twitchy frog" syndrome

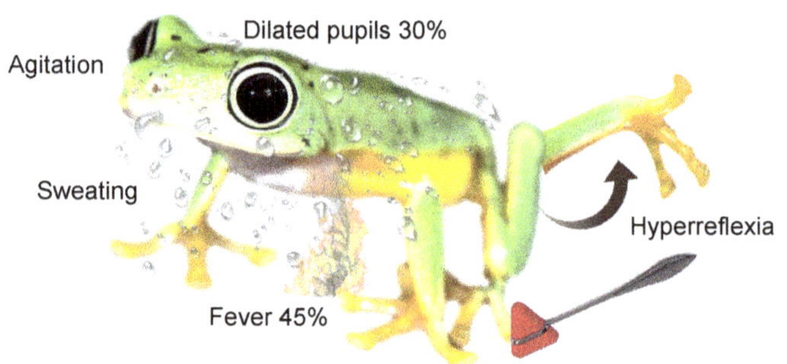

NMS - "can't Bend(er)"

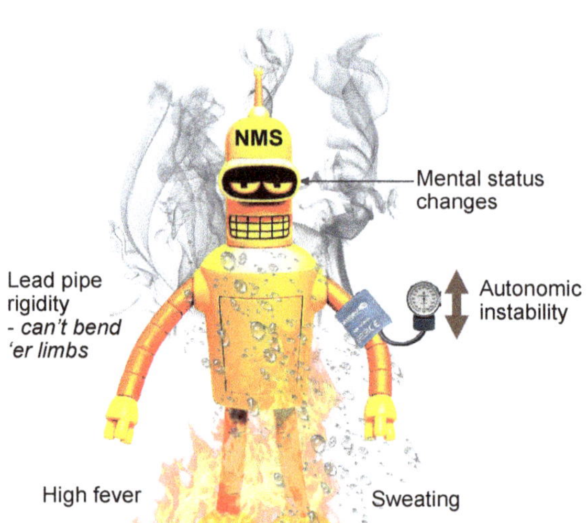

Bender from Futurama

	Serotonin Syndrome	Neuroleptic Malignant Syndrome (NMS)
Mechanism	Serotonin (5-HT) overload in the brain stem	Dopamine blockade in the hypothalamus (fever) and nigrostriatal pathway (rigidity)
Usual onset	Within 24 hours of combining antidepressants (or other serotonergics)	Within 30 days of starting or increasing an antipsychotic (anti-dopaminergic) or stopping a dopaminergic drug
Cardinal features	Myoclonic jerks > 50% Hyperreflexia > 50% Mental status changes > 50% Shivering > 50%	High fever 100% by definition Rigidity 100% by definition Mental status changes 99% Elevated or labile BP most
Fever	45%	Yes; Temp > 40°C (104°F) in 40% of cases
Autonomic instability	35% tachycardia 35% HTN 15% hypotension	99% overall 88% tachycardia 70% labile BP
Mental status change	51% confusion 50% restlessness/hyperactivity/agitation 29% unresponsiveness (may evolve to coma)	Confusion is the first symptom to present in 82% of cases, and may evolve to mutism, profound encephalopathy and coma.
Muscle rigidity	51%, less severe than with NMS	100% by definition; "lead pipe rigidity"
Motor activity	Hyperkinesia (restlessness/hyperactivity)	Bradykinesia (slowness of movement)
Hyperreflexia	52%	No
Clonus	23% - Examine for repetitive dorsiflexion of the ankle in response to one forcible dorsiflexion. Search Google Images for *clonus gif* to see how its done.	No
Tremor	43%	Less prominent
Ataxia	40%	Uncommon
Shivering	> 50%	Uncommon
...with chattering teeth or bruxism	15%	No
Sweating (diaphoresis)	Common	Common
Sialorrhea (hypersalivation)	Often prominent	< 15%
Eyes	30% dilated pupils; 20% unreactive pupils; Ocular clonus is possible. Search Google Images for *ocular clonus gif*	Usually not affected; Search Google Images for *oculogyric crisis gif* to see a manifestation of dystonia which may co-occur with NMS (to contrast with ocular clonus of 5-HT syndrome).

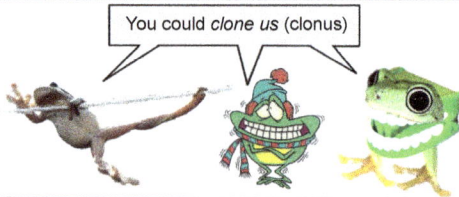

You could *clone us* (clonus)

continued...

	Serotonin Syndrome		Neuroleptic Malignant Syndrome (NMS)	
Nature of syndrome	Can be referred to as serotonin toxicity because it is a true toxidrome, caused by excess serotonin in a concentration-dependent way; Some cases are mild.		An idiosyncratic reaction, not a toxidrome; There is no such thing as a "mild" case of NMS.	
Typical evolution	Rapid onset; May have prodrome of nausea and diarrhea; Serotonin toxicity may be mild to severe.		First: Mental status changes (confusion, mutism, catatonia); Second: Rigidity; Third: Fever and BP lability; Peak severity in as little as 3 days	
Mortality	1% mortality if treated; When fatal, it is usually due to extreme fever, leading to the same complications as seen with NMS.		Fatal if untreated; 10% mortality when treated; Renal failure from rhabdomyolysis, heart attack, respiratory failure (from chest wall rigidity), DVT/pulmonary embolism, dehydration, electrolyte imbalance, disseminated intravascular coagulation (DIC), liver failure, seizures	
Resolution	70% of cases completely resolve within 24 hours.		If not fatal, NMS typically resolves slowly over 1 to 2 weeks.	
Most likely culprits	15% of SSRI overdoses lead to 5-HT toxicity; 50% incidence when overdosing on combo SSRI + MAOI; Clomipramine, imipramine are most likely among TCAs.		High potency 1st gen antipsychotics (FGAs); Haldol is responsible for 44% of cases. Depot antipsychotics (Haldol decanoate, Prolixin decanoate) are higher risk.	
Non-antidepressant/ antipsychotic culprits	LSD ("Acid") MDMA (Ecstasy) Dextromethorphan (DXM) L-Tryptophan Metaxalone (Skelaxin) Linezolid (Zyvox) Ondansetron (Zofran) Amphetamines	St. John's Wort Tramadol (Ultram) Meperidine (Demerol) Buspirone (Buspar) - unlikely Triptans (Imitrex, Maxalt, etc) - highly unlikely	Antiemetics that are D2 blockers: - Metoclopramide (Reglan) - Prochlorperazine (Compazine) - Promethazine (Phenergan) - Trimethobenzamide (Tigan)	Dopamine depleting agents - Reserpine (Serpasil) - Tetrabenazine (Xenazine) - Deutetrabenazine (Austedo) - Valbenazine (Ingrezza)
Lithium?	Lithium may contribute to 5-HT syndrome.		Lithium may contribute to NMS.	
Caused by stopping...	N/A		Stopping a dopaminergic antiparkinson medication (e.g., levodopa) can induce NMS. This variety of NMS is referred to as parkinsonism-hyperpyrexia syndrome or "withdrawal-emergent hyperpyrexia and confusion".	
Relatively low risk medications	Rarely caused by a lone antidepressant; Bupropion and mirtazapine are unlikely contributors.		Low potency 1st gen antipsychotics (Thorazine, Mellaril); 2nd gen antipsychotics (clozapine, quetiapine, olanzapine)	
Leukocytosis	Less prominent		> 75% of cases have WBC > 12,000	
Creatinine kinase (CK) elevation	Less prominent		90% show creatine kinase (CK) over 3x upper limit of normal (ULN). CK of over 5x ULM is diagnostic of rhabdomyolysis (skeletal muscle breakdown), which can lead to renal failure and disseminated intravascular coagulation (DIC). The normal range of CK is 22 to 198 units/Liter. CK is also called creatine phosphokinase (CPK).	
Management	Discontinue the contributing medication(s). Aim to normalize vital signs.		ICU admission, rapid cooling and hydration. Stop the antipsychotic or restart the dopaminergic med.	
Potentially helpful meds	Benzodiazepines for agitation Cyproheptadine (anti-serotonergic antihistamine) Methysergide (anti-serotonergic migraine medication)		Bromocriptine (DA agonist) Amantadine (DA agonist, NMDA antagonist) Dantrolene (direct acting muscle relaxant)	
Risk factors	Combinations of serotonergics, use of street drugs		Iron deficiency, dehydration, catatonia, Lewy body dementia, genetically reduced function of D2 receptors, rapid dose escalation, males under age 40	
Incidence	Severe 5-HT toxicity is rare. Mild toxicity is more common.		Quite rare - About 1 in 5,000 on antipsychotics	
Sequelae	None, although delirium may persist for a few days		Memory problems (although usually temporary)	
Differential diagnosis	Serotonin discontinuation syndrome (withdrawal) in the context of cross-tapering/titrating antidepressants. Anticholinergic toxicity, which manifests as dry, flushed skin ("dry as a bone, red as a beet") rather than diaphoresis.		Alcohol withdrawal, thyrotoxicosis, sepsis, heat stroke, tetanus, acute hydrocephalus, status epilepticus	
Formal diagnosis	Google *Hunter criteria*, which focuses on clonus (spontaneous or inducible), ocular clonus, and hyperreflexia		Defined by DSM 5; Severe rigidity and high fever are both necessary to make the diagnosis.	
Notes	Some experts prefer the term serotonin toxicity to more accurately reflect the condition as a dose-dependent form of 5-HT poisoning.		Neuroleptic, a synonym of antipsychotic, refers to something that "grabs ahold of nerves". Idiopathic NMS (with no identifiable culprit drug) is called malignant catatonia.	

1st and 2nd Generation Antipsychotics

The older antipsychotics came to be known as "typicals" (FGAs) upon the arrival of clozapine (Clozaril), the first "atypical" antipsychotic, in 1990. The atypicals (SGAs) purportedly caused fewer extrapyramidal symptoms (EPS) than the FGAs. Clozapine does not cause EPS, but most of the subsequent atypicals do cause EPS to some extent, which was disappointing. Despite side effects, all available antipsychotic drugs (FGAs and SGAs) are statistically significantly better than placebo for all-cause discontinuation (Leucht et al, 2013). In other words, any antipsychotic is less likely to be stopped than placebo when used to treat schizophrenia.

Class	First Generations Antipsychotics (FGAs)	Second Generation Antipsychotics (SGAs)
Also known as	Typical antipsychotics	Atypical antipsychotics
Mnemonic	The FugGAs, as in "Old fuggers"	The SuGAs, as in "SuGAr diabetes"
Best known for	Extrapyramidal symptoms (EPS) ► Dystonia (muscle rigidity) ► Akathisia (restlessness) ► Pseudo-Parkinsonism - Google *parkinsonism gif* ► Tardive dyskinesia - Google *tardive gif*	Metabolic syndrome ► Weight gain ► Diabetes ► Dyslipidemia
Usual mechanism	D2 dopamine receptor blockade	D2 dopamine receptor blockade and 5-HT_{2A} serotonin receptor blockade; Mnemonic: 2A = **2**nd generation **A**ntipsychotic
Release date	1954 Chlorpromazine (Thorazine) 1956 Prochlorperazine (Compazine) 1957 Perphenazine (Trilafon) 1958 Trifluoperazine (Stelazine) 1960 Fluphenazine (Prolixin) 1967 Haloperidol (Haldol) 1967 Thiothixene (Navane) 1975 Loxitane (Loxapine) 1975 Molindone (Moban) 1978 Thioridazine (Mellaril) 1985 Pimozide (Orap)	1990 Clozapine (Clozaril) 1993 Risperidone (Risperdal) 1996 Olanzapine (Zyprexa) 1997 Quetiapine (Seroquel) 2001 Ziprasidone (Geodon) 2002 Aripiprazole (Abilify)* 2006 Paliperidone (Invega) 2009 Asenapine (Saphris) 2009 Iloperidone (Fanapt) 2010 Lurasidone (Latuda) 2015 Brexpiprazole (Rexulti)* 2016 Cariprazine (Vraylar)* 2017 Pimavanserin (Nuplazid) - does not block DA 2020 Lumateperone (Caplyta) *D2 dopamine receptor partial agonists
Prolactin elevation ► gynecomastia ► galactorrhea ► sexual dysfunction ► osteopenia	Dopamine is also known as "prolactin-inhibiting factor" because it suppresses release of prolactin from the pituitary. All of the FGAs may elevate prolactin, which may result in growth of breast tissue. Hyperprolactinemia is caused by all FGAs because they have a high affinity for the D2 receptor and, once bound, are slow to dissociate from the D2 receptor.	About half of the SGAs increase prolactin, most prominently risperidone and paliperidone. Those SGAs that do not elevate prolactin are those that dissociate quickly from the D2 receptor and easily cross the blood-brain barrier (BBB). The prolactin-elevating effect of antipsychotics occurs outside of the BBB. Risperidone does not cross the BBB easily, so relatively high serum concentrations are necessary to achieve a therapeutic drug level in the central nervous system.
Noteworthy class members	Intermediate potency FGAs have relatively low potential to cause EPS: loxapine (Loxitane), perphenazine (Trilafon), and molindone (Moban)	Lurasidone (Latuda) and ziprasidone (Geodon) do not cause weight gain and may also lower lipids and blood sugar. Aripiprazole (Abilify) suppresses prolactin release.

D2 Receptor Partial Agonists – "Dopamine Stabilizers" **Mnemonic: "ABC"**

D2 partial agonist	~ cost	Weight gain	Akathisia	Somnolence	Advantages
Aripiprazole ABILIFY	$20	+	++	+	Inexpensive as PO. Available in long-acting injectable formulations, which are about $2,000/mo (100x the cost of PO)
Brexpiprazole REXULTI	$1,200	++	+	+/-	Better tolerability and probably anxiolytic properties
Cariprazine VRAYLAR	$1,200	+/-	+++	-	Also a D3 partial agonist, which may contribute cognitive benefits and improvement of negative symptoms

An agonist is a chemical that binds to a receptor and activates it to produce a biological response. Partial agonists can act either as a functional agonist or a functional antagonist, depending on the surrounding levels of naturally occurring neurotransmitters (the full agonist being dopamine, in this case). Partial D2 agonists can serve as "dopamine stabilizers", providing functional antagonism in hyper-DA states and functional agonism in hypo-DA states.

Dopamine Neural Pathways

Dopamine Pathway	Effect of D2 antagonist	Effect of D2 partial agonist
Mesolimbic	↓ DA activity - reduction of positive symptoms of schizophrenia (hallucinations, delusions)	↓ DA activity
Mesocortical	↓ DA - potential worsening of negative symptoms (amotivation, anhedonia, blunting of affect)	↑ DA - potential improvement of negative symptoms; Possibility of hypersexuality or pathologic gambling
Nigrostriatal	↓ DA - EPS, risk of tardive dyskinesia	Akathisia is common, but low risk of tardive dyskinesia
Tuberoinfundibular	↓ DA - increased prolactin, risk of breast growth (gynecomastia)	↑ DA - decreased prolactin, no risk of gynecomastia

D2 receptor blockers

#Rx	Generic/TRADE	Cost	Potency	mg	Minimal effective	FDA 24 hr max	Dose range	Comments
#1	Haloperidol HALDOL	$11	High	0.5 1 2 5 10 20	4 mg total daily dose	100 mg too high	2–10 mg PO BID; 5–10 mg IM q 4 hr PRN; Decanoate 100–300 mg IM q month	Effective and inexpensive. Available as q 4 wk long-acting injectable (LAI), Haldol Decanoate. Short-acting intramuscular Haldol is commonly administered ($2) for acute agitation. Tardive dyskinesia is a major risk at high doses. FDA-approved for Tourette's syndrome. No weight gain. Drug of choice for delirium because it lacks significant anticholinergic effects.
#2	Chlorpromazine THORAZINE	$135	Low	10 25 50 100 200	200 mg total daily dose	1,000 mg too high	25–100 mg PO TID 25–50 IM q 4 hr PRN	Causes sedation, orthostatic hypotension, and photosensitivity. At high doses it can cause blue/grey pigmentation of skin and eyes. Relatively unlikely to cause TD. FDA-approved for intractable hiccups; Available IM.
#3	Perphenazine TRILAFON	$33	Med	2 4 8 16	20 mg total daily dose	64 mg	8–16 mg BID–QID	Perphenazine was the FGA used in the CATIE trial against SGAs. It has low EPS similar to an SGA. It is a vulnerable 2D6 substrate, subject to more interactions than other medium potency FGAs.
#4	Fluphenazine PROLIXIN	$50	High	1 2.5 5 10	4 mg total daily dose	40 mg too high	2.5–5 mg TID; Decanoate 25–50 mg IM q 3–6 wk	Similar to haloperidol. Available as fluphenazine decanoate (Prolixin-D) q 3 to 6 wk long-acting injectable (LAI).
#5	Thiothixene NAVANE	$34	High	1 2 5 10 20	8 mg total daily dose	60 mg too high	2–5 mg BID–TID	Smokers need higher dose because thiothixene is a 1A2 substrate. Antidepressant properties; Minimal anticholinergic effects, as expected for a high potency FGA; Slow onset of tranquilizing effect, 90 minutes.
#6	Loxapine LOXITANE	$16	Med	5 10 25 50	20 mg total daily dose	250 mg	10–50 mg PO TID Adasuve 10 mg inhaled q 24 hr PRN	In addition to blocking D2 receptors, loxapine is the only FGA that blocks serotonin 5-HT_{2A} receptors with sufficient affinity to behave like an SGA. Metabolized to the tetracyclic antidepressant amoxapine. No weight gain and minimal relevant kinetic interactions. Risk of cardiotoxicity and seizures with overdose. Available as ADASUVE inhalation powder since 2014.
#7	Trifluoperazine STELAZINE	$34	High	1 2 5 10	10 mg total daily dose	40 mg too high	2–5 mg BID	Stelazine's marketing slogan was "Calm, but still alert." FDA-approved for schizophrenia and non-psychotic anxiety. Rarely used because, while other high potency FGAs have multiple routes of delivery, Stelazine is only is available PO.
#8	Thioridazine MELLARIL	$19	Low	10 25 50 100	200 mg total daily dose	800 mg too high	50–100 mg TID	Rarely prescribed because it causes the most QT prolongation of all psychotropics. Also, it can cause irreversible retinal pigmentation and degenerative retinopathy > 800 mg. Risk of seizures. It is effective for anxiety, and safe if the dose is kept low.
#9	Pimozide ORAP	$60	High	1 2	4 mg total daily dose	10 mg too high	1–2 mg QD–BID	Approved for Tourette's syndrome only. Risky due to QT prolongation and susceptibility to interactions as a 2D6 and 3A4 substrate.
#10	Molindone MOBAN	$75	Med	5 10 25	20 mg total daily dose	225 mg	10–25 mg TID	Approved for schizophrenia only; Causes weight loss; short half-life of 1.5 hours; Of available antipsychotics, molindone is the least prescribed.

Antiemetics that block D2 receptors

D2 blocking antiemetic	Cost	Potency	mg	Usual dose	Comments
Promethazine PHENERGAN	$8	Low	12.5 25 50	25 mg TID PRN	Much too weak of a D2 blocker to be used as an antipsychotic. Effectiveness as an antiemetic is mostly due to antihistamine activity. Approved for allergic conditions, motion sickness, nausea/vomiting, sedation, and urticaria.
Prochlorperazine COMPAZINE	$8	High	5 10	5–10 mg TID PRN	GoodRx lists Compazine as the #1 prescribed FGA, but today it is almost exclusively prescribed as an antiemetic. High risk of EPS, similar to haloperidol. It has old FDA approvals for schizophrenia and non-psychotic anxiety (12 wk max). Rectal formulation available.
Metoclopramide REGLAN	$6	High	5 10	10 mg QID PRN	High potency D2 blocker but not approved for psychosis. **Black box warning** for tardive dyskinesia. FDA-approved for GERD, diabetic gastroparesis, nausea/vomiting, small bowel intubation, and radiologic exam.

Side effect profile according to potency (of D2 blockade)

Potency	Trade (BRAND)	ACh	QT	↓ BP	↑ PRL	↑ Wt	EPS	NMS	Comments
Low	Chlorpromazine (THORAZINE) Thioridazine (MELLARIL) Promethazine (PHENERGAN)	+++	++	+++	++	++	++	+	Antihistamine properties
Medium	Loxapine (LOXITANE) Molindone (MOBAN) Perphenazine (TRILAFON)	++	-	++	++	-	+	+	EPS risk is similar to 2nd generation antipsychotics (SGAs).
High	Haloperidol (HALDOL) Fluphenazine (PROLIXIN) Pimozide (ORAP) Thiothixene (NAVANE) Trifluoperazine (STELAZINE) Prochlorperazine (COMPAZINE)	+	-	+	++	-	++++	+++	Pimozide causes less EPS than the other high potency FGAs.

Minimal effective = dose per 24 hours considered necessary to adequately treat first-episode schizophrenia; Potency = D2 blockade; LAI = long-acting injectable; ACh = anticholinergic (constipation, urinary retention, dry mouth); QT = QT interval prolongation; ↓ BP = orthostatic hypotension; ↑ PRL = prolactin elevation (gynecomastia, sexual side effects); ↑ Wt = weight gain; NMS = neuroleptic malignant syndrome

#243
1967
$12–$32

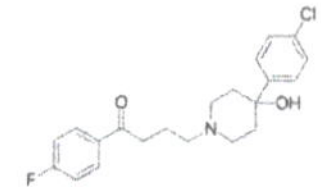

Haloperidol (HALDOL)

hal oh PER i dawl / HAL dawl

"Halo doll"

- ❖ Antipsychotic
- ❖ High potency FGA
- ❖ D2 antagonist

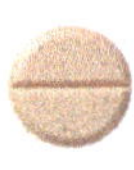

0.5
1
2
5
10
20
mg

FDA-approved for:
- ❖ Psychosis
- ❖ Tourette's disorder

Used off-label for:
- ❖ Agitation/aggression
- ❖ Delirium
- ❖ Mania
- ❖ Gastroparesis

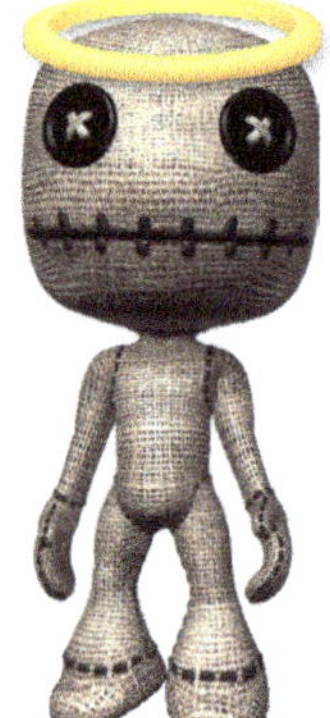

This book uses spooky pictures for antipsychotic medications, because they are used to treat paranoid delusions and hallucinations.

Haloperidol (Haldol) is a High potency 1st generation antipsychotic (FGA), approved in 1967. It remains the most prescribed FGA, mainly used for chronic schizophrenia and acute aggression. Haloperidol is cheap and effective, but it commonly causes extrapyramidal symptoms (EPS). Due to high risk of tardive dyskinesia (TD), it is not a first-line maintenance antipsychotic. It is a reasonable third-line option when two SGAs have failed. Haldol does not cause weight gain. It can be used to augment a 2nd generation antipsychotic (SGA) at low dose.

Intramuscular haloperidol was once essential for treating acute agitation and aggression. IM Haldol is still regarded as a first-line option as a PRN for this purpose. Haloperidol immediate-release injections are inexpensive ($2) and are commonly used in combination with IM lorazepam (Ativan) and/or IM diphenhydramine (Benadryl). Health care professionals widely refer to an injection consisting of Haldol 5 mg and Ativan 2 mg as a "five and two".

A combination of a "five and two" (mixed in one syringe) plus a separate syringe containing Benadryl 50 mg is known as a "B-52". The B-52 is reserved for highly agitated patients who have high tolerance for sedative medication. In addition to sedation, the benzodiazepine (lorazepam) and antihistamine (diphenhydramine) serve to prevent haloperidol-induced akathisia and dystonia. Short-term use of haloperidol does not cause Parkinsonism or TD. Haldol is a drug of choice for acute delirium due to lack of anticholinergic activity.

Prolongation of QT interval with haloperidol can be prominent when administered intravenously. QT prolongation from oral haloperidol is generally insignificant, except in overdose.

The FDA max is 100 mg, which today is considered much too high, and very likely to cause TD with prolonged use. Anyone needing that much haloperidol would be better served by clozapine (Clozaril), which does not cause TD.

To prevent dystonia, the author usually adds the anticholinergic benztropine (Cogentin) 0.5 mg BID (for the short term) if the haloperidol dose is increased to 5 mg BID. EPS is caused by a relative deficiency of dopamine and an excess of acetylcholine in the nigrostriatal pathway. Benztropine may be needed to prevent dystonia because haloperidol has no intrinsic anticholinergic activity. After a month or so, try to taper benztropine or change it to PRN. Long-term use of anticholinergics can increase risk of TD and contribute to negative symptoms (amotivation, anhedonia, blunting of affect).

Dosing:
Haldol 2 mg PO is considered the "minimal effective" daily dose for first-episode psychosis. For multi-episode psychosis, the minimal effective dose is 4 mg. For PO haloperidol for maintenance treatment, the author usually starts 2.5 mg BID, which is half of a 5 mg tab. 10 mg BID is a reasonable maximum dose.

Haloperidol decanoate (Haldol D) is a long-acting injectable (LAI) given every 4 weeks. 100 mg every 4 weeks is equivalent to about 7–10 mg daily oral dose. Don't exceed 100 mg with the first injection and extend the PO dose for a 2-week overlap. FDA max is 450 mg/mo, which is equivalent to about 30–45 mg of a daily PO dose, although it is recommended not to exceed 200 mg monthly. The drug is in a oil suspension, which makes it more painful than other LAIs. It may leave a bump under the skin that can take weeks to resolve. Haloperidol decanoate costs about $50 monthly, much cheaper than the available 2nd generation LAI antipsychotics. See also page 58 for all LAIs.

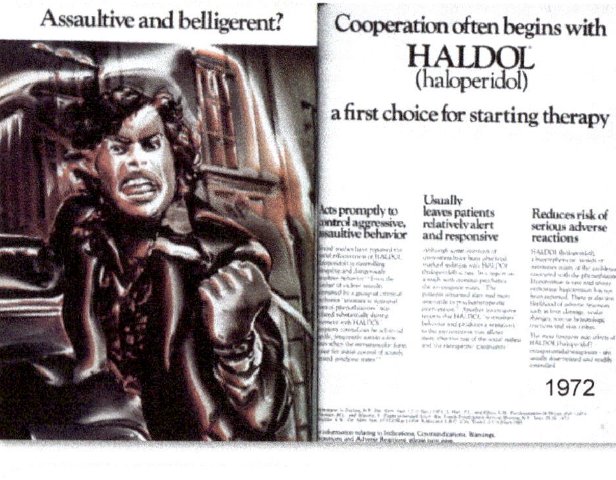

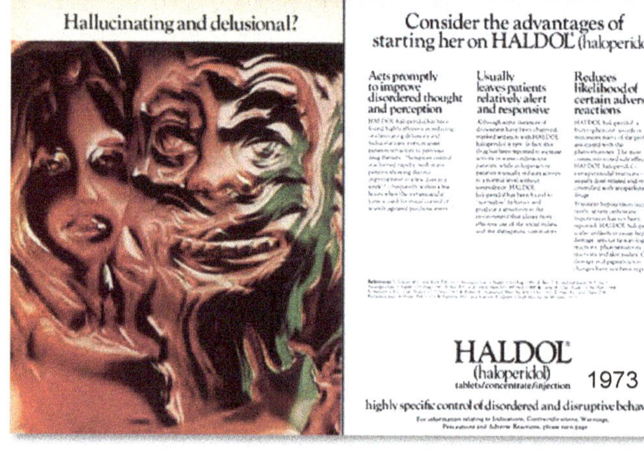

Hallucinating and delusional?
Consider the advantages of starting her on HALDOL (haloperidol)
Acts promptly to improve disordered thought and perception
Usually leaves patients relatively alert and responsive
Reduces likelihood of certain adverse reactions
Assaultive and belligerent?
Cooperation often begins with
HALDOL
(haloperidol)
a first choice for starting therapy
tablets/concentrate/injection
1973
highly specific control of disordered and disruptive behavior

Dynamic interactions:
- ❖ Dopamine antagonist (strong)
- ❖ Extrapyramidal effects (high)
- ❖ Sedation/CNS depression
- ❖ QT prolongation (moderate)
- ❖ Hypotensive
- ❖ Lowers seizure threshold (mild)
- ❖ Prolactin elevating (strong)
- ❖ Hyponatremia
- ❖ Hyperammonemia

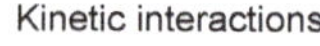

Kinetic interactions:
- ❖ 3A4 substrate
- ❖ 2D6 substrate
- ❖ 1A2 substrate (minor)

page 16

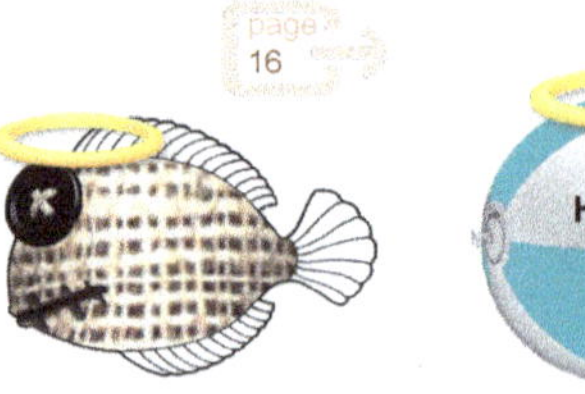

3A4 substrate

page 15

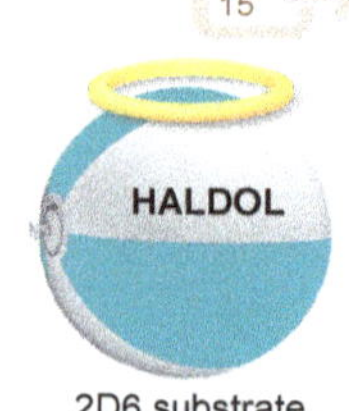

2D6 substrate

page 10

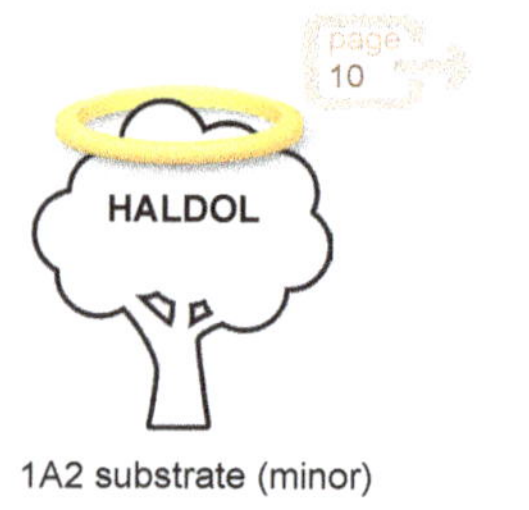

1A2 substrate (minor)

1954
$62–$157

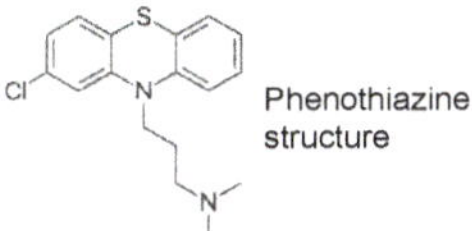

Chlorpromazine (THORAZINE)

klawr PRO muh zeen / THOR a zeen

"Thor's Color promising" (to change)

- ❖ Antipsychotic
- ❖ Low potency FGA
- ❖ D2 antagonist
- ❖ 5-HT_2 antagonist
- ❖ Phenothiazine

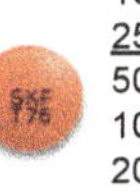

10
25
50
100
200
mg

FDA-approved for:

- ❖ Psychosis
- ❖ Nausea/Vomiting
- ❖ Intractable hiccups
- ❖ Adjunct treatment of tetanus (IM)
- ❖ Acute intermittent porphyria (IM)

Used off-label for:

- ❖ Behavioral disturbance (IM or PO)
- ❖ Impulse control disorders
- ❖ Serotonin Syndrome, adjunct (IM)
- ❖ Anxiety (low dose)
- ❖ Insomnia (low dose)

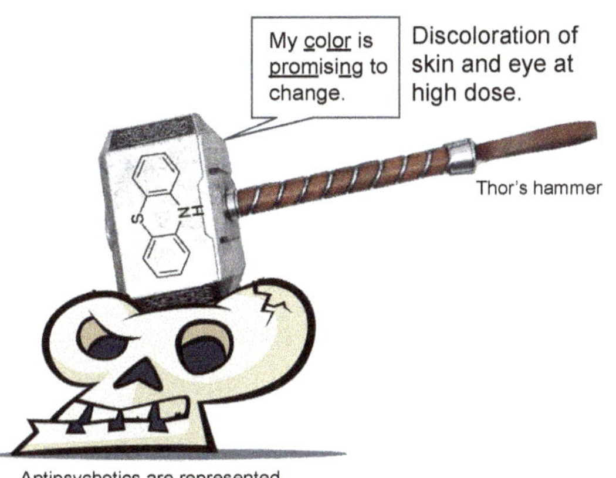

Antipsychotics are represented with spooky mascots.

Specific risks:

- ▶ Photosensitivity (common, phenothiazine class)
- ▶ Pigmentation of skin
- ▶ Pigmentation of eye (benign, unless the retina is involved)
- ▶ Corneal epithelial keratopathy (benign deposits in cornea)
- ▶ Corneal edema (with possible irreversible vision loss)

Phenothiazine structure

page 36

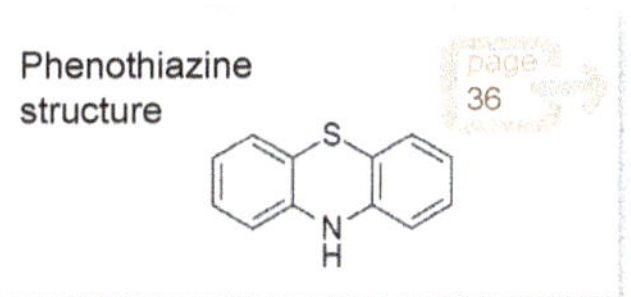

Chlorpromazine (Thorazine) is a low potency FGA—think *ch-lower-promazine*. In 1954, Thorazine revolutionized psychiatry. It largely replaced electroconvulsive therapy, hydrotherapy, psychosurgery (prefrontal lobotomy), and insulin shock therapy. In the 1950s it was used for almost every psychiatric condition, including anxiety and emotional distress associated with almost any medical condition.

Chlorpromazine is an example of a "dirty drug", one that antagonizes several types of receptors (dopaminergic, histaminergic, muscarinic, serotonergic). Thorazine's antihistamine activity contributes prominently to its sedative effect and made it useful in the 1950s for treatment of pruritus and peptic ulcers. Chlorpromazine has been described as possible therapy for serotonin syndrome, based on its antiserotonergic effect.

Although blamed for the "Thorazine Shuffle", chlorpromazine is much less likely to cause Parkinsonism than high potency neuroleptics like haloperidol (Haldol) or fluphenazine (Prolixin). Run a Google image search for *parkinson gait gif* to see what the shuffle looks like.

Currently chlorpromazine is more expensive than the other FGAs. This may be the result of price fixing by the pharmaceutical industry. In 2019, 44 states filed a lawsuit alleging major drug manufacturers conspired to artificially inflate the prices of more than 100 generic drugs. Goodrx.com is a great resource for keeping up with current prices at individual pharmacies.

Dosing: These days, Thorazine is rarely used as monotherapy for schizophrenia. More commonly it is used for anxiety or agitation at low doses (25–100 mg). It is dosed similarly to the SGA quetiapine (Seroquel), which is also a weak antipsychotic that works well for insomnia or anxiety. The FDA max dose is 1,000 mg/day (divided TID–QID), although doses exceeding 400 mg/day may lead to eye problems and skin discoloration.

Chlorpromazine is the only FGA that significantly lowers seizure threshold. There are three SGAs with a higher risk of seizures than chlorpromazine.

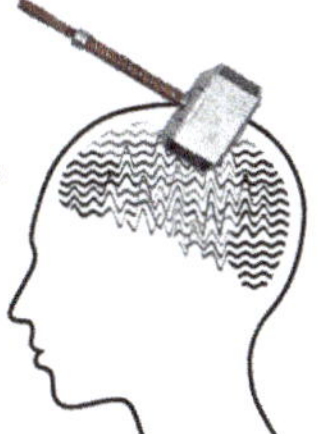

Seizure risk among Antipsychotics (dose-dependent):

#1 Clozapine (Clozaril) up to 10x risk
#2 Olanzapine (Zyprexa) 3x
#3 Quetiapine (Seroquel) 2x
#4 Chlorpromazine (Thorazine) 2x

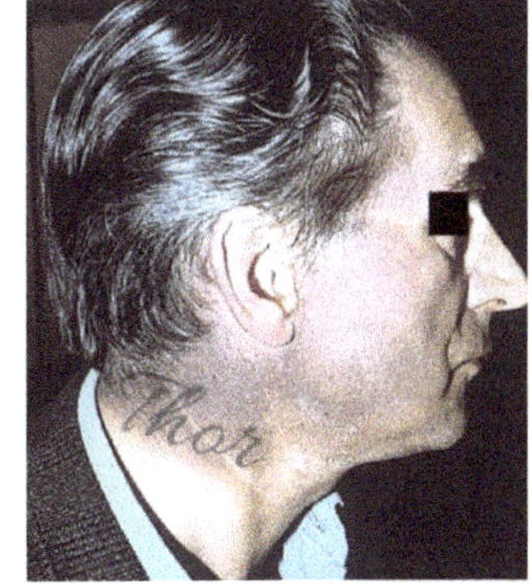

Some patients taking high-dose Thorazine develop a progressive blue-gray or purple discoloration in sun-exposed areas of the skin, with sparing of facial wrinkles. Pigmentation may involve sun-exposed portions of the eye. Thankfully, this condition is reversible.

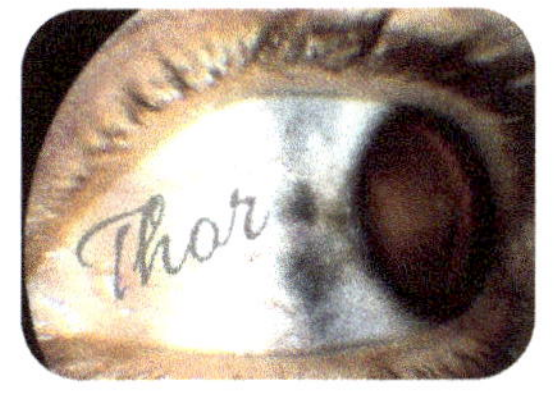

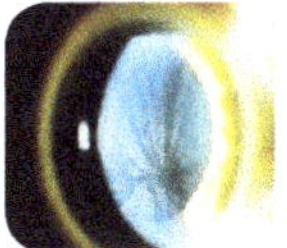

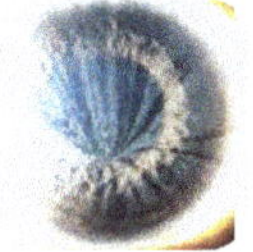

Corneal epithelial keratopathy caused by high dose thorazine. *Cornea verticillata* is the term for the whorl-like deposition of material in the corneal epithelium. The phenomenon is benign and reversible.

Dynamic interactions:

- ❖ Dopamine antagonist
- ❖ Extrapyramidal effects
- ❖ Sedation/CNS depression (strong)
- ❖ QT prolongation (moderate)
- ❖ Hypotensive (strong)
- ❖ Anticholinergic (strong)
- ❖ Lowers seizure threshold (significant)
- ❖ Prolactin elevating
- ❖ Hyponatremia
- ❖ Hyperglycemia
- ❖ Photosensitivity (phenothiazine)

Kinetic interactions:

- ❖ 2D6 substrate, like most phenothiazines
- ❖ 1A2 substrate (minor)
- ❖ 3A4 substrate (minor)

page 15

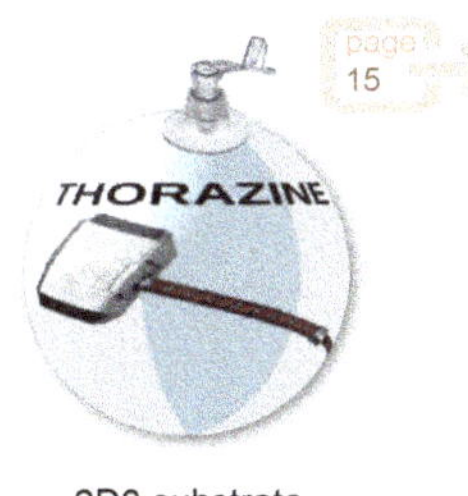

2D6 substrate

Vintage Thorazine ads from physicians' journals

'A fundamental drug in psychiatry' - Smith, Kline & French laboratories

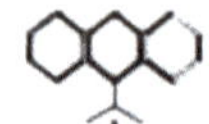

Logo resembling phenothiazine structure

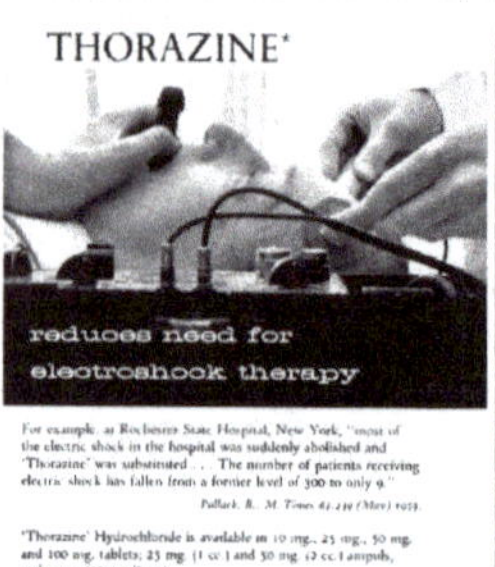

"Thorazine ***reduces need for electroshock therapy.****" 1955*

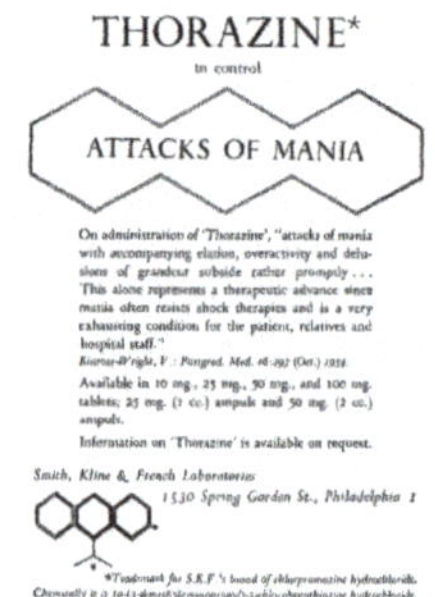

"Thorazine to ***control ATTACKS OF MANIA****...this alone represents a therapeutic advance since mania often resists shock therapies and is a very exhausting condition for the patient, relatives and hospital staff." 1955*

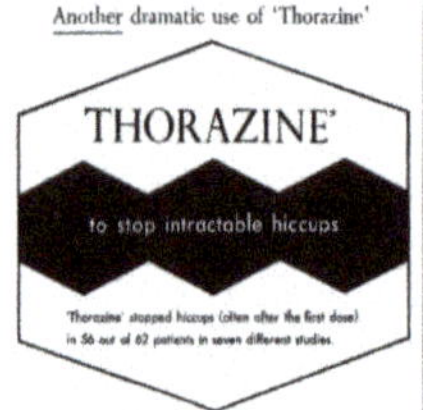

"Another dramatic use of Thorazine...'Thorazine' ***stopped hiccups*** *(often after the first dose) in 56 of 62 patients in seven different studies." 1955*

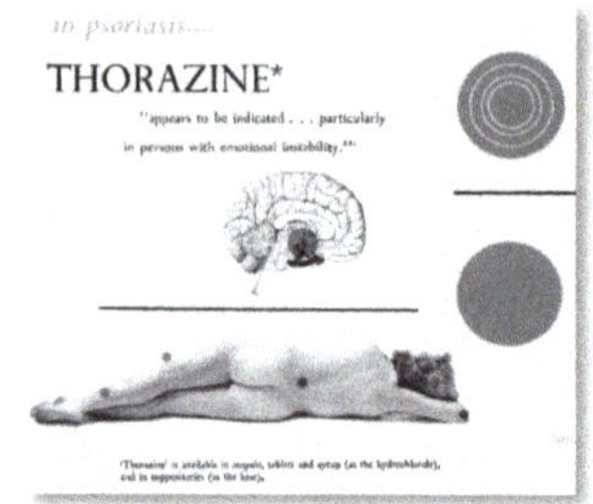

*"****In psoriasis*** *- Thorazine 'appears to be indicated...particularly in persons with emotional instability... the* ***ataractic, tranquilizing effect*** *can do much to relieve the* ***emotional stress*** *that is so often a complicating or even a causative* ***factor in many somatic conditions.****" 1955*

The above ad refers to psoriatic arthritis. Fibromyalgia was not a recognized condition until the 1990s.

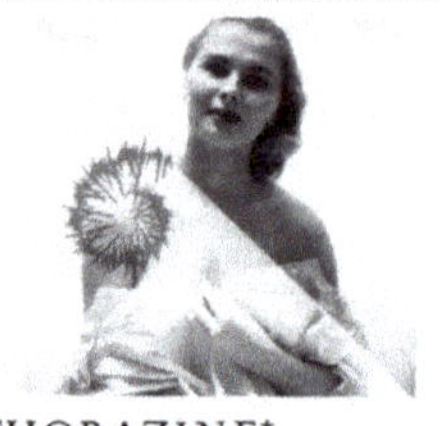

"Thorazine can allay the suffering caused by the pain of ***SEVERE BURSITIS****. The ataractic, tranquilizing action of Thorazine can reduce the anguish and suffering associated with bursitis. Thorazine acts not by eliminating the pain, but by altering the patient's reaction -* ***enabling her to view her pain with a 'serene detachment'****... 'Several of [our patients] expressed the feeling that ['Thorazine'] put a curtain between them and their pain, so that whilst they were aware that the pain existed, they were not upset by it.'" 1956*

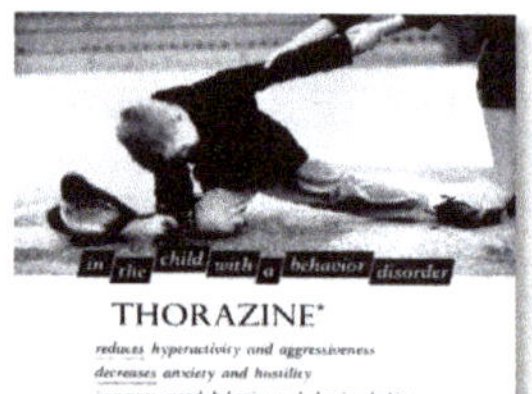

"In the ***child with a behavior disorder*** *Thorazine reduces hyperactivity and aggressiveness; decreases anxiety and hostility; improves mood, behavior and sleeping habits;* ***establishes*** *accessibility to guidance or psychotherapy;* ***increases amenability to supervision****...bear in mind- 'Thorazine' may give the impression of a cure, simultaneous supportive counseling and guidance are necessary... 'Thorazine' should be administered discriminantly." 1956*

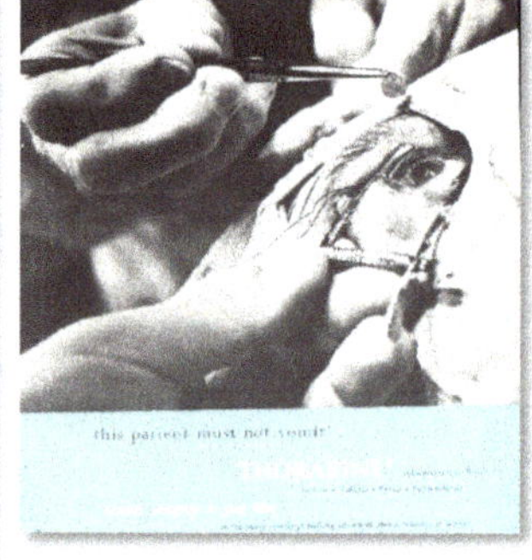

*"****This patient must not vomit!*** *Ocular surgery is just one of the many emesis-provoking situations and conditions...drugs, radiation, disease, pregnancy..." 1956*

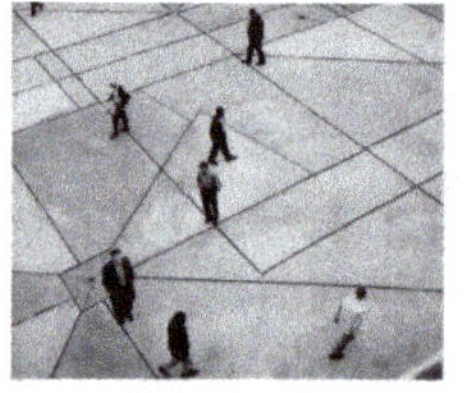

"Thorazine helps ***keep more patients out of mental hospitals****...more patients can be treated in the community, at clinics or in the psychiatrist's office without being hospitalized at all." 1956*

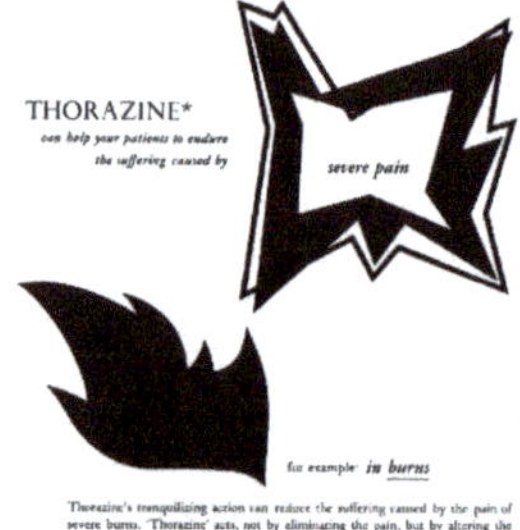

"Thorazine's ***tranquilizing action*** *can reduce the suffering caused by the pain of severe burns... Thorazine produced 'a* ***quiet, phlegmatic acceptance of pain.****'" 1956*

The combination of Thorazine & Dexedrine (dextroamphetamine) is no longer available. Anxious depression is no longer treated with an antipsychotic plus a Schedule II stimulant. Such combinations (as separate pills) are still used for hyperactive ADHD. The most prescribed antipsychotic for behaviorally disordered children is now risperidone (Risperdal). Dexedrine is similar to Adderall (mixed amphetamine salts).

"When the patient's anxiety is complicated by depression... both symptoms often respond to THORA-DEX, a combination of a specific ***anti-anxiety agent, 'Thorazine'****, and* ***a standard antidepressant, 'Dexedrine'****. The preparation is of unusual value in mental and emotional disturbances and in somatic conditions complicated by emotional stress - especially when depression occurs together with anxiety, agitation or apprehension. The patient treated with 'Thora-Dex' is generally both calm and alert...with normal interest, activity and capacity for work...Thora-Dex should be administered discriminantly." 1957*

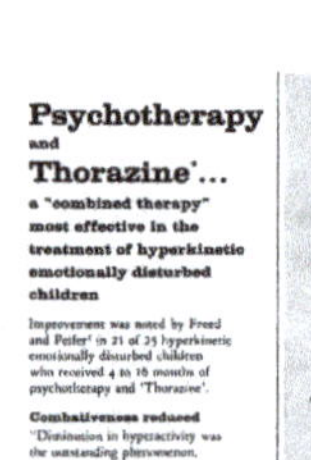

"Psychotherapy and Thorazine...a 'combined therapy' most effective in the treatment of ***hyperkinetic emotionally disturbed children****...Diminution in hyperactivity was the outstanding phenomenon." 1957*

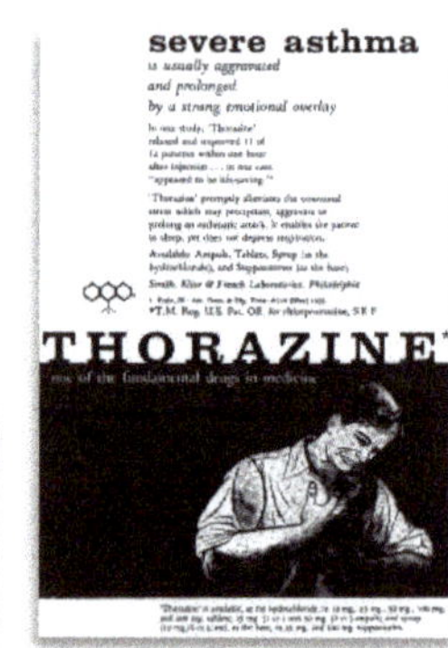

*"****Severe asthma*** *is usually aggravated and prolonged by a strong emotional overlay... Thorazine promptly alleviates the emotional stress which may precipitate, aggravate or prolong an asthmatic attack. It enables the patient to sleep, yet does not depress respiration". 1958*

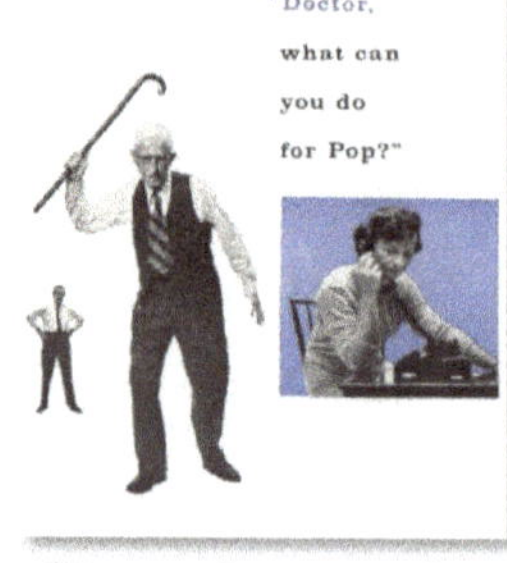

"Doctor, what can you do for Pop?" 1957

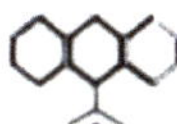

Vintage Thorazine ads from physicians' journals

'One of the fundamental drugs in medicine' - Smith, Kline & French laboratories

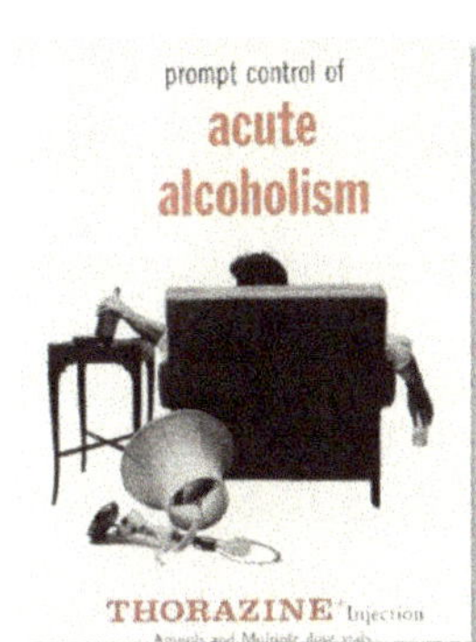

"Prompt control of acute alcoholism. Thorazine injection." 1959

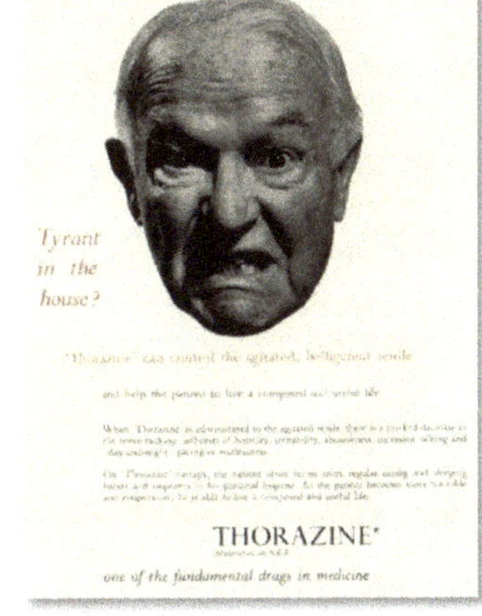

*"**Tyrant in the house?** Thorazine can control **the agitated, belligerent senile** and help the patient to **live a composed and useful life.** Thorazine, one of the fundamental drugs in medicine". 1959*

All antipsychotics now have a black box warning: "Not approved for dementia-related psychosis; **increased mortality risk in elderly dementia patients**."

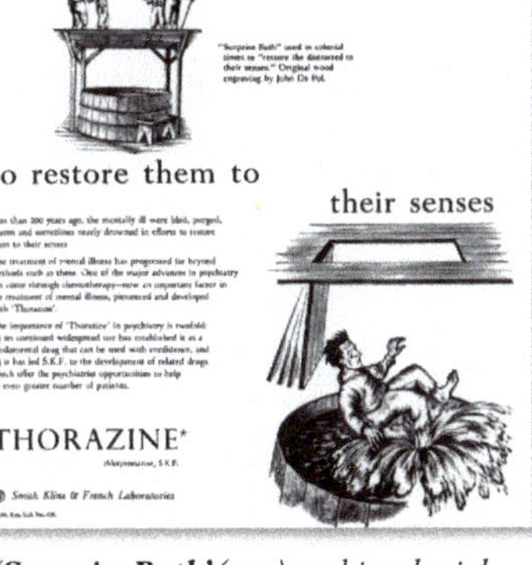

*"**'Surprise Bath'** (was) used in colonial times to **'restore the distracted to their senses.'** Less than 200 years ago, the mentally ill were bled, purged, beaten and sometimes nearly drowned...the treatment of mental illness has progressed far beyond...with chemotherapy... pioneered and developed with Thorazine." 1959*

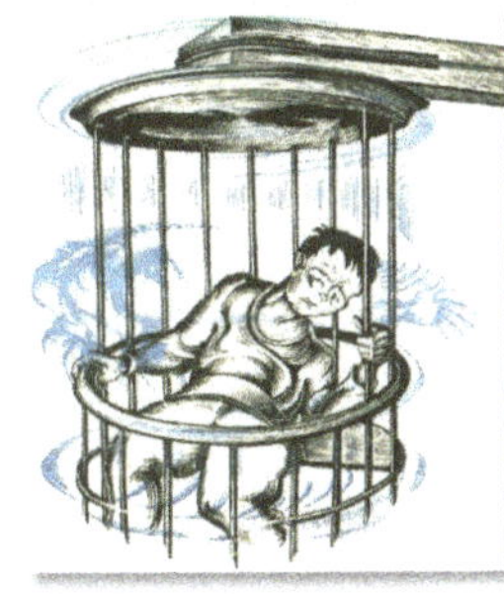

*"**To free the mind from madness** - in nineteenth century psychiatry, **the 'rotator'** was a major therapeutic device. Today, psychopharmacologic therapy, pioneered and developed with Thorazine, is one of the most important methods used in the treatment of mental illness." 1959*

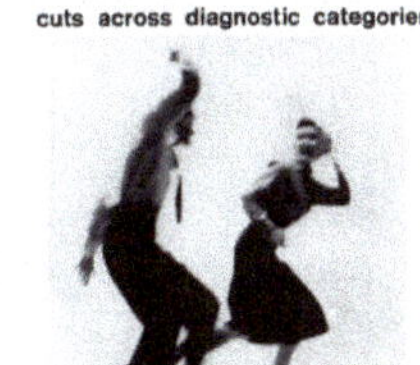

*"To control **agitation**—a symptom that cuts across diagnostic categories...Thorazine, a fundamental drug in psychiatry...Because of its **sedative** effect, Thorazine is especially useful in controlling hyperactivity, irritability and hostility." 1960*

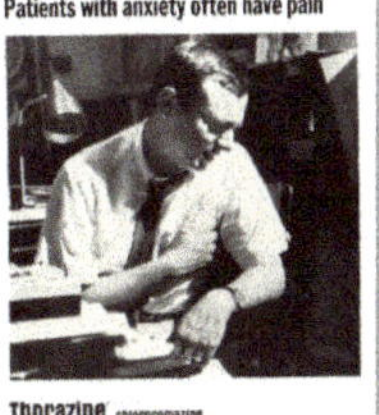

*"Patients with pain often have anxiety. Patients with anxiety often have pain. Thorazine helps **reduce reaction to pain, relieves anxiety.**" 1960*

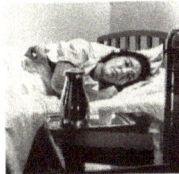

Today, the antiepileptic drug gabapentin (Neurontin) is used for various co-presentations of pain and anxiety.

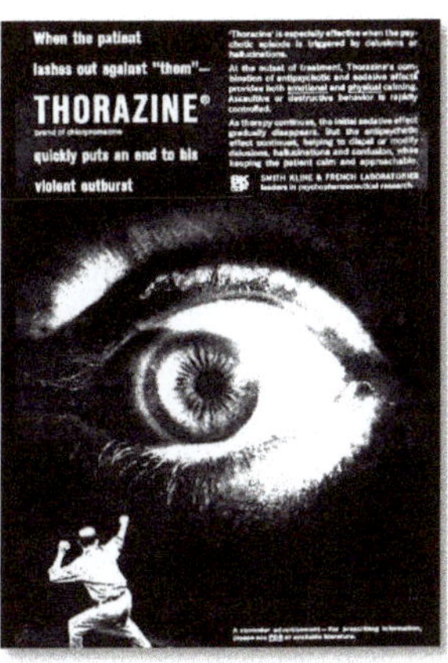

*"**When the patient lashes out against 'them'**— Thorazine quickly puts an end to his violent outburst." 1962*

*"For your **cancer patients**, at home or in the hospital. Thorazine **improves mental outlook.** The **unique tranquilizing effect** of Thorazine helps the cancer patient to overcome his manifold fears and anxieties, thus improving his mental outlook and making him easier to care for...Thorazine reduces his suffering." 1961*

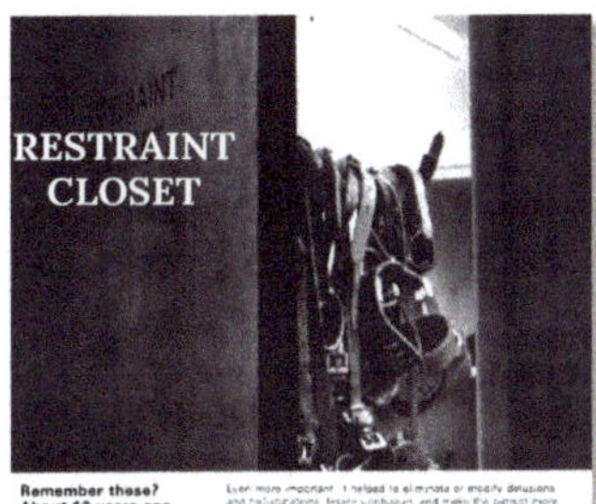

*"**Restraint Closet - remember these?** About 13 years ago, Thorazine helped make them obsolete. In psychiatry, Thorazine remains **today's most widely prescribed ataractic**... Contraindication: Comatose states or the presence of large amounts of C.N.S. depressant; Precaution: Antiemetic effect may mask signs of overdosage of toxic drugs or obscure diagnosis of other conditions; Side Effect: **Parkinsonism-like symptoms on high dosages (in rare instances, may persist).**" 1967*

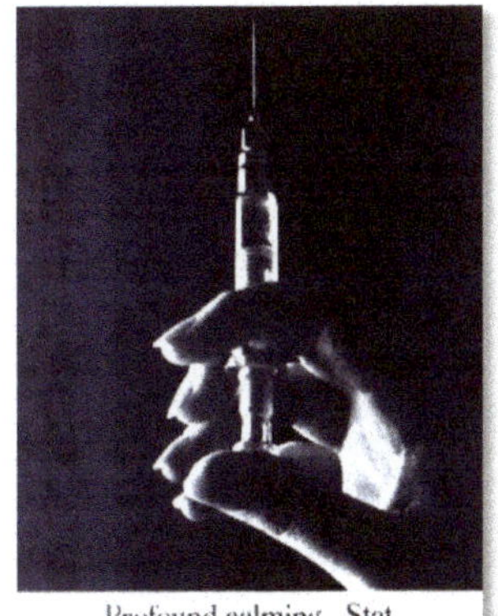

*"**Profound calming**...Stat." 1968*

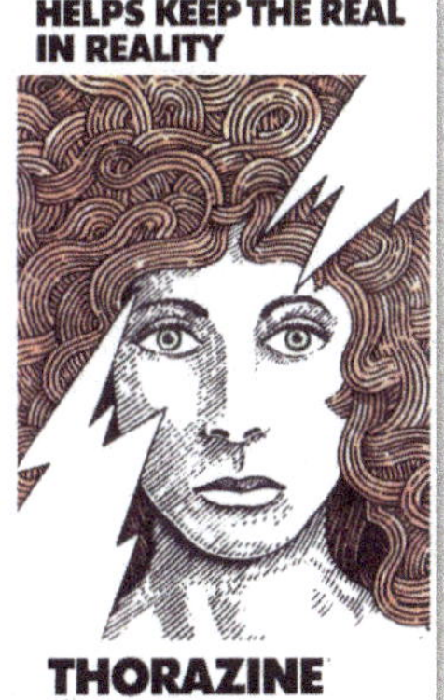

"Helps keep the real in reality." 1973

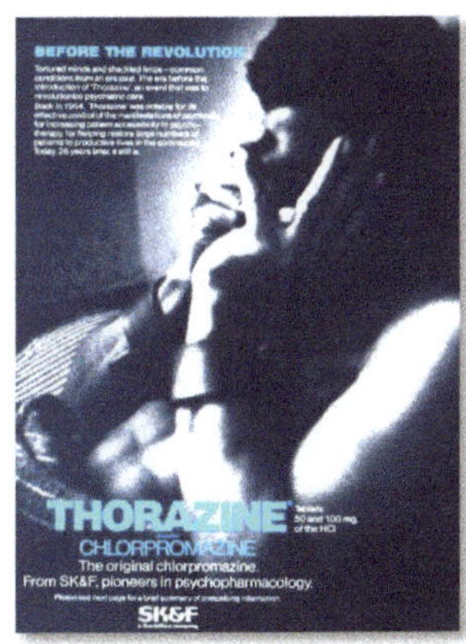

*"**Before the revolution...** Tortured minds and shackled limbs—common conditions from an era past. The era before the introduction of Thorazine, an event that was to revolutionize psychiatric care." 1982*

1957
$31–$115

Phenothiazine structure

Perphenazine (TRILAFON)

per FEN uh zeen / TRIL uh fon

"Perple Trial phone"

- ❖ Antipsychotic
- ❖ Medium potency FGA
- ❖ D2 antagonist
- ❖ Phenothiazine

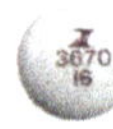

2
4
8
16
mg

FDA-approved for:

- ❖ Schizophrenia
- ❖ Nausea/vomiting

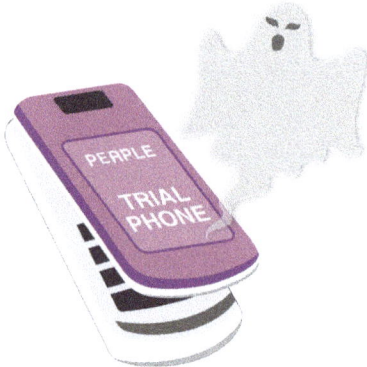

Antipsychotics are represented with spooky mascots.

Perphenazine (Trilafon) was the first generation antipsychotic (FGA) included in the CATIE schizophrenia trial (Lieberman et al, 2005), which compared it to several second generation antipsychotics (SGAs)—olanzapine (Zyprexa), risperidone (Risperdal), quetiapine (Seroquel), and ziprasidone (Geodon). Perphenazine showed comparable effectiveness and caused no more EPS than these SGAs. Perphenazine was no less effective in improving cognitive performance than the SGAs. Although these four SGAs are now affordable, they were much more expensive when the CATIE trial was conducted. Olanzapine, risperidone, and quetiapine are now cheaper than perphenazine.

When choosing a medium potency FGA, the author prefers loxapine (Loxitane) over perphenazine because loxapine has fewer relevant kinetic interactions. Perphenazine is such a susceptible 2D6 substrate that the FDA recommends 2D6 genotype testing before it is started, because levels will be increased 3-fold for 2D6 poor metabolizers.

Even though perphenazine's half-life is about 10 hours, maintenance dosing can be once daily. For antipsychotics in general, continuous dopamine D2 receptor blockade is not necessary to sustain antipsychotic response (Takeuchi et al, 2014).

Dosing: Suggested starting dose is 4 mg BID or TID. For maintenance treatment, once daily dosing is equally effective to BID–TID dosing. In the CATIE trial, patients received between 8–32 mg/day. FDA max is 24 mg/day for non-hospitalized patients. For hospitalized patients, the FDA max is 64 mg/day. Smokers and African Americans may need higher doses due to increased rate of clearance (Jin et al, 2010).

Perphenazine is available in a fixed-dose combo with the antidepressant amitriptyline (Elavil), branded as TRIAVIL. The combo is FDA-approved for (1) depression with anxiety and (2) psychosis with depression. Available since 1963, it is rarely used today.

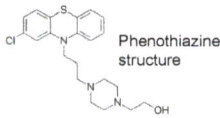

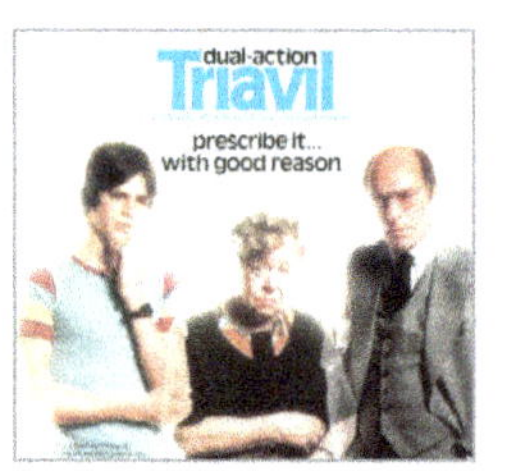
dual-action
Triavil
prescribe it...
with good reason

Dynamic interactions:

- ❖ Dopamine antagonist
- ❖ Extrapyramidal effects
- ❖ Sedation/CNS depression
- ❖ Hypotensive
- ❖ Anticholinergic (moderate)
- ❖ Lowers seizure threshold (mild)
- ❖ Prolactin elevating
- ❖ Hyponatremia
- ❖ Hyperglycemia
- ❖ Photosensitivity (phenothiazine)

Kinetic interactions:

- ❖ 2D6 substrate, like most phenothiazines
- ❖ FDA recommends 2D6 genotyping prior to starting perphenazine, levels of which are increased 3-fold for 2D6 poor metabolizers

page 15

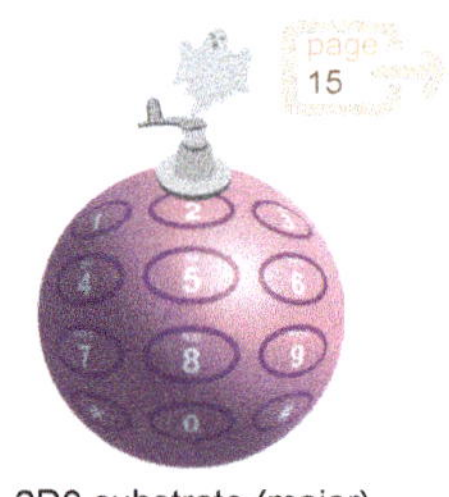

2D6 substrate (major)

1960
$21–$233

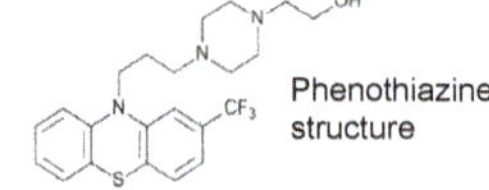

Phenothiazine structure

Fluphenazine (PROLIXIN)

flu FEN uh zeen / pro LIK sin

"Prolix Floppy hen"

- ❖ Antipsychotic
- ❖ High potency FGA
- ❖ D2 antagonist
- ❖ Phenothiazine

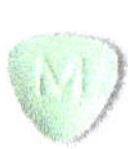

1
2.5
5
10
mg

FDA-approved for:

- ❖ Psychosis.

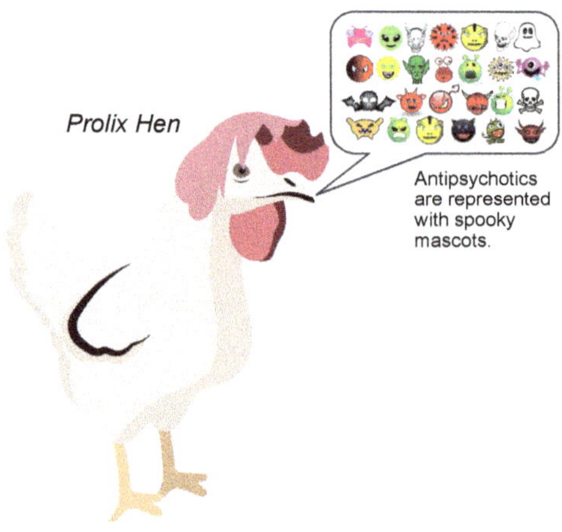

Prolix Hen

Antipsychotics are represented with spooky mascots.

prolix (adjective): given to speaking or writing at great or tedious length; long and wordy, redundant

"Prolix hen"—Prolixin (fluphenazine) is a high potency FGA. Prolixin's only FDA-approved indication is psychosis. It is very similar to haloperidol (Haldol). As a high potency D2 blocker, fluphenazine causes significant EPS including risk of tardive dyskinesia.

As with haloperidol, fluphenazine is available as a decanoate long-acting injectable (LAI). Fluconazole decanoate (Prolixin D) is given IM q 3 to 6 wk. It is also available as an oral liquid and immediate-release injectable.

Dosing: Start 1 mg TID. FDA max is 40 mg total daily dose, which is too high in most circumstances due to risk of tardive dyskinesia. A reasonable maintenance dose is 2.5 mg TID—5 mg TID. Stop if absolute neutrophil count (ANC) drops below 1,000. See page 58 for dosing of the long-acting injectable.

Dynamic interactions:

- ❖ Dopamine antagonist (strong)
- ❖ Extrapyramidal effects (high)
- ❖ Sedation/CNS depression
- ❖ Hypotensive
- ❖ Anticholinergic (moderate)
- ❖ Lowers seizure threshold (mild)
- ❖ Prolactin elevating (strong)
- ❖ Hyponatremia
- ❖ Hyperglycemia
- ❖ Photosensitivity (phenothiazine)

Kinetics interactions:

- ❖ 2D6 substrate, like most phenothiazines
- ❖ Relatively few relevant kinetic interactions

page 15

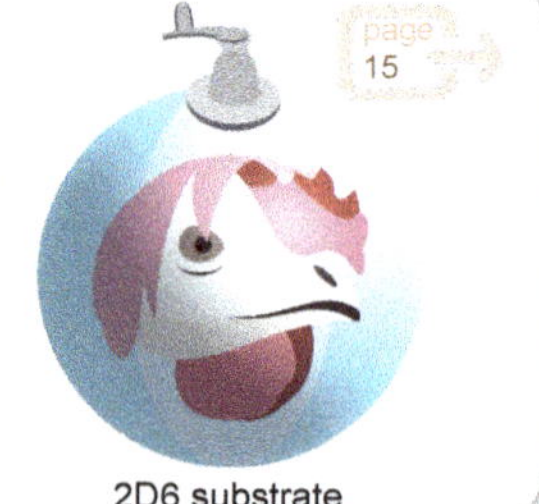

2D6 substrate

1967
$57 - $147

Thiothixene (NAVANE)

thye oh THIX een / NAH vane

"Thighs thick to Navel"

- Antipsychotic
- High potency FGA
- D2 antagonist

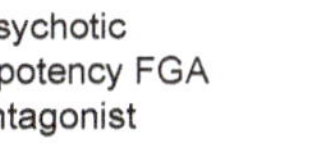

1
2
<u>5</u>
10
mg

FDA-approved for:
- Schizophrenia

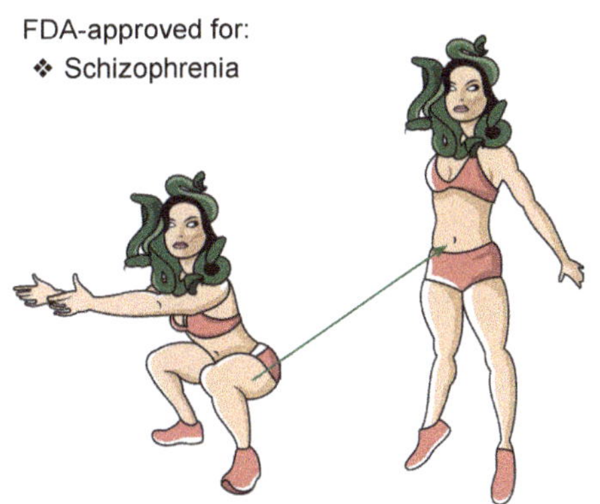

Antipsychotics are represented with spooky mascots.

Thiothixene (Navane) is a seldom prescribed first generation antipsychotic (FGA). It is <u>only available orally</u>, as a capsule. <u>High potency</u> FGA alternatives Haloperidol (Haldol) and fluphenazine (Prolixin) are each available in several formulations, including long-acting injectables. Thiothixene is not ideal for acute agitation because it takes 90 minutes to produce tranquilizing effect, which is slower than haloperidol or loxapine. When developed in the 1960s, thiothixene was also found to work as an antidepressant, but it is not used for that purpose. The only FDA-approved indication is for schizophrenia.

Dosing: According to the label, target dose is 2–5 mg BID–TID; The "minimal effective" dose to adequately treat first-episode schizophrenia is 8 mg/day; The label instructs to start 2 mg TID if mild/moderate psychosis; If severe psychosis, start 5 mg BID; FDA max is 60 mg/day, which is too high due to risk of tardive dyskinesia); It is best not to exceed 20 mg/day; Discontinue if absolute neutrophil count (ANC) drops below 1,000.

Agitation and hostility rapidly controlled

Navane (thiothixene)(thiothixene HCl)

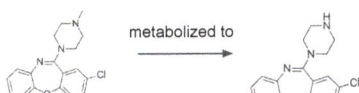

Dynamic interactions:
- Dopamine antagonist (strong)
- Extrapyramidal effects (high)
- Sedation/CNS depression
- Hypotensive
- Anticholinergic (mild)
- Lowers seizure threshold (mild)
- Prolactin elevating (strong)
- Hyponatremia

Kinetic interactions:
- 1A2 substrate
- Tobacco (1A2 in<u>D</u>ucer) lowers levels of thiothixene

page 10

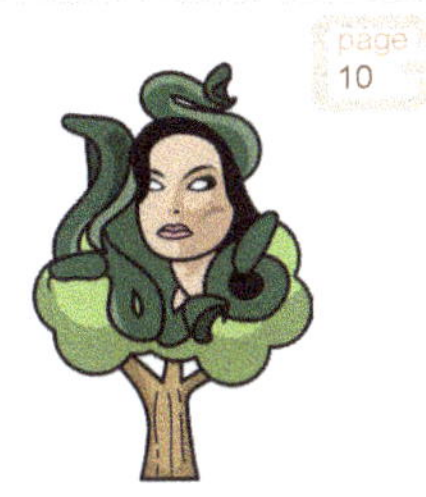

1A2 substrate

1975
$21–$48

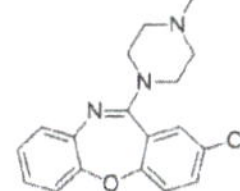

Loxapine (LOXITANE)

LOX a peen / LOX i tane

"Lots a' ping, Lots o' Tang"

- Antipsychotic
- Medium potency FGA
- D2 antagonist - ⇩ DA
- 5-HT_{2A} antagonist - ⇧ DA

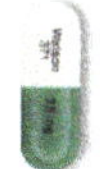

5
10
<u>25</u>
50
mg

FDA-approved for:
- Psychosis

Used off-label for:
- Bipolar mania

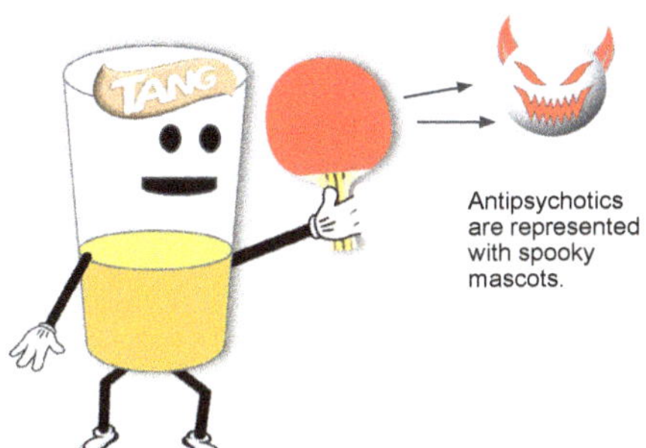

Antipsychotics are represented with spooky mascots.

Loxapine (Loxitane) is a typical (1st generation) antipsychotic with atypical characteristics. In addition to blocking D2 receptors, loxapine <u>blocks serotonin 5-HT_{2A} receptors as if it were a second generation</u> antipsychotic (SGA). Loxapine binds with higher affinity to <u>D4 receptors</u> than other dopaminergic receptors, similarly to clozapine. At high doses, loxapine has an adverse effects profile comparable to other FGAs. Loxapine <u>does not cause weight gain</u>. It is involved in fewer *clinically significant* interactions than most FGAs. Loxapine is metabolized to the tetracyclic antidepressant amoxapine (Asendin), which makes it more cardiotoxic in overdose than the average antipsychotic. In overdose, loxapine is likely to induce a seizure.

Loxapine is the only psychotropic medication available <u>by inhalation</u>. ADASUVE, released in 2014, is a single-use disposable inhaler containing 10 mg of loxapine powder <u>approved for agitation</u> related to schizophrenia or bipolar I disorder. Adasuve has a black box warning of bronchospasm leading to respiratory distress and respiratory arrest. The inhaled product is rarely prescribed.

Dosing: The label instructs starting at 10 mg PO BID and titrating over 7-10 days; Severely disturbed patients may require starting dose of 25 mg BID; The "minimal effective dose" to adequately treat first-episode schizophrenia is 20 mg/day. FDA maximum total daily dose is 250 mg.

loxapine (antipsychotic) — metabolized to → amoxapine (antidepressant)

Dynamic interactions:
- Sedative
- Anticholinergic (moderate)
- Antidopaminergic (moderate)
- Extrapyramidal effects
- Hypotensive
- Prolactin elevating

Kinetic interactions:
- Substrate of 1A2, 2D6 and 3A4 (multi-CYP)
- Significant kinetic interactions are unlikely

page 18

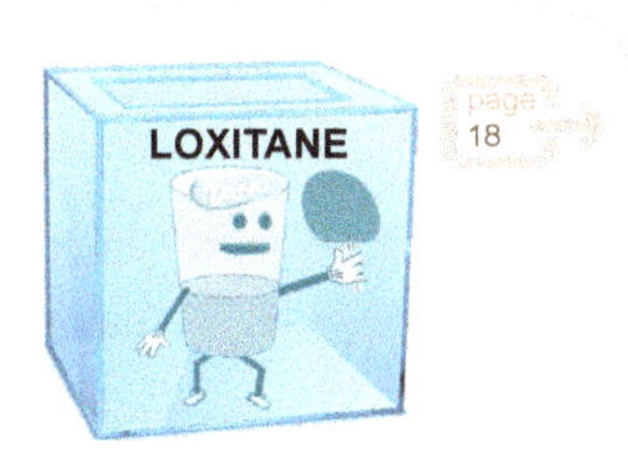

in a box - relevant kinetic interactions are possible, but unlikely

1958
$64–$180

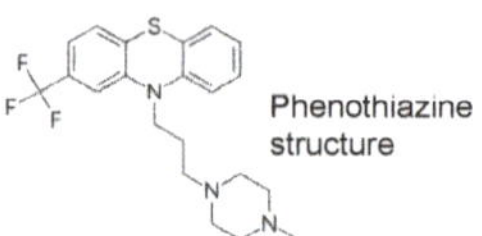

Phenothiazine structure

Trifluoperazine (STELAZINE)

try floo uh PER uh zeen / STEL a zine

"Tri-flowered Stellation"

- ❖ Antipsychotic
- ❖ High potency FGA
- ❖ D2 antagonist
- ❖ 5-HT_2 antagonist
- ❖ Phenothiazine

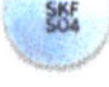

1
<u>2</u>
5
10
mg

FDA-approved for:

- ❖ Schizophrenia
- ❖ Anxiety

Antipsychotics are represented with spooky mascots.

Trifluoperazine (Stelazine) is a <u>high potency antipsychotic like haloperidol</u>. Stelazine never gained much of a market share. It is only available as an oral tablet—no liquid or injectable formulations.

Stelazine was marketed to physicians in the 1970's as treatment for "<u>chronic neurotic anxiety</u>", a phrase which is out of use. The ads shown below imply doctors can prescribe Stelazine to "needy" patients in order to stop being bothered.

It was also marketed as "activating" and relatively non-sedating.

Due to risk of tardive dyskinesia, trifluoperazine is no longer prescribed for anxiety. Half-life is 18 hours.

Dosing: For any indication, start 1–2 mg BID; The "minimal effective dose" to adequately treat first-episode schizophrenia is 10 mg/day. For psychosis, the FDA maximum dose is 40 mg/day (which is too strong given the risk of tardive dyskinesia); For non-psychotic anxiety the max is 6 mg/day for 12 weeks; Discontinue if absolute neutrophil count (ANC) drops < 1,000.

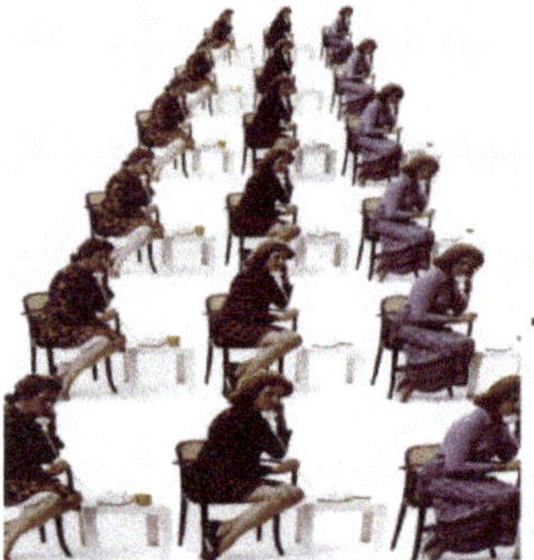

*"If she calls you morning...noon...and night, day after day after day. To **allay her chronic neurotic anxiety**, try her on Stelazine". 1973*

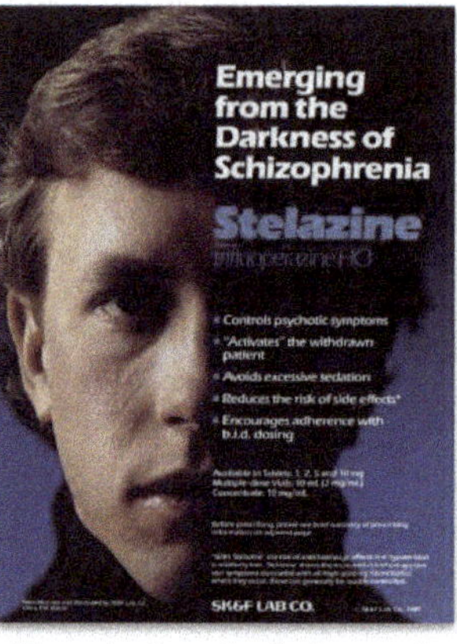

*"Emerging from the Darkness of Schizophrenia…Controls psychotic symptoms, **'Activates' the withdrawn patient**, Avoids excessive sedation." 1989*

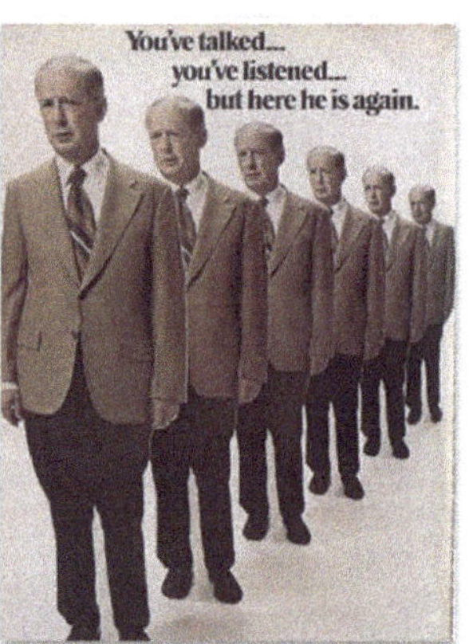

*"You've talked...you've listened, **but here he is again**. To allay his chronic neurotic anxiety, try him on Stelazine." 1973*

The phenothiazines: drugs derived from phenothiazine

- ❖ Chlorpromazine (Thorazine)
- ❖ Flu<u>ph</u>enazine (Prolixin)
- ❖ Per<u>ph</u>enazine (Trilafon)
- ❖ Prochlorperazine (Compazine)
- ❖ Promethazine (<u>Ph</u>energan)
- ❖ Thioridazine (Mellaril)
- ❖ Trifluoperazine (Stelazine)

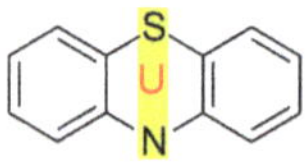

S
U
N

⇒ <u>P</u>henothiazines cause <u>p</u>hotosensitivity. <u>P</u>henothiazines cause <u>p</u>hotosensitivity. We added *U* to the to phenothiazine chemical structure to spell *SUN*.
⇒ Most are 2D6 substrates (not trifluoperazine)
⇒ Most are antipsychotics (not promethazine)

Dynamic interactions:

- ❖ Dopamine antagonist (strong)
- ❖ Extrapyramidal effects
- ❖ Sedation/CNS depression
- ❖ Hypotensive
- ❖ Anticholinergic (strong)
- ❖ Lowers seizure threshold (mild)
- ❖ Prolactin elevating (strong)
- ❖ Hyponatremia
- ❖ Hyperglycemia
- ❖ <u>Ph</u>otosensitivity (<u>ph</u>enothiazine)

page 10

Kinetic interactions:

- ❖ 1A2 substrate (minor)

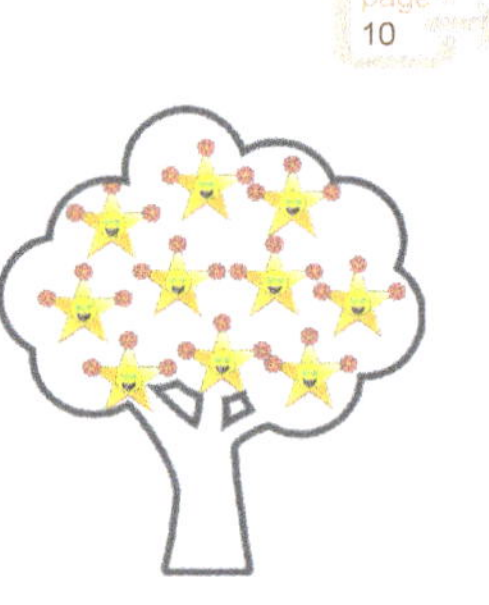

1A2 substrate (minor)

1978
$13–$16

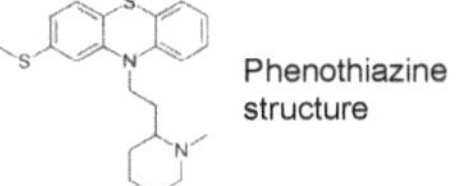

Phenothiazine structure

Thioridazine (MELLARIL)

thi uh RID uh zeen / MEL uh ril

"Mellow & Tired daze"

- ❖ Antipsychotic
- ❖ Low potency FGA
- ❖ D2 antagonist
- ❖ Phenothiazine

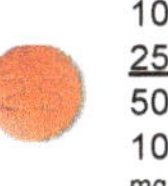

10
<u>25</u>
50
100
mg

FDA-approved for:

- ❖ <u>Refractory</u> schizophrenia

Used off-label for:

- ❖ Anxiety (low dose)

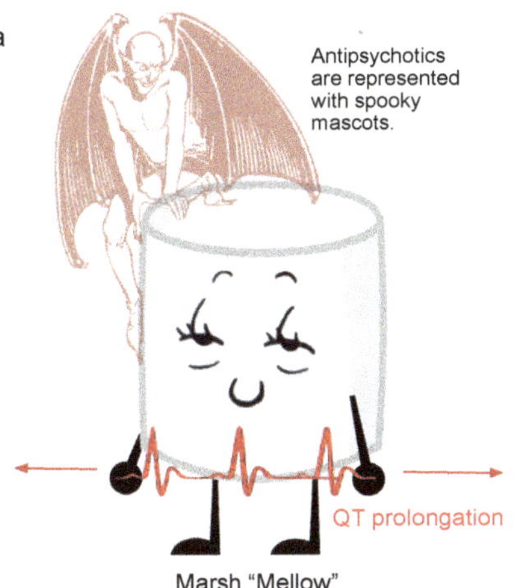
Antipsychotics are represented with spooky mascots.
QT prolongation

Marsh "<u>Mell</u>ow"

Thioridazine (Mellaril) is approved for <u>refractory schizophrenia</u> only. Thioridazine is rarely prescribed due to the risk of cardiac arrhythmias. It has the <u>highest risk of QT prolongation</u> among all psychotropic medications.

Mellaril is also the antipsychotic known for irreversible retinal pigmentation/degenerative <u>retinopathy</u>, a risk at high doses. Contrast this with chlorpromazine (Thorazine) which causes corneal deposits but rarely affects the retina.

Mellaril works well for anxiety and can be prescribed safely at low doses.

The other medication FDA-approved for refractory schizophrenia is clozapine (Clozaril), which is more effective than thioridazine.

<u>CYP2D6 genotyping</u> is recommended prior to starting Mellaril, as explained below.

Dosing: For refractory schizophrenia, the target dose range is 200–800 mg divided BID–QID; Start 50–100 mg TID; Max is 800 mg/day; Check electrocardiogram (EKG) for QT prolongation before and during treatment; Stop if absolute neutrophil count (ANC) < 1000.

"Why take the risk of dystonic reactions…"

In the 1980s thioridazine was marketed as an atypical antipsychotic, despite having a conventional phenothiazine structure.

Low potency D2 blockers are less likely to cause EPS, as touted in this 1983 ad.

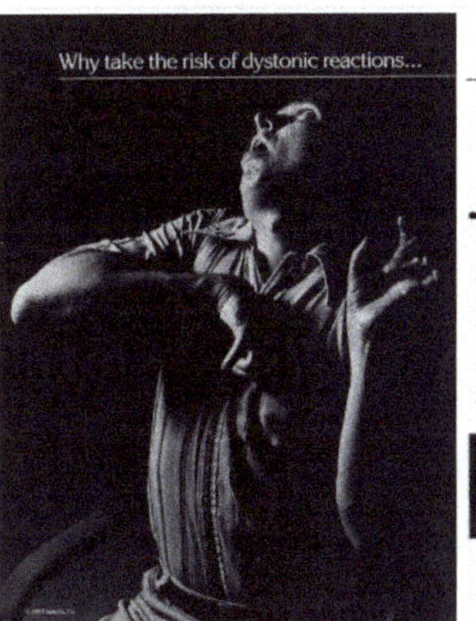
Why take the risk of dystonic reactions...

when you can often avoid them with

MELLARIL
(thioridazine)

MELLARIL (thioridazine)
Keeps the risk of extrapyramidal side effects to a minimum

The phenothiazines:
drugs derived from phenothiazine

- ❖ Chlorpromazine (Thorazine)
- ❖ Flu<u>ph</u>enazine (Prolixin)
- ❖ Per<u>ph</u>enazine (Trilafon)
- ❖ Prochlorperazine (Compazine)
- ❖ Promethazine (<u>Ph</u>energan)
- ❖ Thioridazine (Mellaril)
- ❖ Trifluoperazine (Stelazine)

S
U
N

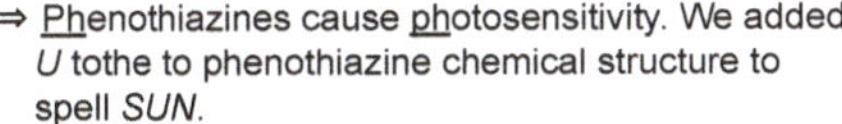

- ⇒ <u>Ph</u>enothiazines cause <u>ph</u>otosensitivity. We added *U* tothe to phenothiazine chemical structure to spell *SUN*.
- ⇒ Most are 2D6 substrates (not trifluoperazine)
- ⇒ Most are antipsychotics (not promethazine)

Dynamic interactions:

- ❖ Dopamine antagonist
- ❖ Extrapyramidal effects
- ❖ Sedation/CNS depression (strong)
- ❖ QT prolongation (high risk)
- ❖ Hypotensive
- ❖ Anticholinergic (strong)
- ❖ Lowers seizure threshold (mild)
- ❖ Prolactin elevating
- ❖ Hyponatremia
- ❖ Hyperglycemia
- ❖ <u>Ph</u>otosensitivity (<u>ph</u>enothiazine)

Kinetic interactions:

- ❖ 2D6 substrate (major)

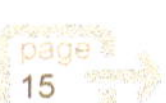
page 15

2D6 genotyping is recommended prior to starting Mellaril, a susceptible 2D6 substrate. 2D6 poor metabolizers (PM) have 4-fold increased levels of this medication (10% of the population). Mellaril is contraindicated for 2D6 PMs. For this same reason, Mellaril is also contraindicated in combination with strong 2D6 inhibitors.

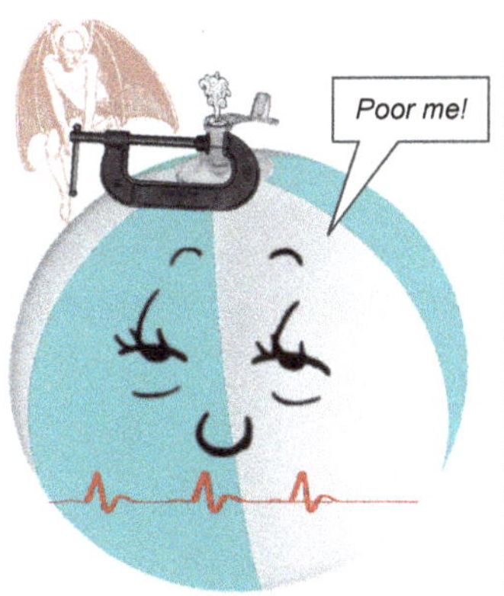
Poor me!

2D6 poor metabolizer (PM)

2D6 ultra-rapid metabolizers (UM) are likely to be nonresponders to Mellaril (3% of population).

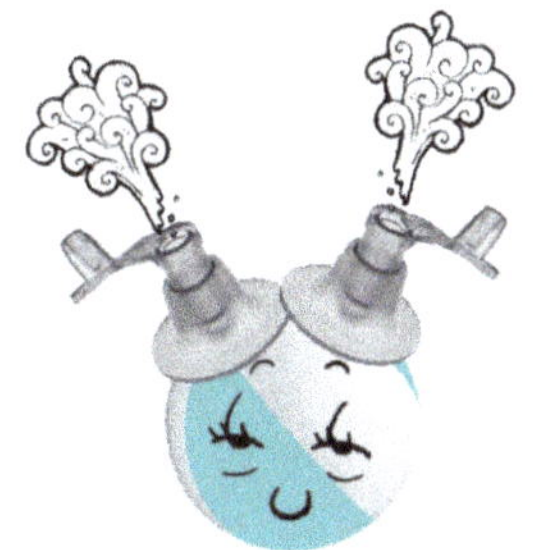

2D6 ultrarapid metabolizer (UM)

1985
$34–$72

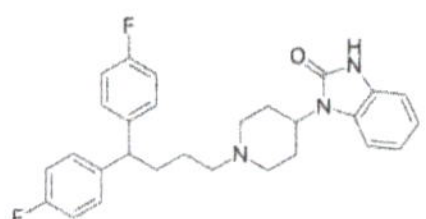

Pimozide (ORAP)

PIM o zide / OH rap

"Ol' rappin' Pimp"

- ❖ Antipsychotic
- ❖ High potency FGA
- ❖ D2 antagonist

1
2
mg

FDA-approved for:

- ❖ Tourette syndrome, severe

Used off-label for:

- ❖ Schizophrenia

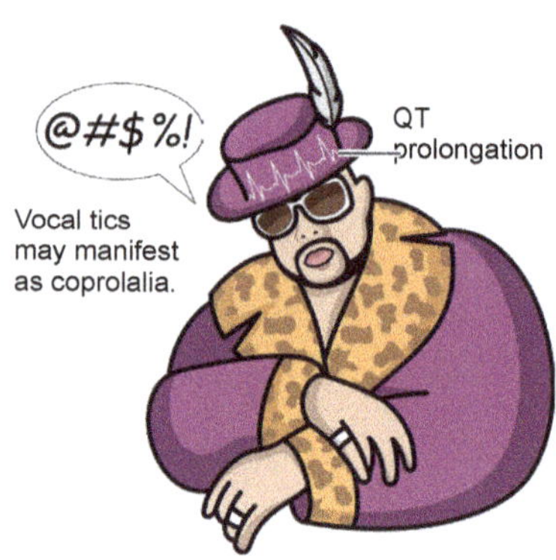

Pimozide (Orap) is a 1st generation antipsychotic that was FDA-approved in 1985 as an orphan drug for the treatment of Tourette's syndrome. It is only to be used for tics that severely compromise daily life function and do not respond to standard treatment. The standard medications include alpha-2 agonists (clonidine, guanfacine) and antipsychotics less likely to prolong QT interval (haloperidol, risperidone, ziprasidone).

DSM-5 defines Tourette's Disorder as a neurodevelopmental motor disorder characterized by both (1) multiple motor tics and (2) one or more vocal tics, without onset prior to age 18. These tics characteristically wax and wane, can be suppressed temporarily, and are typically preceded by an unwanted urge or sensation in the affected muscles. Some common tics are eye blinking, coughing, throat clearing, sniffing, and facial movements. An example of a vocal tic is coprolalia. This is the production of obscenities as an abrupt, sharp bark or grunt utterance which lacks the prosody of similar inappropriate speech observed in human interactions.

Adult dosing: Check CYP2D6 genotype if planning to exceed 4 mg/day; Target dose is 2–10 mg either QD or divided BID; Start at 1 mg QD or 1 mg BID; May increase dose every 2 days (every 2 weeks for a 2D6 poor metabolizer; Max is 0.2 mg/kg/day up to 10 mg/day (max of 4 mg/day for 2D6 poor metabolizer); Check EKG for QT prolongation; Taper gradually to discontinue; Stop if absolute neutrophil count (ANC) drops below 1,000.

Dynamic interactions:

- ❖ Dopamine antagonist
- ❖ Extrapyramidal effects
- ❖ Sedation/CNS depression
- ❖ QT prolongation (high risk)
- ❖ Anticholinergic (moderate)
- ❖ Lowers seizure threshold (mild)

Kinetic interactions:

- ❖ 2D6 substrate
- ❖ 3A4 substrate

2D6 genotyping is recommended for doses over 4 mg/day to check for 2D6 poor metabolizer (PM) genotype.

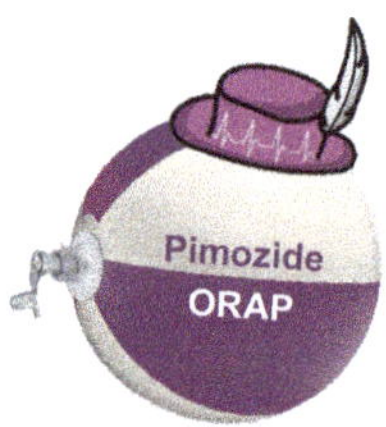

2D6 substrate

Pimozide is contraindicated in combination with many medications, including QT prolongers and 3A4 inhibitors. Sudden death has occured when the antibiotic clarithromycin (Biaxin) was added to ongoing pimozide therapy.

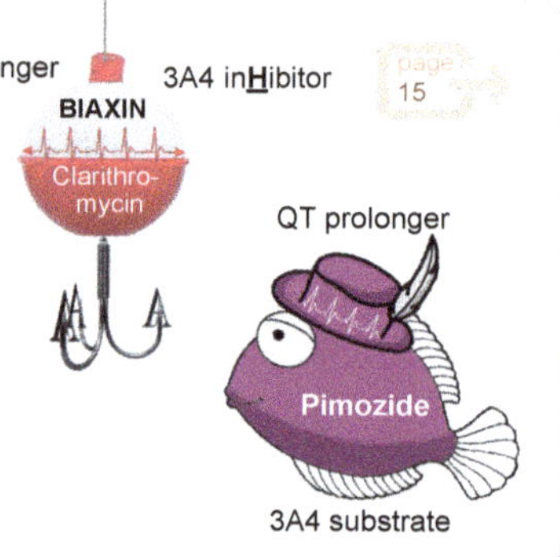

page 15

1975
$24–$42

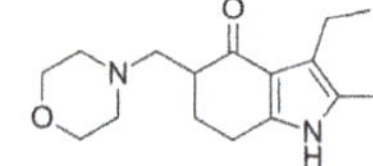

Molindone (MOBAN)

mol in dohn / MO ban

"Mole Dome Mole ban"

- ❖ Antipsychotic
- ❖ Medium potency FGA
- ❖ D2 antagonist

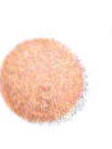

5
10
25
mg

FDA-approved for:

- ❖ Schizophrenia

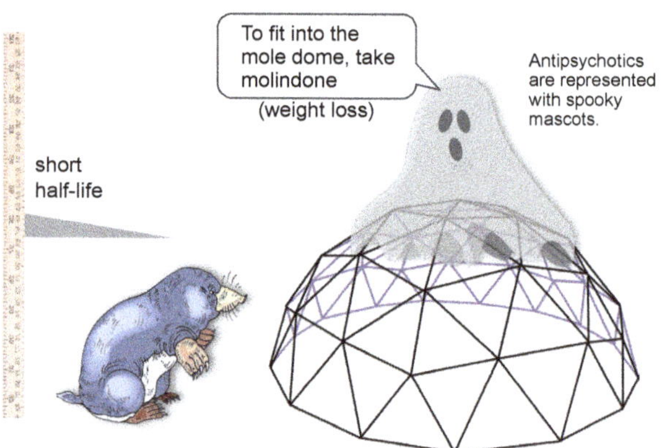

Dosing: Target dose for schizophrenia is 5–50 mg divided TID–QID; Start 50–75 mg/day divided TID–QID; May increase to 100 mg/day (25 mg QID) after 3–4 days; Max is 225 mg/day; Stop if absolute neutrophil count (ANC) drops below 1,000.

Molindone (Moban) is a rarely prescribed intermediate potency FGA, discontinued by the original manufacturer in 2010. It is still available, but you're unlikely to see it in the wild.

Molindone has a short half-life 1.5 hours but pharmacological effect from a single dose persists for 24–36 hours due to several active metabolites.

Molindone is associated with weight loss, averaging 7.6 kg after 3 months, with most of the loss occurred during the first month (among 9 schizophrenic patients, Gardos & Cole, 1977). Envision the mole being able to squeeze through the triangles of the dome as he loses weight.

Dynamic interactions:

- ❖ Dopamine antagonist
- ❖ Extrapyramidal effects
- ❖ Sedation/CNS depression
- ❖ Anticholinergic (moderate)
- ❖ Lowers seizure threshold (mild)
- ❖ Prolactin elevation (moderate)

Kinetic interactions:

- ❖ None significant

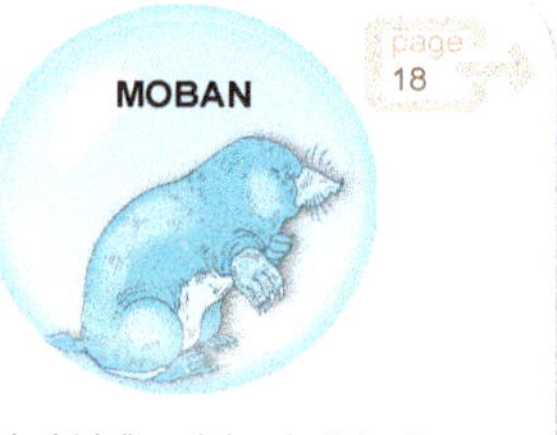

"in a bubble" - minimal clinically significant kinetic interactions

page 18

An antiemetic is a drug effective against nausea and vomiting (emesis). Some antiemetics work by blocking dopamine D2 receptors, which is the same mechanism employed by antipsychotics. The antiemetic effect is mediated by D2 blockade in the vomiting center of the brainstem, whereas the antipsychotic effect is mediated by D2 blockade in the mesolimbic pathway.

Other dopamine antagonists that work as off-label antiemetics include olanzapine (Zyprexa), haloperidol (Haldol), and chlorpromazine (Thorazine). Not all antipsychotics decrease nausea. In fact, the D2 partial agonists such as aripiprazole (Abilify) are likely to induce nausea.

In addition to being triggered by dopamine, the vomiting center in the brainstem is triggered by serotonin, histamine, and acetylcholine. Anti-serotonergics, antihistamines and anticholinergics work as antiemetics. Serotonergic antidepressants and cholinergic Alzheimer's medications have the opposite effect of inducing nausea. Unsurprisingly, dopaminergic medications for Parkinson's disease such as ropinirole (Requip) are likely to cause nausea.

Antiemetics that do not block dopamine receptors include:

- ▶ **Ondansetron (Zofran)** - blocks serotonin 5-HT_3 receptors in the brainstem's vomiting center and in the GI tract
- ▶ **Scopolamine (Transderm Scōp)** - anticholinergic effect in the brainstem and GI tract
- ▶ **Diphenhydramine (Benadryl)** - blocks H_1 histamine receptors in the brain, plus anticholinergic effects
- ▶ **Aprepitant (Emend)** - substance P antagonist (SPA) that mediates its effect by blocking the neurokinin 1 (NK1) receptor in the brain

As a side note, nausea is one of the most common reasons patients stop medications prematurely. Nausea tends to be a transient side effect that usually resolves spontaneously. Nausea can often be avoided altogether with slow titration. Another tip for medication-induced nausea is to take the pill after food—not with food, immediately after a meal. Also effective for nausea is ginger extract (one 550 mg capsule) taken 1 hour before a meal, for a maximum of 3 caps/day (Bodagh et al, 2019; Rajnish Mago, MD; The Carlat Psychiatry Report, Jun/Jul 2019). Ginger ale does not suffice.

D2 blocking antiemetic	Potency of D2 blockade	Antipsychotic?
Prochlorperazine (Compazine)	High	Yes
Metoclopramide (Reglan)	High	No
Promethazine (Phenergan)	Low	No
Trimethobenzamide (Tigan)	Low	No

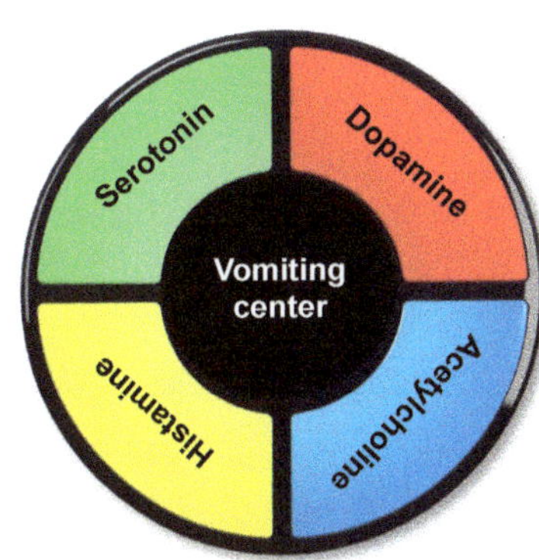

When the brainstem is overloaded by any of these 4 neurotransmitters, the vomiting center thinks the body is being poisoned. Blocking these neurotransmitters relieves nausea.

#288
1956
$9–$23

Phenothiazine structure

Prochlorperazine (COMPAZINE)

pro klor PEAR a zeen / COM pa zeen

"Procure, pear! (a Compass)"

- ❖ Antiemetic/Antipsychotic
- ❖ High potency FGA
- ❖ D2 antagonist
- ❖ Antihistamine
- ❖ Phenothiazine

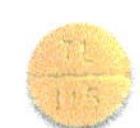

5
10
mg

FDA-approved for:
- ❖ Nausea/vomiting, severe
- ❖ Schizophrenia
- ❖ Non-psychotic anxiety

Used off-label for:
- ❖ Migraines
- ❖ Status migrainosus (IV)

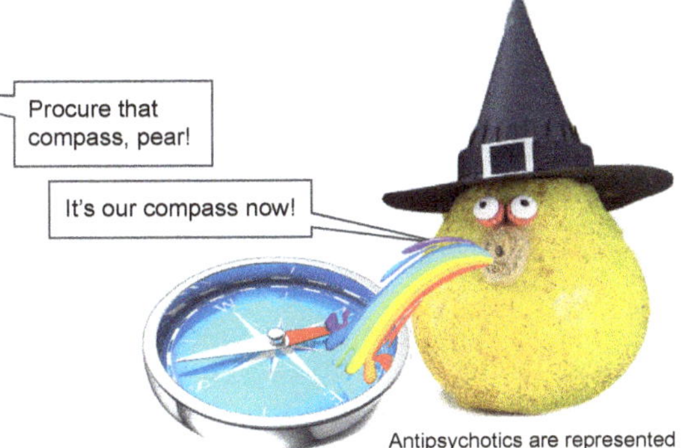

Antipsychotics are represented with spooky mascots (witch hat)

Recommendation: Rather than prescribing a D2 blocking antiemetic, choose **ondansetron (Zofran)**. It works by blocking serotonin 5-HT_3 receptors, does not cause EPS, and carries no risk of tardive dyskinesia.

Although approved for schizophrenia, prochlorperazine (Compazine) is now almost exclusively used as an antiemetic. Psychiatrists rarely prescribe it.

The antiemetic effect of prochlorperazine is brought about by blocking D2 receptors in the vomiting center of the brainstem. Its antipsychotic effect is through blocking D2 receptors in the mesolimbic pathway.

Since Compazine is a high potency FGA, it can cause EPS including akathisia and dystonia with short-term use, and tardive dyskinesia with long-term use. It has the potential to cause neutropenia and should be stopped if there is an unexplained decrease in white blood cell count.

Dosing: For severe nausea/vomiting, use 5–10 mg q 6–8 hr; For anxiety, use 5 mg q 6–8 hr for a maximum of 12 weeks; For schizophrenia, start 5 mg TID; FDA max for schizophrenia is 150 mg/day, but this is too high due to risk of tardive dyskinesia.

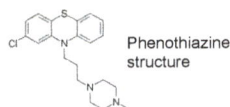

Dynamic interactions:
- ❖ Dopamine antagonist (strong)
- ❖ Extrapyramidal effects (high)
- ❖ Sedation/CNS depression
- ❖ QT prolongation (mild)
- ❖ Hypotensive
- ❖ Anticholinergic (moderate)
- ❖ Lowers seizure threshold (mild)
- ❖ Prolactin elevating
- ❖ Hyponatremia
- ❖ Hyperglycemia
- ❖ Photosensitivity (phenothiazine)

Kinetic interactions:
- ❖ Minimal clinically significant kinetic interactions (in a bubble)

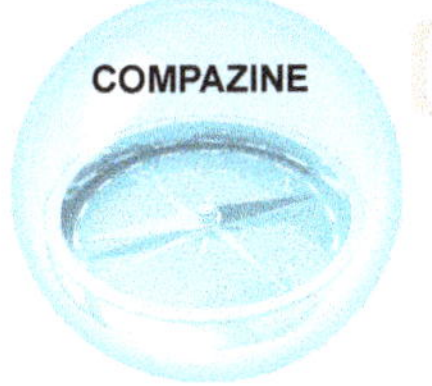

page 18

#160
1951
$3–$19

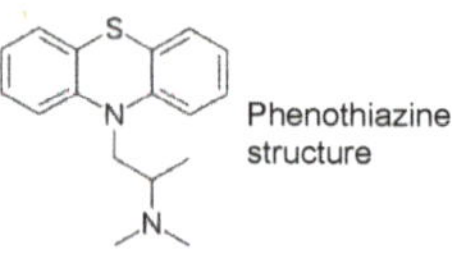

Promethazine (PHENERGAN)

proh METH uh zeen / FIN er gan

"Finnegan's Prom hazing"

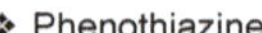

- Weak D2 antagonist
- Antihistamine
- Antiemetic
- Phenothiazine

12.5
25
50
mg

Not an antipsychotic

FDA-approved for:

- Allergic conditions
- Urticaria
- Motion sickness
- Nausea/vomiting
- Sedation

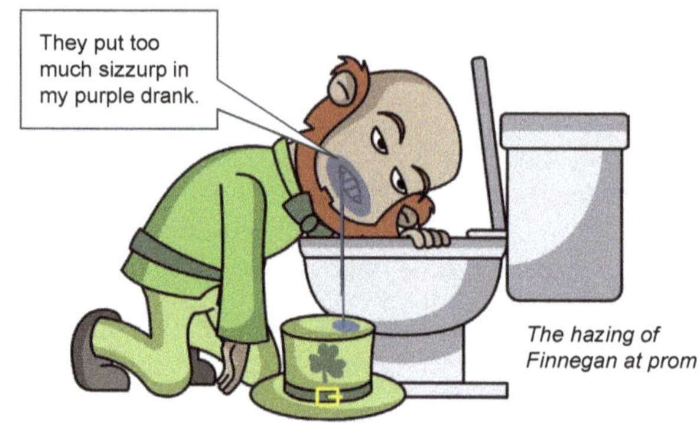

The hazing of Finnegan at prom

Phenergan is a phenothiazine. Promethazine (Phenergan) was the original antihistamine that revolutionized the treatment of allergies in the 1950s. This monograph would likely reside in the antihistamine/anticholinergic chapter if not for the phenothiazine structure.

Promethazine is the only available medication with a phenothiazine structure that is not useful as an antipsychotic. Today it is commonly prescribed as an antiemetic, but not for allergies. As with all first generation antihistamines, promethazine is highly sedating and strongly anticholinergic.

Like other phenothiazines, promethazine antagonizes D2 receptors, although weakly. Promethazine blocks D2 receptors at 10% potency of the antipsychotic chlorpromazine (Thorazine), which itself is low potency. Extrapyramidal effects are highly unlikely with such a weak D2 blocker, in contrast to the antiemetics metoclopramide (Reglan) and prochlorperazine (Compazine) which are high potency D2 blockers.

Promethazine is available IM, IV, and as a rectal suppository for occasions when vomiting would make the PO route ineffective. It is one of the few drugs that can turn urine green, apropos to this mnemonic.

Promethazine has two black box warnings, for respiratory depression and risk of severe tissue injury/gangrene—*"gang-green"*—with parenteral administration. Avoid co-administering with other respiratory depressants. Promethazine injection can cause severe chemical irritation and tissue damage including burning, thrombophlebitis, tissue necrosis, and gangrene when given IM or IV, but more likely with the IV route due to potential perivascular extravasation (unintentional leaking into the surrounding tissue). It should be injected into a large muscle to avoid unintentional intra-arterial insertion.

Promethazine is a component of prescription cough syrup with the opioid codeine. Promethazine is the antihistamine—as an alternative to diphenhydramine (Benadryl)—for sneezing, rhinorrhea, and watery eyes. The codeine component serves antitussive and analgesic purposes. The promethazine/codeine combo is not recommended and has nine (!!) black box warnings.

Promethazine is commonly misused by recovering opioid addicts to potentiate the high caused by methadone.

A concoction of promethazine/codeine syrup mixed with Sprite (and sometimes grape Jolly Ranchers candy) is known as "purple drank", sizzurp or "lean". The euphoria from sizzurp is derived from codeine, which is metabolized by 2D6 to morphine. The sedative "lean" (as in leaning against a wall) is from promethazine.

Dosing: For nausea, the recommended dose is 12.5–25 mg PO or IM q 4–6 hr PRN; Max is 50 mg/dose PO/IM (25 mg IV) and 100 mg/day; Product labeling states that promethazine may be given by slow IV push, but IM administration into a large muscle is preferred over IV due to risk of serious tissue injury with the IV route.

The phenothiazines:
drugs derived from phenothiazine

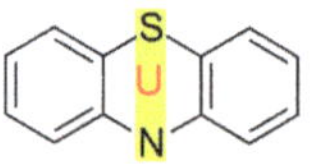

- Chlorpromazine (Thorazine)
- Fluphenazine (Prolixin)
- Perphenazine (Trilafon)
- Prochlorperazine (Compazine)
- Promethazine (Phenergan)
- Thioridazine (Mellaril)
- Trifluoperazine (Stelazine)

⇒ Phenothiazines cause photosensitivity. We added *U* to the chemical structure to spell *SUN*.
⇒ Most are 2D6 substrates (not trifluoperazine)
⇒ Most are antipsychotics (not promethazine)

Green urine can be caused by:

- Promethazine (Phenergan)
- Metoclopramide (Reglan)
- Amitriptyline (Elavil)
- Cimetidine (Tagamet)
- Propofol (Diprivan)
- Methylene blue

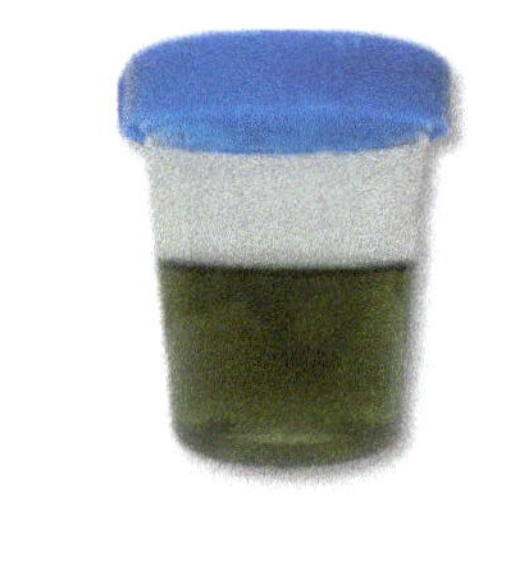

Dynamic interactions:

- Dopamine antagonist (weak)
- Extrapyramidal effects (mild)
- Sedation/CNS depression (strong)
- Respiratory depression
- QT prolongation (mild)
- Hypotensive
- Anticholinergic (strong)
- Lowers seizure threshold (mild)
- Prolactin elevating
- Hyponatremia
- Hyperglycemia
- Photosensitivity (phenothiazine)

Kinetic interactions:

- 2D6 substrate

page 15

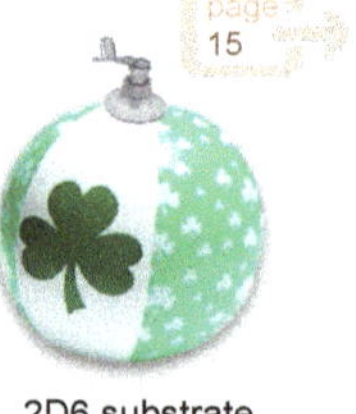

2D6 substrate

1979
$4–$11

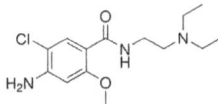

Metoclopramide (REGLAN)

met o KLOH pra mide / REG lan

"Ronald Reglan Met a clopper"

❖ Antiemetic
❖ High potency D2 antagonist

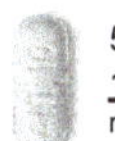

5
10
mg

Not an antipsychotic

FDA-approved for:

❖ GERD
❖ Diabetic gastroparesis
❖ Nausea/vomiting prevention (chemotherapy; postoperative)
❖ Small bowel intubation
❖ Radiologic exam

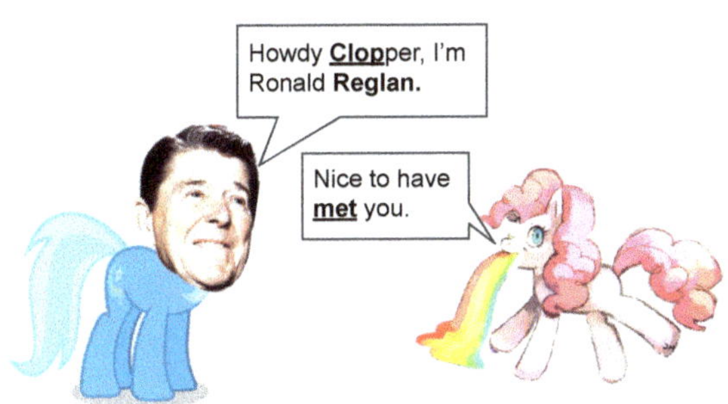

Howdy Clopper, I'm Ronald Reglan.
Nice to have met you.

Metoclopramide, introduced in 1979, is the <u>only FDA-approved treatment for gastroparesis</u>. It is useful after gastric surgery and for treatment of hyperemesis gravidarum (severe nausea and vomiting of pregnancy).

Metoclopramide is a dopamine D2 receptor antagonist. It exerts its effect in the vomiting center of the <u>brain stem</u>. It also antagonizes dopamine on gastrointestinal smooth muscle, which causes an indirect <u>cholinergic effect</u>, and can lead to the SLUDGE symptom diarrhea. The drug enhances gastric emptying, which is believed to minimize stasis that precedes vomiting.

Despite being a D2 blocker, you won't see metoclopramide in the antipsychotic section of most textbooks. Metoclopramide <u>lacks antipsychotic efficacy</u> except at a high dose, so it is not used for psychiatric purposes. Unsurprisingly, metoclopramide can cause <u>sedation</u>.

Metoclopramide can cause adverse effects like the antipsychotic class, including akathisia, hyperprolactinemia, neuroleptic malignant syndrome (NMS), and <u>tardive dyskinesia</u> (TD). <u>It may be the most common cause of drug-induced movement disorders</u>. It carries a **black box warning** <u>not to exceed 12 weeks</u> of treatment due to risk of TD. There are still thousands of active tardive dyskinesia lawsuits against the manufacturers of metoclopramide.

An off-label alternative treatment for gastroparesis is the cholinergic medication bethanechol (Urecholine), which does not cause tardive dyskinesia.

Dosing: 10–15 mg PO, IM, or IV 4x daily PRN; Use 5 mg for elderly patients; Maximum is 60 mg/day (30 mg/day for 2D6 poor metabolizers).

page 15

Dynamic interactions:

❖ Dopamine antagonist (strong)
❖ Extrapyramidal effects (high)
❖ Sedation/CNS depression
❖ Anticholinergic (moderate)
❖ Prolactin elevation

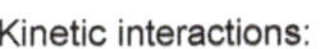

Kinetic interactions:

❖ 2D6 substrate

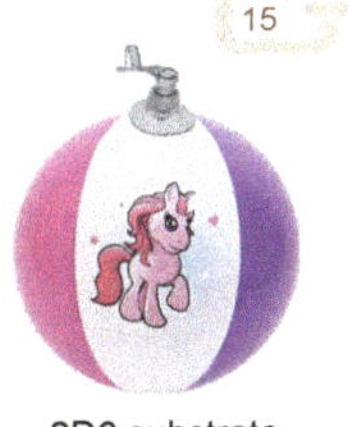

2D6 substrate

1974
$39–$174

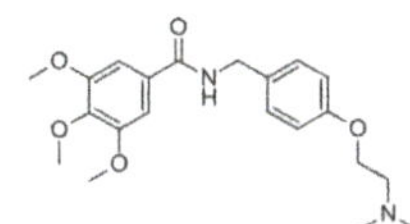

Trimethobenzamide (TIGAN)

try METH oh BENZ a mide / TEE gan

"Trim bendy Tigger"

❖ Antiemetic
❖ Low potency D2 antagonist

300
mg

Not an antipsychotic

FDA-approved for:

❖ Nausea/vomiting

Used off-label for:

❖ Suppression of gag reflex in surgery

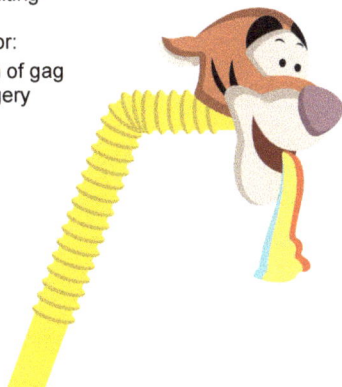

Trimethobenzamide (Tigan) has been shown to block the emetic reflex <u>without causing sedation</u>, hypotension or other undesirable side effects produced by other D2-blocking antiemetics. Tigan has weak antidopaminergic activity. When used parenterally for surgery, it has the added benefit of <u>gag reflex suppression</u>.

Tigan has a niche for the treatment and prevention of nausea caused by apomorphine (Apokyn) in rescue treatment of Parkinson's disease "off" episodes. Ondansetron (Zofran) is contraindicated with apomorphine because the combination can cause severe hypotension.

Dosing: For nausea/vomiting (PO route) give 300 mg TID–QID; For IM route give 200 mg TID–QID.

Dynamic interactions:

❖ Dopamine antagonist (weak)
❖ Extrapyramidal effects (mild)
❖ Sedation/CNS depression
❖ Hypotension (IM use)
❖ Lowers seizure threshold (mild)

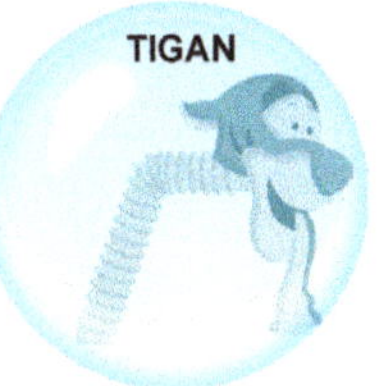

TIGAN

page
15

Kinetic interactions:

❖ Minimal clinically significant kinetic interactions (in a bubble)

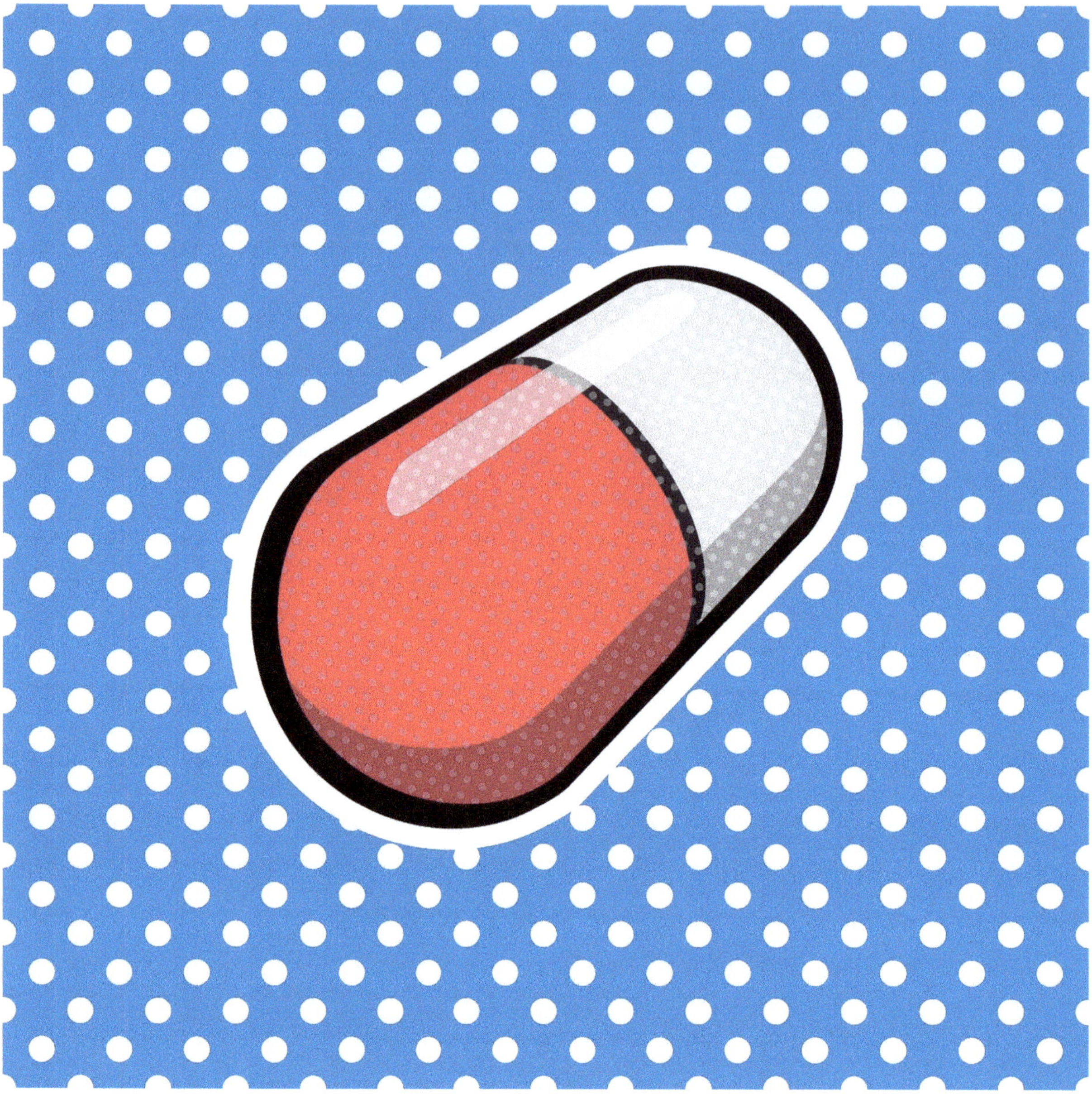

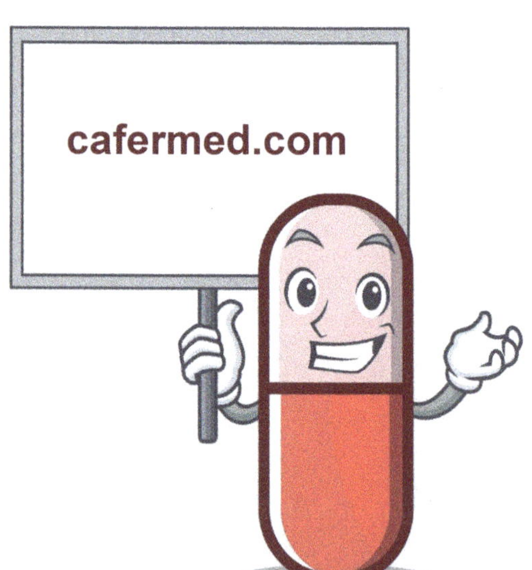
cafermed.com

All antipsychotics introduced after 1990 are classified as second generation antipsychotics (SGAs), also known as atypical antipsychotics. As a class, SGAs have a lower risk of EPS and a higher risk of weight gain and diabetes compared to first generation antipsychotics (FGAs). The FGA/SGA distinction is based more on convention than science. The best approach is to consider the properties of each antipsychotic individually.

What really distinguishes SGAs from FGAs is, with SGAs, therapeutic effects can usually be achieved at a dose lower than would cause EPS. If FGAs are dosed carefully as to avoid EPS, evidence suggests there is no overall advantage of SGAs over FGAs. In general, SGAs have more potential for metabolic disturbance (obesity, hyperlipidemia and diabetes), though there are exceptions (lurasidone, ziprasidone).

Patients taking SGAs need routine monitoring of weight, lipids and hemoglobin A1c.

Unopposed blockade of D2 dopamine receptors in the nigrostriatal pathway is what causes EPS. The prototypical FGA is just a D2 blocker. Most SGAs block D2 receptors and 5-HT**2A** serotonin receptors. Mnemonic: ***2nd** generation **A**ntipsychotic*. 5-HT2A blockade indirectly increases dopamine in the basal ganglia, making EPS less likely.

It has become apparent that SGAs are safe during pregnancy, except risperidone and paliperidone—these two are associated with a small increase in congenital malformations (Huybrechts et al, 2016). Risperidone and paliperidone are also the two SGAs that prominently elevate prolactin levels.

Here are the SGAs available in the US, ranked by number of prescriptions:

Rx	Generic TRADE	Cost/ month	Weight gain	Sedation	Akathisia	Involuntary movement risk*	Prolactin elevation	Constip-ation	Comments
#1	Quetiapine SEROQUEL	$10	+++	++++	-	-	-	+	A weak antipsychotic, more often prescribed for mood disorders than for schizophrenia. Orthostatic hypotension is common with the first few doses. Slight potential for recreational abuse.
#2	Aripiprazole ABILIFY	$20	+/-	+/-	++	-	-	-	D2 partial agonist. 1st line for schizophrenia and bipolar. Few side effects other than akathisia. Long half-life of 3 to 6 days. Risk of compulsive behaviors (gamling, etc). Two long-acting injectable brands: ARISTADA and Abilify MAINTENA.
#3	Risperidone RISPERDAL	$10	++	+	++	++	+++	-	2nd line for men due to risk of gynecomastia. 1st line option for women (although galactorrea possible). Titration needed. EPS at doses > 6 mg. Several pediatric indications including autism-associated irritability for ages 5+. LAI Risperdal CONSTA q 2 wk IM, PERSERIS q 4 wk sub-Q
#4	Olanzapine ZYPREXA	$20	++++	++	+/-	+/-	+	++	#2 most effective for schizophrenia. #1 weight gain and DM risk. The least likely antipsychotic to be stopped (all-cause) because it is effective with minimal side effects, other than weight gain and blood glucose elevation.
#5	Lurasidone LATUDA	$1200	-	++	++	++	-	-	Approved for schizophrenia and bipolar depression. Poorly absorbed unless taken with food, at least 350 calories. Dosed once daily, usually with the evening meal. Weight loss is more likely than weight gain. Improves Hgb A1c. Highly susceptible 3A4 substrate, contraindicated with Tegretol
#6	Ziprasidone GEODON	$30	-	+++	+	+	+	-	Less effective than Risperdal. Take BID with meals for adequate absorption. Shortest half-life of SGAs, 2.5 hours. Most QT prolongation among the SGAs, although not extreme. IM available for acute agitation. Risk of DRESS syndrome (Drug Reaction with Eosinophilia and Systemic Symptoms) which is rare but serious. Similar to lurasidone.
#7	Clozapine CLOZARIL	$100 + labs	++++	++++	-	-	-	++++	#1 most effective for schizophrenia. Risks of severe neutropenia, myocarditis, seizures. Weekly CBC for the first 6 months (neutropenia). No EPS. Constipation and hypersalivation can be severe. Titrate slowly (hypotension).
#8	Brexpiprazole REXULTI	$1200	+	+/-	+	+	-	-	D2 partial agonist similar to aripiprazole and cariprazine. Approved for schizophrenia and as an adjunct to antidepressant for major depressive disorder.
#9	Cariprazine VRAYLAR	$1200	-	+/-	+++	+	-	-	D2 partial agonist. Approved for schizophrenia and bipolar maintenance. Activating rather than sedating. Possible benefit for cognitive difficulties and negative symptoms of schizophrenia. Akathisia is common. Longest half-life of antipsychotics at 14 days.
#10	Paliperidone INVEGA	$300	++	+/-	+	++	+++	-	Active metabolite of risperidone. Cleared renally, suitable for those with liver problems. Long-acting injectable (LAI) Invega SUSTENNA q 4 wk and Invega TRINZA q 3 mo.
#11	Asenapine SAPHRIS	$600	++	+++	++	+	+	+	The only sublingual (SL) antipsychotic. FDA: schizophrenia, bipolar. Risk of serious allergic reactions (rare).
#12	Iloperidone FANAPT	$500	+++	+/-	-	-	+	-	Titrate dose to avoid orthostatic hypotension. "No EPS", marketed for those sensitive to akathisia. #3 among antipsychotics for weight gain.
#13	Pimavanserin NUPLAZID	$2000	-	+/-	-	-	-	+/-	For hallucinations and delusions of Parkinson's disease. 5-HT2A serotonin receptor inverse agonist. The only available antipsychotic that does not act at dopamine receptors. May cause edema. Caution with heart conditions.
NEW	Lumateperone CAPLYTA	$1300	+/-	+++	-	-	-	-	Modulates glutamate in addition to the usual SGA mechanisms, with low D2 receptor occupancy. 42 mg is the only recommended dose. Causes modest weight loss but modest elevation of hemoglobin A1c and lipids.

* There may be small risk of tardive dyskinesia from antipsychotics designated (-). Antipsychotics are not always to blame for involuntary movements presumed to be tardive dyskinesia. In the pre-antipsychotic era, 4% of individuals developed spontaneous dyskinesia with the first psychotic episode (Fenton, 2013).

#86
1997
$3–$124

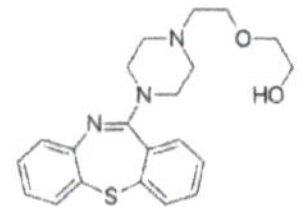

Quetiapine (SEROQUEL)

kwe TYE a peen / SER o kwel

"Sera, Quit typing!"

- Antipsychotic (SGA)
- D2 antagonist (weak) - ⇩ DA
- 5-HT_{2A} antagonist - ⇧ DA
- NE reuptake inhibitor (metabolite)

25 mg
50
100
200
300
400

FDA-approved for:

- Schizophrenia
- Bipolar, manic episode
- Bipolar, depressive episode - XR formulation
- Adjunct (to antidepressant) for major depressive disorder

Used off-label for

- "Racing thoughts"
- Anxiety
- Insomnia
- Behavioral disturbance
- Coming down from meth binge

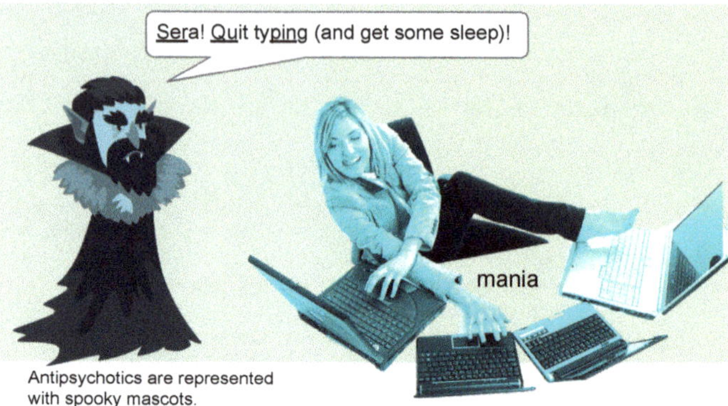

Antipsychotics are represented with spooky mascots.

"Quetiapine quiets the voices of schizophrenia". Quetiapine (Seroquel), FDA-approved in 1997, is arguably the weakest antipsychotic, often not very effective for schizophrenia. It is widely used for bipolar disorder, and is the #1 most prescribed antipsychotic (#86 prescribed drug overall) in the US. Quetiapine is calming and great for coming down from a manic episode or methamphetamine binge. Although not a controlled substance, quetiapine has some potential for abuse and has modest street value, nicknamed "Susie Q". It can contribute to fatality if taken at high doses in combination with other sedatives, likely due to respiratory depression.

Quetiapine can cause weight gain and diabetes, but the risk is substantially less than with olanzapine (Zyprexa). Quetiapine can be highly sedating, especially with first few doses.

Quetiapine has minimal risk of causing EPS because it is a weak D2 receptor blocker with a high 5-HT_{2A}/D_2 blockade ratio. It was the drug of choice for treatment of delusions and hallucinations associated with Parkinson's disease until the arrival of pimavanserin (Nuplazid). Among SGAs, quetiapine and clozapine have the lowest incidence of akathisia. Anticholinergic effects with quetiapine are minimal. At low dose, quetiapine is a common choice for elderly patients who need an antipsychotic due to low anticholinergic effects and low incidence of EPS.

Quetiapine has a relatively short half-life of 6 hours. The package insert recommends twice daily dosing. However, for antipsychotics in general, there is no compelling efficacy argument for maintaining consistent blood levels throughout the day. Seroquel is commonly dosed once daily at bedtime. The Seroquel XR formulation is intended for once daily dosing and may be a bit less sedating than immediate-release quetiapine dosed twice daily.

The author usually prescribes the immediate-release (IR) formulation which is cheaper than XR. Maintenance dosing at HS is better tolerated than BID. The minimal effective dose for first-episode psychosis is 150 mg. For multi-episode psychosis, 300 mg is the minimal effective dose.

Dosing: Start 25–50 mg BID or HS and titrate to target dose over 4 days to avoid orthostatic hypotension; For schizophrenia, the target dose 150–750 mg/day divided BID–TID; For bipolar mania, start 50 mg BID, then increase by 100 mg/day to achieve 200 mg BID by day four; For bipolar depression, the target is 300 mg HS, although lower doses are often used; The maximum daily dose is 800 mg. It may cause respiratory depression at higher doses.

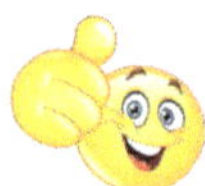

The augmenting agents with best evidence for treatment-resistant unipolar depression (added to an antidepressant):

- Lithium
- **Quetiapine (Seroquel)**
- Aripiprazole (Abilify)
- Risperidone (Risperdal)

Antipsychotics approved for bipolar depression (2019):

Second generation antipsychotic (SGA)	Number needed to treat (for one patient to respond)
Olanzapine/fluoxetine combo (Symbyax)	4
Lurasidone (Latuda)	5
Quetiapine XR (Seroquel XR)	6
Cariprazine (Vraylar)	7

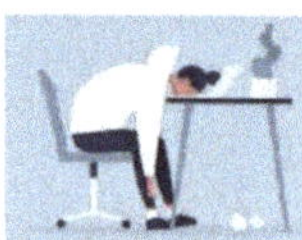

Sedation among SGAs, ranked:

1. Clozapine (Clozaril) - by far the most sedating
2. **Quetiapine (Seroquel)**
3. Ziprasidone (Geodon)
4. Olanzapine (Zyprexa)
5. Asenapine (Saphris)
6. Risperidone (Risperdal)
7. Lurasidone (Latuda)
8. Aripiprazole (Abilify) - minimal sedation
9. Iloperidone (Fanapt) - minimal sedation
10. Paliperidone (Invega) - the least sedating

Seizure risk among SGAs

1. Clozapine (Clozaril) - 10-fold
2. Olanzapine (Zyprexa) - 3-fold
3. **Quetiapine (Seroquel) - 2-fold**
4. Minimal risk with all others

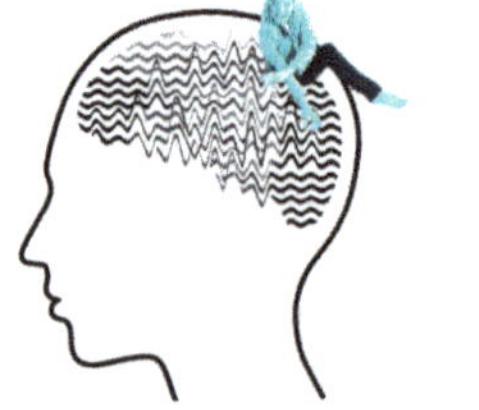

Dynamic interactions:

- Antidopaminergic (weak)
- EPS (low)
- Anticholinergic (mild)
- Sedation (strong)
- Hypotensive effects (strong)
- Lowers seizure threshold
- Prolactin elevation (weak)
- QT prolongation (low/mod)
- Hyperglycemia (moderate)
- Weight gain (moderate)

Kinetic interactions:

- Dosing adjustments are often necessary with 3A4 inhibitors/inducers

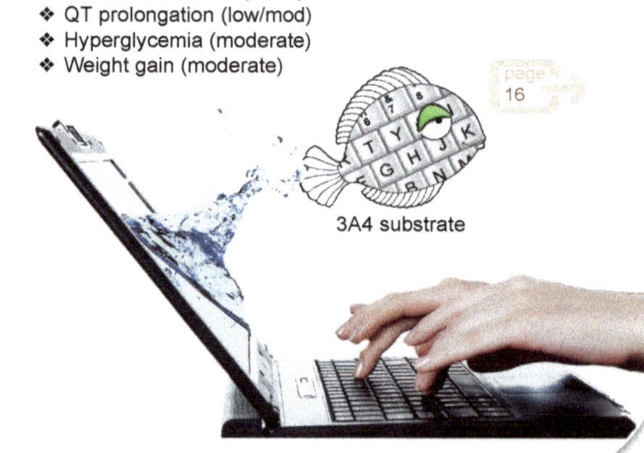

page 16

#131
2002
$21–$755

Aripiprazole (ABILIFY)

ar i PIP ra zole / a BIL e fy

"A ripped peep (is) Able to fly"

- ❖ Antipsychotic (SGA)
- ❖ D2 partial agonist - ⇔ DA
- ❖ $5\text{-}HT_{1A}$ partial agonist - ⇔ DA
- ❖ $5\text{-}HT_{2A}$ antagonist - ⇧ DA

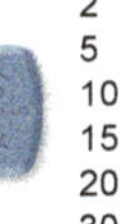

2
5
10
15
20
30 mg

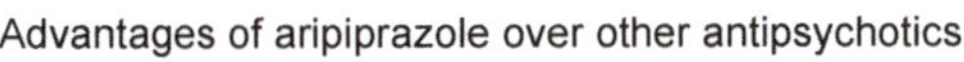

FDA-approved for:
- ❖ Schizophrenia
- ❖ Bipolar mania
- ❖ Depression (adjunct)
- ❖ Irritability in autism
- ❖ Tourette's disorder

Used off-label for:
- ❖ Bipolar depression
- ❖ Adjunct to olanzapine (Zyprexa) to minimize weight gain
- ❖ Adjunct to risperidone or paliperidone to normalize prolactin levels

generally non-sedating

aripiprazole treatment

no gyneco-mastia

Antipsychotics are represented with spooky mascots.

"weight neutral" (some people lose, some people gain)

Advantages of aripiprazole over other antipsychotics:
- ► Generally non-sedating (usually taken in morning)
- ► "Weight neutral" (although some gain weight; others lose weight)
- ► Relatively low risk of diabetes
- ► No risk of gynecomastia (decreases prolactin levels)
- ► Low risk of irreversible movement disorders
- ► Fewer sexual side effects than other antipsychotics
- ► Insignificant QT prolongation
- ► Several long-acting injectable (LAI) options

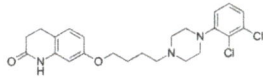

Aripiprazole (Abilify) was released in 2002 as the first dopamine receptor partial agonist, known colloquially as a "dopamine stabilizer". It is available in several formulations for many FDA-approved indications, including pediatric. Abilify is a good first-line antipsychotic due to a favorable side effect profile. However, an individual's response to aripiprazole is less predictable than with other antipsychotics. Agitation, insomnia, and compulsive behavior may occur due to increased dopamine activity. Serum levels are less predictable due to the possibility of the individual being a 2D6 ultra-rapid (3%) or poor metabolizer (10%). Several kinetic interactions must be considered. High doses are no more effective than moderate doses.

Contrast aripiprazole with olanzapine (Zyprexa) which is predictably effective and more so at higher doses, though at the expense of weight gain and elevated blood sugar. Consider olanzapine for short-term use and aripiprazole for long-term use.

The main troublesome side effect of Abilify is akathisia, which is a feeling of inner restlessness and inability to keep still. Akathisia is usually short-lived, and more common for those treated for mood disorders compared to those treated for schizophrenia. Akathisia is easily addressed with addition of propranolol or a low dose benzodiazepine. Some patients experience nausea, headache, or insomnia.

Aripiprazole has been associated with new onset of impulse-control problems such as pathological gambling, compulsive eating, compulsive shopping, and hypersexual behavior. These problems may be related to increased dopamine activity in patients with low baseline dopamine tone.

There is no risk of gynecomastia with aripiprazole because it decreases prolactin levels, which is the opposite of many antipsychotics. Aripiprazole has a long half-life of 3 to 6 days.

There are two competing aripiprazole long-acting injectable (LAI) products—ARISTADA and ABILIFY MAINTENA. The Aristada injection, administered every 4 to 8 weeks, is more painful than Abilify Maintena, which is given every 4 weeks. After the first injection, oral aripiprazole needs to be continued for 2 weeks (Maintena) to 3 weeks (Aristada). With Aristada, as an alternative to the 3-week PO overlap, a single injection of ARISTADA INITIO can be be administered (deltoid) simultaneously with the first Aristada injection (gluteal), along with a one time 30 mg PO dose.

Dosing: For schizophrenia and bipolar the recommended starting dose of 10 mg is the same as the recommended maintenance dose. The FDA maximum is 30 mg, but exceeding 15 mg is rarely more effective. Adjunctively for depression, start 2 mg or 5 mg QD, with maintenance dose 5–10 mg QD. If sedation is an issue with AM dosing, change to HS. Since akathisia is common with initiation of treatment, consider splitting the starting dose in half for the first couple days. Adjust dose for the kinetic interactions described below. See page 58 for dosing of long-acting injectable (LAI) formulations.

Dynamic interactions:
- ❖ Antidopaminergic (balanced)
- ❖ EPS (low, other than akathisia)
- ❖ CNS depression (minimal)
- ❖ Hypotensive effects (mild)
- ❖ Hyperglycemia (possible)
- ❖ Weight gain (possible)

Kinetic interactions:
- ❖ 2D6 substrate (major)
- ❖ 3A4 substrate (major)

As a substrate of 2D6 and 3A4, Abilify is subject to victimization by many kinetic interactions.

Consider dosing aripiprazole at 50% strength if the patient is taking a 2D6 inHibitor such as:
- ► Fluoxetine (Prozac)
- ► Paroxetine (Paxil)
- ► Bupropion (Wellbutrin)
- ► Duloxetine (Cymbalta)

It is recommended to use a double strength dose of Abilify in the presence of a strong 3A4 inDucer such as:
- ► Carbamazepine (Tegretol)
- ► Phenytoin (Dilantin)
- ► Phenobarbital (Luminal)

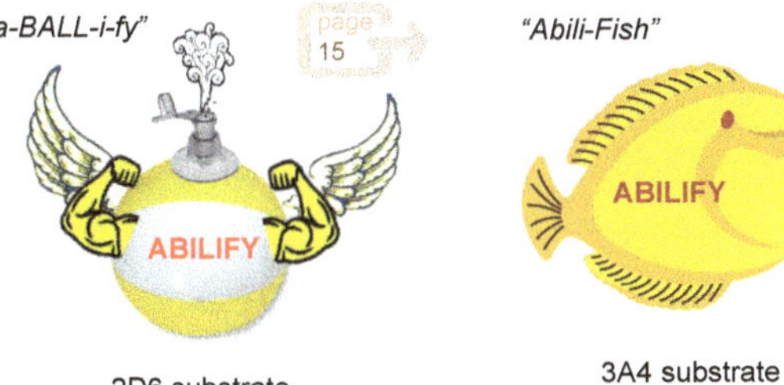

2D6 substrate

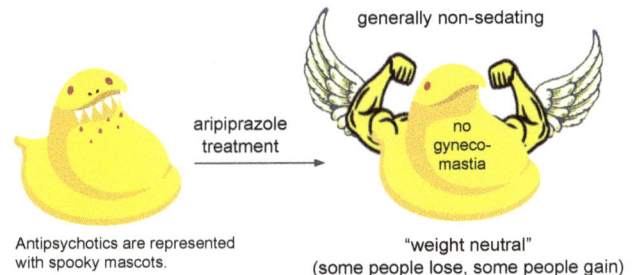

3A4 substrate

If the patient is taking a 2D6 inHibitor (or is 2D6 PM) and taking a 3A4 inHibitor, prescribing ¼ of the usual dose is recommended, and it is worthwhile to check a serum aripiprazole level.

Known 2D6 poor metabolizers (PM) should be given aripiprazole at 50% strength. 2D6 genotyping can be ordered for about $200, but testing is generally not needed to prescribe Abilify. Consider starting at a low dose of 5 mg to account for the possibility of the patient being a 2D6 PM.

#159
1993
$4–$66

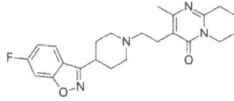

Risperidone (RISPERDAL)

ris PER i dohn / RIS per dal

"Breast-perdal"

- Antipsychotic (SGA)
- D2 antagonist - ⇩ DA
- 5-HT_{2A} antagonist - ⇧ DA
- Alpha-adrenergic antagonist

0.25
0.5
1
2
3
4 mg

FDA-approved for:

- Schizophrenia > 13 years old
- Bipolar > 10 years old
- Irritability of autism > 5 years old

Used off-label for:

- Treatment-resistant depression
- Tourette's disorder
- Aggression
- Agitation of dementia
- PTSD

Risperidone (Risperdal) was the second of the second generation antipsychotics (SGAs) to be released (1993), following clozapine (1990). It is one of the few antipsychotics approved for use in children. In *Memorizing Pharmacology,* Dr. Tony Guerra nicknamed the medication "whisper-dal" because it *quiets the whispers* of auditory hallucinations. Risperidone is relatively non-sedating because it has low affinity for blocking D4 receptors.

Risperidone causes increased release of prolactin from the pituitary, potentially leading to galactorrhea in women and gynecomastia in men. In the book *Memorable Psychopharmacology*, Dr. Jonathan Heldt offers a mnemonic about *rise-pair-idone* giving *"rise to a pair"* of breasts. The prolactin-elevating effect of antipsychotics occurs outside of the blood-brain barrier (BBB). Risperidone does not cross the BBB easily because it is pumped out by the P-glycoprotein (P-gp)—*"Pumpers gonna pump"*. Hence, relatively high serum concentrations of risperidone are necessary to achieve therapeutic levels in the brain. Those SGAs that cross the BBB easily are much less likely to elevate prolactin at therapeutic doses. Prolactin elevation may also cause sexual side effects. Retrograde ejaculation (into the bladder) is possible, although this is due to alpha-1 adrenergic receptor antagonism.

As an antipsychotic, risperidone has been found to be less effective than olanzapine, but more effective than ziprasidone and quetiapine. Risperidone can be regarded as a first-line antipsychotic for women, but second- or third-line for men. Risperidone commonly elevates prolactin levels, making gynecomastia common.

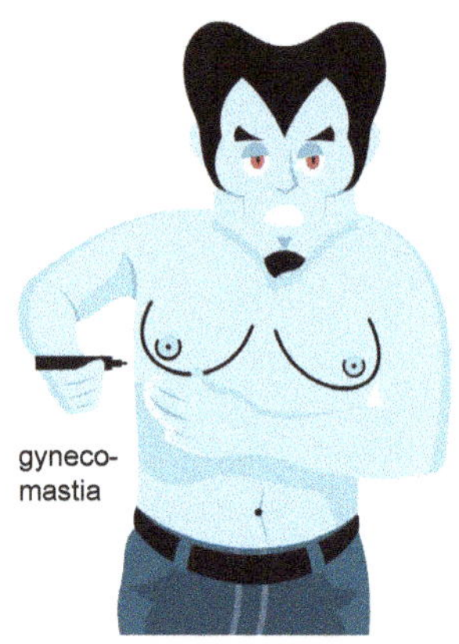

Antipsychotics are represented with spooky mascots.

If a man is doing well on risperidone (or paliperidone) but is concerned about the risk of gynecomastia, check a fasting prolactin level in early morning. If the prolactin level is substantially elevated, offer to stop or switch the medication. If prolactin level is below 20 ng/mL, reassure the patient that there is no risk of risperidone-induced gynecomastia.

Risperidone is available as a q 2 week long-acting injectable (LAI) called RISPERDAL CONSTA. Two weeks between injections is more frequent than the other antipsychotic LAIs—*you're getting shots CONSTAntly*. In 2019 a subcutaneous LAI was announced, called PERSERIS for q 4 week administration. Perseris is the only available subcutaneous LAI antipsychotic.

An active metabolite of risperidone, hydroxy-risperidone (OH-risp) is available as paliperidone (Invega), as featured on page 53. If the patient has liver problems, it is best to prescribe paliperidone. Otherwise, choose risperidone over paliperidone because risperidone is much less expensive. The liver converts risperidone to paliperidone (OH-risp) anyhow, mostly by CYP2D6.

Serum risperidone level can be checked, but results may take several days to arrive from an outside laboratory. The lab will report the level of risperidone and, separately, OH-risperidone.

Both risperidone and the OH-metabolite are biologically active, and therapeutic range is defined by the sum of the two chemicals. The relevant result is "risperidone and metabolite". 2 mg/day is expected to produce a combined level of 14 ng/mL. 16 mg/day produces a mean of 110 ng/mL. Risperdal/OH-risp serum ratio is usually < 1. An inverted ratio (> 1) means the patient is likely a CYP2D6 ultrarapid metabolizer (UM).

Adult dosing: For an acute manic episode, start 2 mg QD then titrate by 1 mg q 24 hr, to a max of 6 mg. For schizophrenia, start either 0.5 mg BID or 1 mg HS and increase in about a week to 1 mg BID or 2 mg HS. The "minimal effective dose" of risperidone for first episode psychosis is 2 mg. For multi-episode psychosis, the minimal effective dose is 4 mg. Doses > 4 mg/day are rarely more effective for schizophrenia. At doses above 6 mg risperidone behaves more like a first generation antipsychotic, i.e., carries a significant risk of EPS, including the possibility of tardive dyskinesia with long-term use. At risperidone's FDA maximum dose of 16 mg, it has no advantage over the FGAs in terms of EPS. The 0.25 mg tab is for pediatric use. See page 58 for dosing of the risperidone long-acting injectables (LAIs)—Risperdal Consta (q 2 wk IM) and Perseris (q 4 wk SQ).

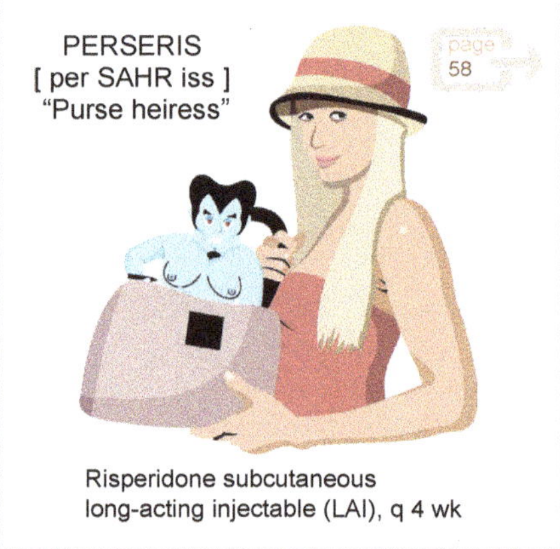

Risperidone subcutaneous long-acting injectable (LAI), q 4 wk

Prolactin elevation among SGAs, most to least (approximate):

- Paliperidone (Invega) - high, equal to risperidone
- Risperidone (Risperdal) - high, equal to paliperidone
- Lurasidone (Latuda) - mild, ⅛ the extent of risperidone
- Ziprasidone (Geodon) - mild
- Iloperidone (Fanapt) - mild
- Olanzapine (Zyprexa) - minimal
- Asenapine (Saphris) - minimal
- Clozapine (Clozaril) - does not increase prolactin
- Quetiapine (Seroquel) - does not increase prolactin
- Aripiprazole (Abilify) - decreases prolactin

Note that all first generation antipsychotics (FGAs) elevate prolactin.

Dynamic interactions:

- Antidopaminergic (moderate)
- EPS (dose dependent)
- Sedation (mild)
- Hypotensive effects
- Prolactin elevation (strong)
- Hyperglycemia (moderate)
- Weight gain (moderate)
- QT prolongation (low/mod)

Kinetic interactions:

- 2D6 substrate
- 3A4 substrate

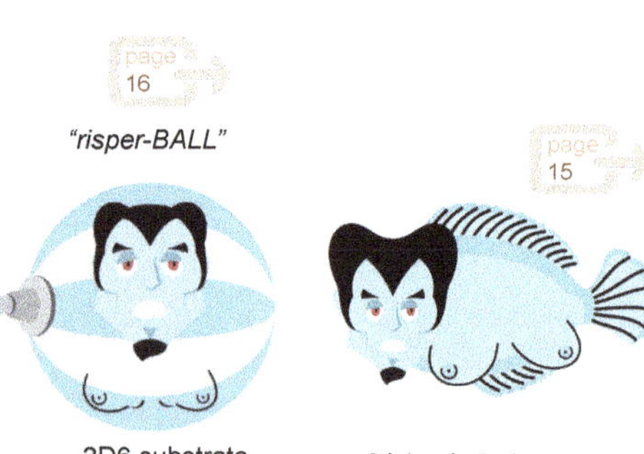

#225
1996
$5–$400 tab
$20–$500 ODT

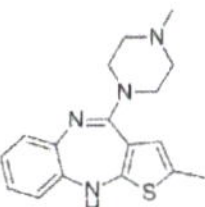

Olanzapine (ZYPREXA)

o lan za peen / zy PREX a

"Owl lands upon (cra)Zy pretzel"

- Antipsychotic (SGA)
- D2 antagonist - ⇩ DA
- 5-HT_{2A} antagonist - ⇧ DA

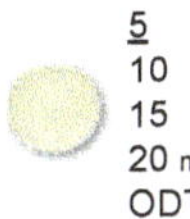

5
10
15
20 mg
ODT

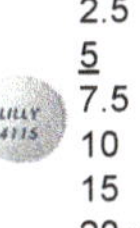

2.5
5
7.5
10
15
20 mg

FDA-approved for:

- Schizophrenia
- Bipolar mania
- Bipolar maintenance
- Bipolar depression (with fluoxetine)
- Treatment-resistant depression (with fluoxetine)
- Acute agitation of mania (IM route)

Used off-label for:

- Behavioral disturbance
- Nausea/vomiting
- Anorexia nervosa

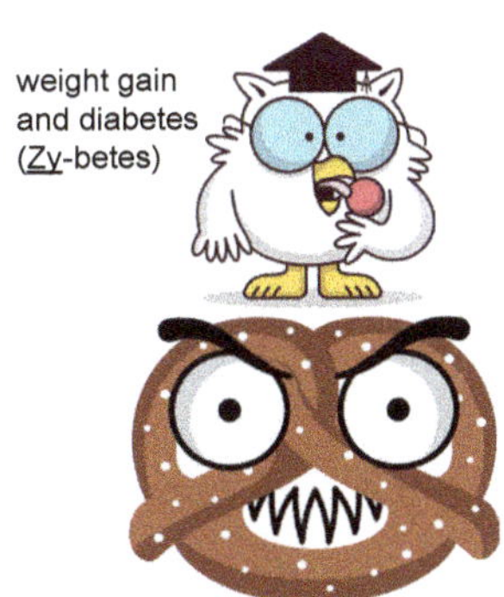

Antipsychotics are represented with spooky mascots.

The first thing to know about the SGA olanzapine (Zyprexa) is its potential to cause type II diabetes and substantial weight gain. It is #1 among all psychotropic medications for causing these problems. This is unfortunate because olanzapine is highly effective and has minimal side effects otherwise. Among antipsychotics, olanzapine is the #2 most effective treatment for schizophrenia (after clozapine) available in the US. Amisulpride, an antipsychotic available in other countries, was ranked #2, with olanzapine #3 (Leucht, 2013). Olanzapine is the antipsychotic most similar to clozapine in terms of molecular structure, efficacy, weight gain, and low EPS. Risk of seizures with olanzapine is greater than other antipsychotics, but much less than with clozapine. Single-drug overdoses of olanzapine are rarely lethal.

Olanzapine is a reasonable first-line antipsychotic for schizophrenia and acute mania. The dose can be titrated quickly. Although olanzapine is FDA-approved for bipolar maintenance, there are other effective options with less potential for weight gain.

Beyond diet and exercise, there are several options for ameliorating olanzapine-induced weight gain. Metformin is a great add-on to minimize weight gain and elevation of blood glucose. Aripiprazole (Abilify) ameliorates weight gain as an adjunct to olanzapine (Henderson et al, 2009). Melatonin and the antiepileptic drug topiramate (Topamax) have also been used.

Olanzapine is an effective antiemetic comparable to promethazine (Phenergan). It is modestly effective for promoting weight gain with anorexia nervosa, but also half of anorexic patients discontinue it.

Half-life is 21 to 54 hours. IM olanzapine generally reaches maximum concentration in 15 to 45 minutes, compared with 4 hours after an oral dose.

IM Zyprexa, FDA-approved for acute agitation in schizophrenia or bipolar, is contraindicated in combination with IM lorazepam (Ativan) due to risk of respiratory depression. However, Evidence of risk with the IM olanzapine/benzodiazepine combination is lacking (Williams et al, 2018).

Zyprexa RELPREVV is the long-acting injectable (LAI) formulation. It is rarely used because the patient must be monitored for at least three hours post-injection due to risk of post-injection delirium/sedation syndrome.

SYMBYAX is a branded fixed-dose combination of olanzapine (6–12 mg) and fluoxetine (Prozac), FDA-approved for acute depression in bipolar I disorder and treatment-resistant unipolar depression.

The FDA maximum is 20 mg/day, but higher doses are well-tolerated and associated with better efficacy. This is not the case with most other antipsychotics. High-dose olanzapine may be a safer alternative to clozapine for refractory psychosis. The main side effects at high dose are anticholinergic (page 59–60).

Therapeutic blood level monitoring for olanzapine may be useful, more so than with most antipsychotics. The therapeutic serum range is about 20–80 ng/mL, but higher concentrations may be necessary. There is no need to check olanzapine levels if the patient is doing well at modest doses (≤ 20 mg). Olanzapine level > 700 ng/mL is considered toxic and associated with QT prolongation.

PO Dosing: For schizophrenia, starting dose is usually 5–10 mg HS. FDA max is 20 mg/day, but for treatment-resistant cases, 30 mg or 40 mg total daily dose (typically divided BID) is commonly necessary. The author occasionally goes as high as 60 mg/day divided 30 mg BID. Stahl (2017) regards doses up to 90 mg/day as occasionally justifiable for short-term treatment. **For acute mania or psychosis** in the inpatient setting, the author generally starts 10 mg HS or BID, plus 5–10 mg PRN.

Oral dose does not need to be adjusted for renal impairment. Use a lower dose with moderate/severe hepatic impairment. As with most antipsychotics, treatment should be suspended if absolute neutrophil count (ANC) drops below 1,000 or if Drug Rash with Eosinophilia and Systemic Symptoms (DRESS syndrome) is suspected.

IM Dosing: The recommended initial injection for acute agitation is 10 mg. A second injection can be given after 2 hours, with no more than 3 injections within 24 hours.

Seizure risk among antipsychotics:

#1 Clozapine (Clozaril) 10x risk at high dose
#2 **Olanzapine (Zyprexa)** 3x
#3 Quetiapine (Seroquel) 2x
#4 Chlorpromazine (Thorazine) 2x

Risk is minimal for other antipsychotics. Risperidone (Risperdal), haloperidol (Haldol), fluphenazine (Prolixin), and thiothixene (Navane) are especially safe.

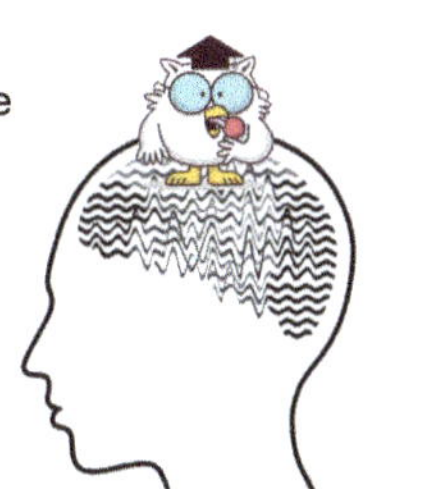

Weight gain among 2nd gen antipsychotics (SGAs), approximate rank:

1. **Olanzapine (Zyprexa)** - large weight gain, may be extreme
2. Clozapine (Clozaril) - nearly as much as olanzapine
3. Iloperidone (Fanapt) - higher than quetiapine
4. Quetiapine (Seroquel) - similar to risperidone
5. Risperidone (Risperdal)
6. Paliperidone (Invega) - equal to risperidone
7. Brexpiprazole (Rexulti)
8. Asenapine (Saphris) - low potential for weight gain
9. Aripiprazole (Abilify) - minimal
10. Cariprazine (Vraylar)
11. Ziprasidone (Geodon) - possible weight loss
12. Lurasidone (Latuda) - possible weight loss

Dynamic interactions:

- Antidopaminergic
- EPS (low)
- Anticholinergic (moderate)
- Sedation (moderate)
- Hypotensive effects (moderate)
- Lowers seizure threshold
- Prolactin elevation (weak)
- Hyperglycemia (high)
- Weight gain (high)

Kinetic interactions:

- 1A2 substrate
  - Smokers may need a higher dose of olanzapine due to 1A2 inDuction by tobacco. Nicotine replacement products (gum, patches) do not induce 1A2.
  - Use lower doses of olanzapine if co-administered with a 1A2 inhibitor such as fluvoxamine (Luvox).

page 10
1A2 substrate

Most women are slow at metabolizing 1A2 substrates. Expect a woman's olanzapine blood level to be up to double that of a man taking the same dose.

#227
2010
$1,212–$1,490

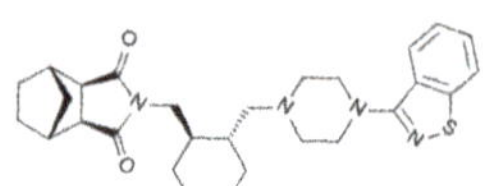

Lurasidone (LATUDA)

loo RAS i dohn / la TUDE a

"Lured (to the) Latitude"

❖ Antipsychotic (SGA)
❖ D2 antagonist - ⇩ DA
❖ 5-HT_{2A} antagonist - ⇧ DA

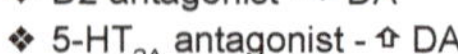

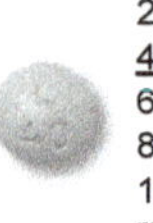

20
40
60
80
120
mg

FDA-approved for:

❖ Schizophrenia
❖ Bipolar I depressive episode - monotherapy
❖ Bipolar depression as adjunct to lithium or valproate (Depakote, Depakene)—but contraindicated with carbamazepine (Tegretol)

Used off-label for:

❖ Bipolar maintenance

Among antipsychotics, lurasidone (Latuda) is the most metabolically favorable. Weight loss is more likely than weight gain, and lurasidone actually *improves* Hgb A1c! The same can be said about ziprasidone (Geodon), which is the antipsychotic most similar to lurasidone.

Half-life of lurasidone is 18 to 40 hours. It is dosed once daily with at least 350 calories, usually with the evening meal. Food is necessary for absorption. Compare this to ziprasidone, which must be given with food for the same reason, but ziprasidone has a shorter half-life, necessitating twice daily dosing. Another advantage of lurasidone (over ziprasidone) is lack of QT prolongation. Most other antipsychotics prolong QT interval to some extent.

Despite these advantages, patients with schizophrenia in clinical trials were likely to discontinue treatment with Latuda, due to either lack of benefit and/or side effects. In the real world, Latuda is even more likely to be stopped due to cost.

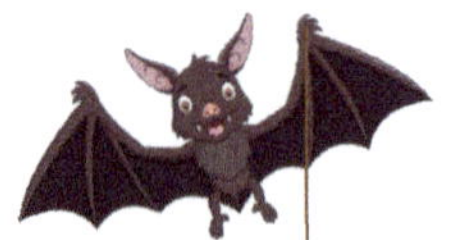

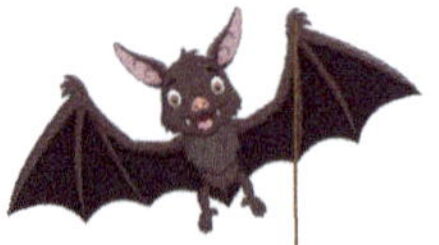

Antipsychotics are represented with spooky mascots.

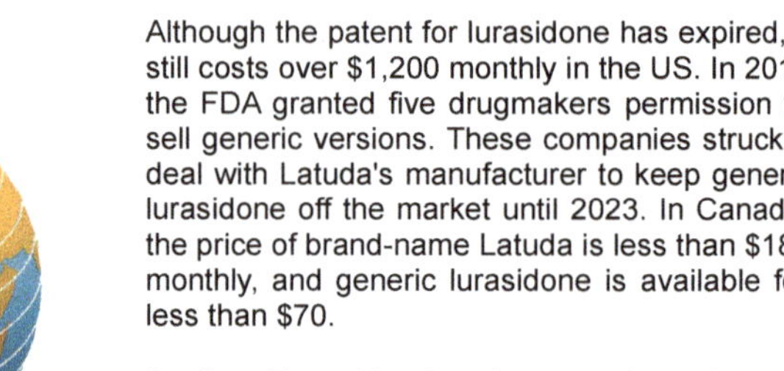

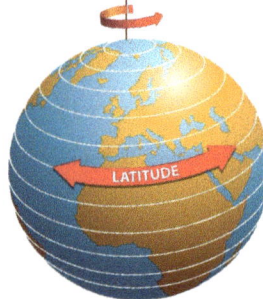

It is noteworthy that the SGAs that do not cause weight gain (Latuda and Geodon) are the most likely to be stopped, while those causing the most weight gain (Zyprexa and Clozapine) are the most likely to be continued.

Lurasidone is relatively more likely than other SGAs to cause extrapyramidal symptoms (EPS).

Lurasidone is almost exclusively metabolized by CYP3A4, making it highly vulnerable to kinetic interactions. With most substrate medications, interactions can be handled by adjusting the dose. With lurasidone, 3A4 interactions are of such high consequence that it is contraindicated with strong 3A4 inducers or inhibitors.

Although the patent for lurasidone has expired, it still costs over $1,200 monthly in the US. In 2019 the FDA granted five drugmakers permission to sell generic versions. These companies struck a deal with Latuda's manufacturer to keep generic lurasidone off the market until 2023. In Canada, the price of brand-name Latuda is less than $180 monthly, and generic lurasidone is available for less than $70.

Dosing: For schizophrenia, start 40 mg QD with evening meal, max 160 mg/day; For bipolar depression, start 20 mg QD with evening meal, max 120 mg/day. Decrease dose for hepatic insufficiency.

Antipsychotics approved for bipolar depression (2020), listed in order of apparent effectiveness:

Second generation antipsychotic	NNT*
Olanzapine/fluoxetine combo (Symbyax)	4
Lurasidone (Latuda)	5
Quetiapine XR (Seroquel XR)	6
Cariprazine (Vraylar)	7

*NNT = Number Needed to Treat, i.e., number of patients you need to treat for one patient to respond. The lower the NNT, the more effective the medication.

All-cause discontinuation of SGAs in clinical trials for schizophrenia, approximate rank from most to least likely to be stopped by doctor or patient:

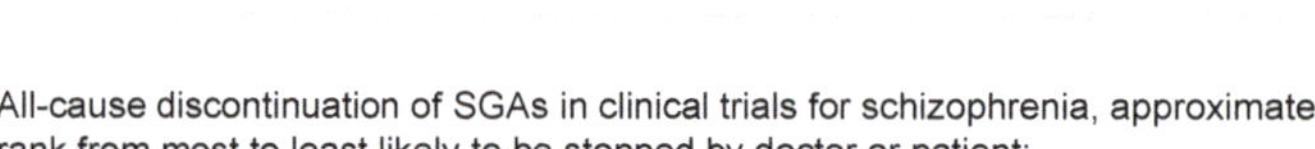

❖ **Lurasidone (Latuda)** - most likely to be stopped
❖ Ziprasidone (Geodon) - slightly fewer discontinuations than lurasidone
❖ Iloperidone (Fanapt)
❖ Asenapine (Saphris)
❖ Quetiapine (Seroquel)
❖ Aripiprazole (Abilify)
❖ Risperidone (Risperdal)
❖ Paliperidone (Invega)
❖ Clozapine (Clozaril) - despite side effects and inconveniences, patients continue it because it is effective
❖ Olanzapine (Zyprexa) - effective and usually no issues other than weight gain and diabetes

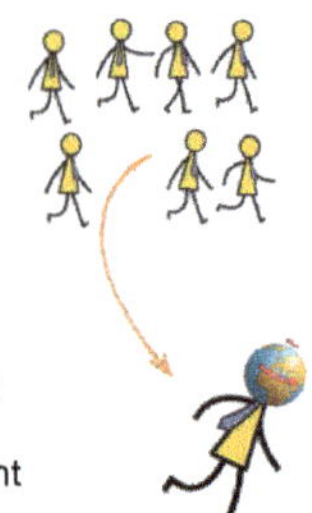

The fish (our symbol for 3A4 substrate) is big because with lurasidone 3A4 interactions are a very big deal.

Lurasidone is **contraindicated** with strong 3A4 in**D**ucers, because lurasidone will be useless due to rapid clearance, reducing lurasidone levels by about **6-fold:**

❖ Carbamazepine (Tegretol)
❖ Phenytoin (Dilantin)
❖ Phenobarbital (Luminal)
❖ St. John's wort
❖ Rifampin

Lurasidone is also **contraindicated** with strong 3A4 in**H**ibitors due to radically increased lurasidone levels, up to **8-fold**:

❖ Fluconazole and other -azole antifungals
❖ Clarithromycin (antibacterial)
❖ Ritonavir (antiretroviral for HIV)

The minimal effective daily dose for schizophrenia is 40 mg. If coadministered with a **moderate** 3A4 in**D**ucer, lurasidone may need to be titrated to a higher dose. If used with a moderate 3A4 in**H**ibitor, give half of the usual dose.

Dynamic interactions:

❖ Antidopaminergic
❖ Extrapyramidal effects
❖ Sedation (moderate)
❖ Hypotensive effects
❖ Prolactin elevation (mild)

Kinetic interactions:

❖ 3A4 substrate (major)

page 16

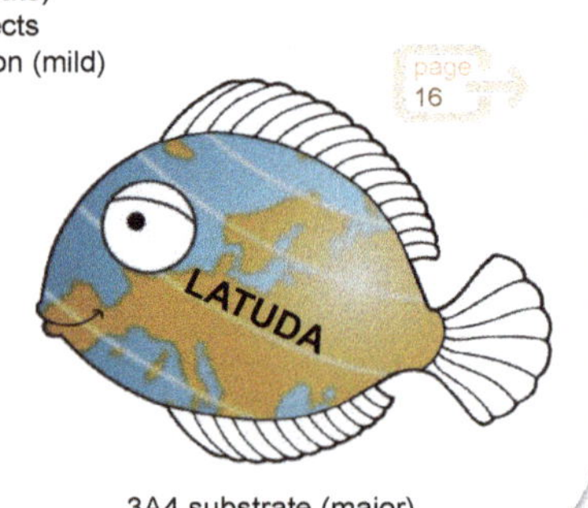

3A4 substrate (major)

2001
$32–$292

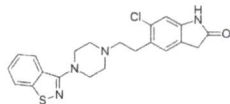

Ziprasidone (GEODON)

zi PRAY si dohn / GEE o don

"Geode Don's Zipper"

- Antipsychotic (SGA)
- D2 antagonist - ⇩ DA
- 5-HT_{2A} antagonist - ⇧ DA

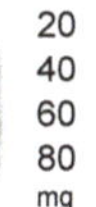

20
40
60
80
mg

FDA-approved for:

- Schizophrenia
- Bipolar mania
- Schizophrenia-associated agitation (IM)

Used off-label for:

- Bipolar maintenance
- Impulse control disorders
- Delirium
- Agitation of any type (IM)

For this antipsychotic, think *"Geo-down"*, as in bringing a psychotic or manic patient down to earth.

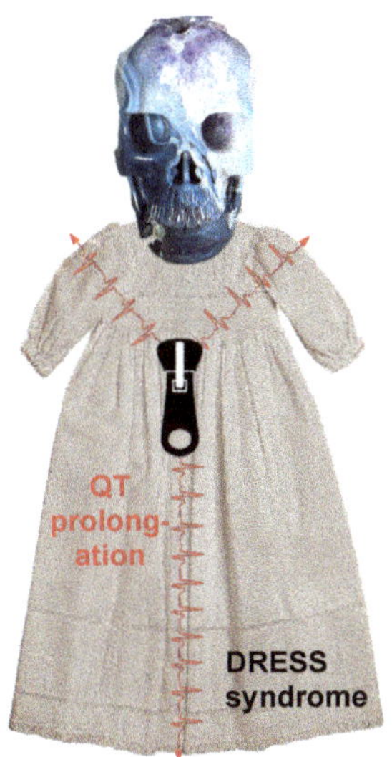

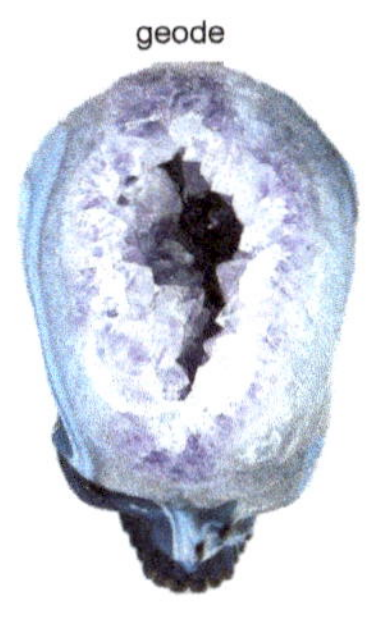

Antipsychotics are represented with spooky mascots.

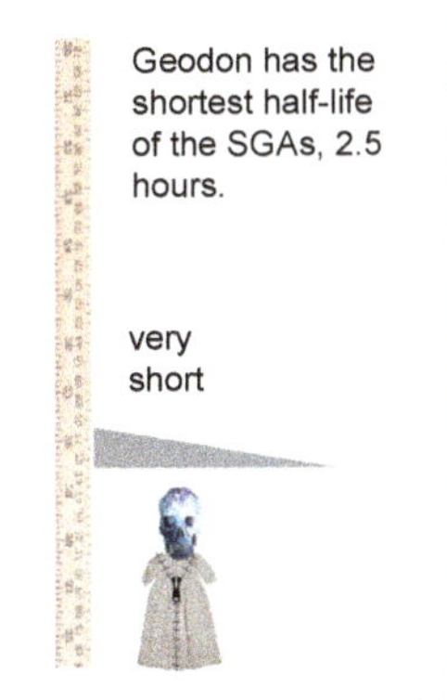

Geodon has the shortest half-life of the SGAs, 2.5 hours.
very short

Ziprasidone (Geodon) is recognized as the SGA most likely to prolong QT interval. At the maximum approved dose of 160 mg/day, ziprasidone is expected to prolong QTc by 10 msec. However, *clinically significant* QT prolongation (QTc > 500 msec) at 160 mg does not exceed placebo (Klein-Schwarz et al, 2007). QT prolongation with ziprasidone can be dangerous with overdose or polypharmacy. It is advisable to check an EKG before exceeding the FDA maximum dose or when combining ziprasidone with other QT prolonging drugs (page 23).

Ziprasidone has a benign metabolic profile, potentially having a positive impact on lipids and blood sugar. Patients may even have a modest weight loss with ziprasidone. Unfortunately, it is not as effective for schizophrenia as the more fattening SGAs like olanzapine (Zyprexa), risperidone (Risperdal), and clozapine (Clozaril). It is to be taken BID with meals, which is necessary for adequate absorption. The most similar antipsychotic to ziprasidone is lurasidone (Latuda), which may also improve metabolic parameters and must be taken with food for absorption. Ziprasidone is dosed BID, while lurasidone is QD.

Immediate-release IM ziprasidone is among first-line choices for acute psychotic agitation. IM ziprasidone is suitable for agitation associated with acute delirium because it lacks significant anticholinergic effects. IM ziprasidone can be prepared quickly, with a 30 second shake of the vial. There is no long-acting Injectable (LAI) formulation.

DRESS syndrome (Drug Reaction with Eosinophilia and Systemic Symptoms) is a rare but potentially fatal illness associated with ziprasidone. DRESS begins as a rash and progresses to swollen lymph nodes, fever, and inflammation of multiple organs. The heart, liver, kidneys, and pancreas may be damaged. Be especially vigilant for rash with ziprasidone and be quick to stop the medication if DRESS is suspected. Other medications that may rarely cause DRESS are the antipsychotic olanzapine (Zyprexa), modafinil (Provigil), several antibiotics, and several anticonvulsants including gabapentin (Neurontin).

PO Dosing: Titrate quickly for mania, starting 40 mg BID with meals for one day (2 doses) then increase to the target dose of 60–80 mg BID. FDA maximum dose is 160 mg/day (80 BID), although safety data exists for up to 320 mg/day (160 mg BID); Check EKG before exceeding the FDA max; Titrate slowly for schizophrenia, starting at 20 mg BID. For schizophrenia "doses > 40 mg/day (20 mg BID) are rarely more effective". As with most antipsychotics, discontinue if absolute neutrophil count (ANC) drops below 1,000.

IM Dosing: For schizophrenia-associated agitation (or off-label for any kind of agitation) may give 10 mg IM q 2 hours PRN or 20 mg IM q 4 hours PRN; Max is 40 mg/day x 3 days. The author uses the 20 mg dose unless the patient is small, elderly or medically compromised.

QT prolongation among SGAs:

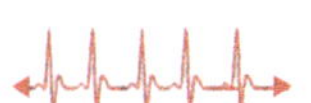

page 23

Risk	Second Generation Antipsychotic
Mod/High	Ziprasidone (Geodon)
Moderate	Iloperidone (Fanapt)
Low/Mod	Asenapine (Saphris), Clozapine (Clozaril), Quetiapine (Seroquel), Risperidone (Risperdal)
Low	Paliperidone (Invega), Pimavanserin (Nuplazid)
Essentially none	Lumateperone (Caplyta), Lurasidone (Latuda), Olanzapine (Zyprexa); **All D2 partial agonists:** Aripiprazole (Abilify), Brexpiprazole (Rexulti), Cariprazine (Vraylar)

The 3 psychotropic medications that must be taken **with food** for adequate absorption - the *DONE-nuts*.

- Vilazodone (VIIBRYD) - antidepressant
- Ziprasidone (GEODON) - antipsychotic
- Lurasidone (LATUDA) - antipsychotic

Without food, absorption is decreased by 50%.

page 18

Dynamic interactions:

- Antidopaminergic
- EPS
- Sedation (strong)
- QT prolongation
- Hypotensive effects
- Prolactin elevation (mild)

Kinetic interactions:

- Metabolized in liver primarily by aldehyde oxidase, with small contribution from several CYP enzymes

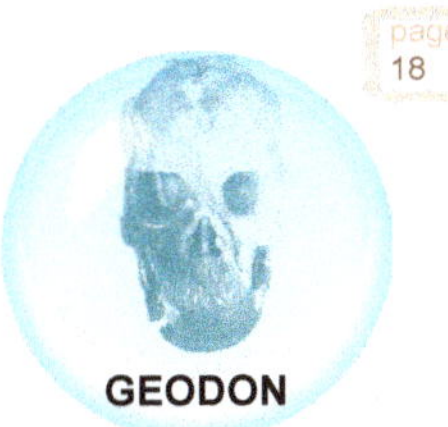

in a bubble - minimal clinically significant kinetic interactions

1990
$42–$184 + labs

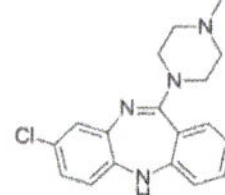

Clozapine (CLOZARIL)

KLOE za peen / KLOE za ril

"Clothes pin"

- ❖ Antipsychotic (SGA)
- ❖ D2 antagonist - ⇩ DA
- ❖ $5\text{-}HT_{2A}$ antagonist - ⇧ DA
- ❖ Alpha-adrenergic antagonist

25
50
<u>100</u>
200
mg

FDA-approved for:
- ❖ <u>Treatment-resistant</u> schizophrenia
- ❖ Prevention of schizophrenia-associated <u>suicide</u>

Used off-label for:
- ❖ Treatment-resistant aggression
- ❖ Psychosis with tardive dyskinesia
- ❖ Psychosis with Parkinson's disease

Neutrophil

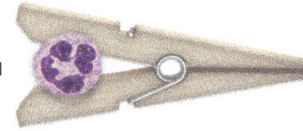

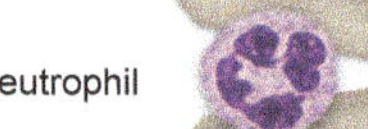

Clozapine, released in 1990 as <u>the first atypical</u> (2nd generation) antipsychotic, is clearly the <u>most effective treatment for schizophrenia</u>. Clozapine can be a <u>miracle drug</u> when nothing else works. It is the only antipsychotic approved specifically for treatment-resistant schizophrenia. Clozapine is the most effective medication for <u>reduction of suicide</u> associated with schizophrenia. It is a truly atypical antipsychotic in that it does not cause EPS, which is a beautiful thing considering the population being treated with clozapine, i.e., individuals with severe psychosis who would otherwise be at high risk of tardive dyskinesia (TD) from high doses of other antipsychotics.

Although several SGAs do not cause EPS above placebo (olanzapine, quetiapine, iloperidone, pimavanserin, lumateperone), with clozapine the <u>risk of EPS is *less than* placebo</u> (Leucht et al, 2013). Clozapine <u>*improves* tardive dyskinesia</u>. Clozapine is an antipsychotic of choice for those with Parkinson's disease (along with quetiapine and pimavanserin).

Unfortunately, clozapine is plagued by <u>serious risks</u> and <u>severe side effects</u>. Of all available psychiatric medications, clozapine is <u>#2 for weight gain</u>, a close second to olanzapine. Clozapine is <u>#1 for constipation</u> and <u>#1 for sialorrhea</u> (salivation) due to <u>anticholinergic effect on the colon</u> and <u>cholinergic effect on salivary glands</u>, respectively. The S in the cholinergic SLUDGE mnemonic stands for salivation (page 59). Clozapine does not elevate prolactin levels.

Despite clozapine's superiority for treatment-resistant schizophrenia, only 5% of patients who would benefit from clozapine are prescribed it (Olfson et al, 2016). Many psychiatrists are understandably reluctant to prescribe clozapine, given the health risks and time/effort involved in the initial titration, which often includes <u>tapering off sedatives</u>, anticholinergics and other antipsychotics. All prescribers must certify in the Clozapine Risk Evaluation and Mitigation Strategy (REMS) program, which takes less than an hour. *The Clozapine Handbook* by Meyer & Stahl is recommended for prescribers of this complicated medication.

Clozapine increases the probability of <u>seizures</u> up to 10-fold. Clozapine is the only psychotropic drug with a **black box warning** for lowering seizure threshold. Since seizure risk is dose-dependent, consider adding a prophylactic antiepileptic (valproate or lamotrigine) when exceeding 600 mg/day. Other **black box warnings** concern severe <u>neutropenia</u>, orthostatic <u>hypotension</u>/bradycardia/syncope, <u>myocarditis</u>/cardiomyopathy/mitral valve incompetence and (applicable to all antipsychotics) mortality in dementia-related psychosis.

Risk of life-threatening neutropenia (agranulocytosis) necessitates frequent blood draws. <u>Absolute neutrophil count</u> (ANC) must be checked <u>weekly</u> for the first 6 months, twice monthly for the next 6 months, then monthly *ad infinitum*. Pharmacies will not dispense clozapine unless ANC values are current in the national clozapine REMS database, which trademarked the slogan "No Blood, No Drug" (apropos to our vampire mascot). Clozapine treatment should be interrupted if <u>ANC drops below 1,000</u> unless the patient had low baseline ANC as seen in some individuals of African descent, a condition known as Benign Ethnic Neutropenia (BEN).

A majority of patients on clozapine become <u>constipated</u>. Although agranulocytosis may be fatal, patients are more likely to die from clozapine-related <u>bowel obstruction</u>, which may progress to toxic megacolon and bowel rupture. It is wise to start senna and docusate when initiating clozapine. <u>Avoid anticholinergics</u>. Encourage hydration and physical activity to ameliorate constipation.

Half-life of clozapine is 12 hours. Clozapine must be <u>slowly titrated</u> to avoid orthostatic <u>hypotension</u> and <u>sedation</u>. If the patient becomes <u>febrile</u> within 6 weeks, <u>suspect myocarditis</u> and order EKG, C-reactive protein (CRP), and troponin. As clozapine is being titrated, it is often possible to taper off most of the patient's other psychotropic medications. Extreme caution should be used if combining clozapine with benzodiazepines, opioids, or other drugs that may depress respiration.

Dosing: BID dosing; AM and HS doses may be unequal with HS > AM dose. Consolidate to HS if sedation is problematic. <u>Tobacco</u> users may need double the dose due to 1A2 induction. Initial <u>outpatient titration</u> (non-smokers): 12.5 mg HS (days 1–2), 25 mg/day (days 3–5), 50 mg/day (days 6–8), 75 mg/day (9–11), 100 mg/day (days 12–14), 125 mg/day (days 15–17), 150 mg/day (days 18–20); 175 mg/day (days 21–23); 200 mg/day (days 24 onward). For initiation in <u>inpatient setting</u>, 200 mg/day can be achieved in 1–2 weeks; <u>Target dose</u> is 300–600 mg/day with max of 900 mg/day, guided by blood levels and clinical response. Check <u>clozapine blood level</u> 4 days after establishment of the full-strength dose. The target blood level for clozapine is <u>≥ 350</u> ng/ml, **not** including the norclozapine metabolite. It is less effective at blood level > 700 ng/ml; High seizure risk > 1200 ng/ml; Toxic > 1500 ng/ml.

In addition to neutropenia, major risks and side effects of clozapine include:

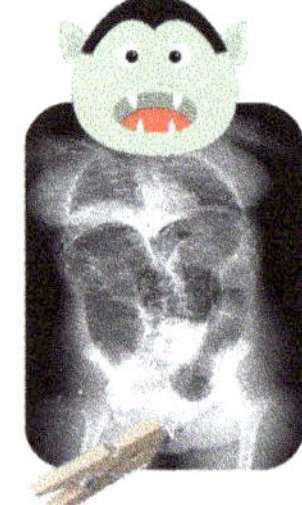

Severe constipation, which can lead to toxic megacolon and bowel rupture. Mechanism of constipation is anticholinergic and anti-serotonergic.

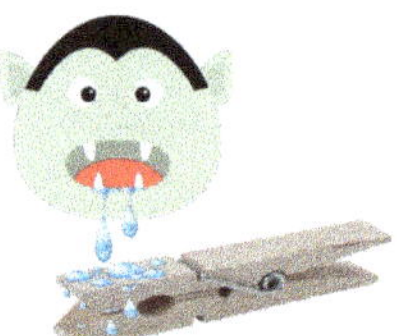

Hypersalivation by cholinergic mechanism (the S in SLUDGE)

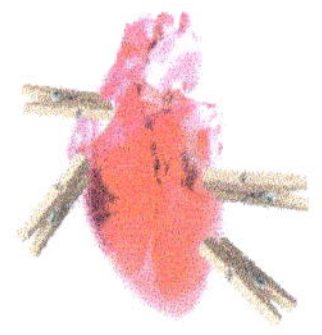

Potentially fatal myocarditis

Weight gain

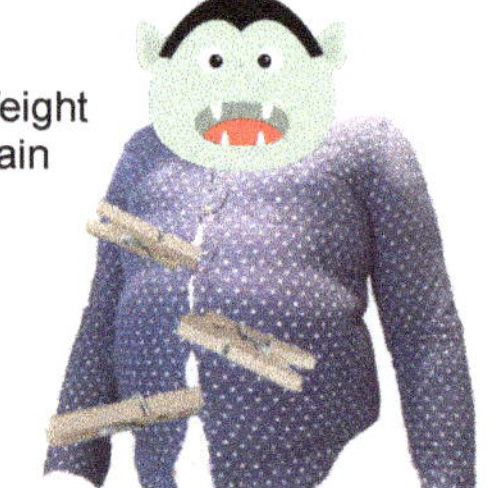

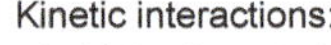

Antipsychotics are represented with spooky mascots.

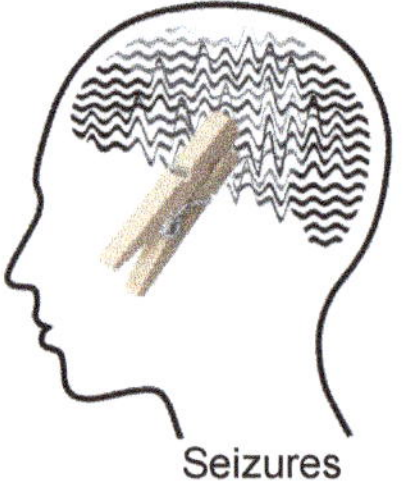

Seizures

By in<u>D</u>ucing 1A2, tobacco decreases serum clozapine levels by about 50%. Smokers require a double dose.

As a potent in<u>H</u>ibitor of 1A2, fluvoxamine (Luvox) increases clozapine levels 3-fold on average (but up to 10-fold in some cases). As a less potent 1A2 in<u>H</u>ibitor, ciprofloxacin increases clozapine exposure about 2-fold. See page 11 for important nuances of the fluvoxamine interaction.

Major inflammations, infections with fever or female gender (estrogen) may increase clozapine levels 2-fold (page 11).

Dynamic interactions:
- ❖ Antidopaminergic
- ❖ Anticholinergic (constipation)
- ❖ Sedation (strong)
- ❖ Hypotensive effects (strong)
- ❖ Lowers seizure threshold (high)
- ❖ Hyperglycemia (high)
- ❖ Weight gain (high)
- ❖ QT prolongation (low/moderate)
- ❖ Myelosuppression
- ❖ Respiratory suppression with benzos

Kinetic interactions:
- ❖ 1A2 substrate (major)
- ❖ 3A4 substrate (minor)

pages 10-11

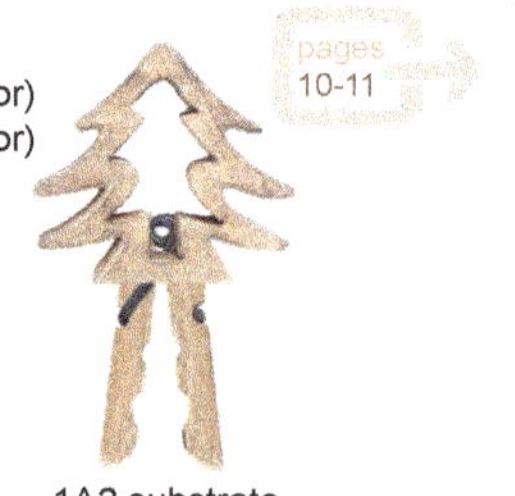

1A2 substrate

2015
$1,154–$1,351

Brexpiprazole (REXULTI)

brex PIP ra zole / rex UL tee

"Bee-Rex (Rex-salty)"

- Antipsychotic (SGA)
- D2 partial agonist - ⇔ DA
- $5\text{-}HT_{1A}$ partial agonist - ⇔ DA
- $5\text{-}HT_{2A}$ antagonist - ⇧ DA

0.25
0.5
1
2
3
4 mg

FDA-approved for:

- Schizophrenia
- Adjunct for major depression

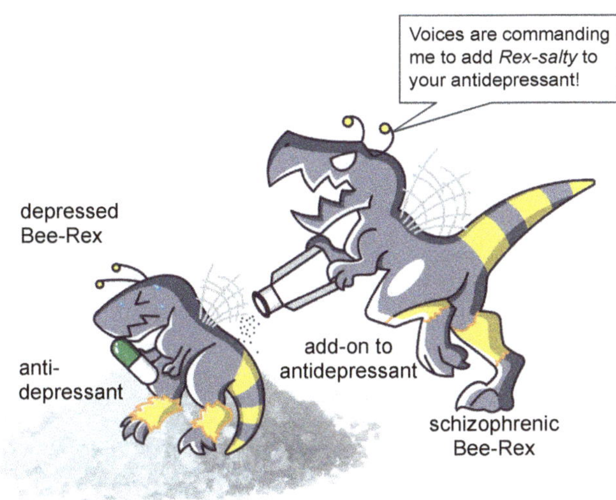

Brexpiprazole (Rexulti) was released in 2015 by the makers of aripiprazole (Abilify) as Abilify's patent was expiring. Rexulti has the same mechanism of action—dopamine D2 partial agonist, serotonin $5\text{-}HT_{1A}$ partial agonist and serotonin $5\text{-}HT_{2A}$ antagonist. It has been described as a Serotonin-Dopamine Activity Modulator.

Compared to Abilify, Rexulti has lower affinity for D2 receptors, thereby causing significantly less akathisia than Abilify. Rexulti has much higher affinity for $5\text{-}HT_{1A}$ and $5\text{-}HT_{2A}$ receptors, which may improve tolerability and contribute some anxiolytic effect.

Rexulti is FDA-approved for schizophrenia and as an adjunct to antidepressants for treatment of major depressive disorder (MDD).

Like Abilify, Rexulti is not expected to cause sedation.

Rexulti may be associated with more weight gain than Abilify. It does not lower prolactin (as does aripiprazole) but does not elevate prolactin to a clinically significant extent. Other side effects may include nausea, headaches, and dizziness.

Dosing: The recommended dose of Rexulti depends on the indication. For schizophrenia, the dose is higher, and the titration is faster than if augmenting an antidepressant. See below for details. It can be taken at morning or night, with or without food. As with most antipsychotics, discontinue if absolute neutrophil count (ANC) drops below 1,000.

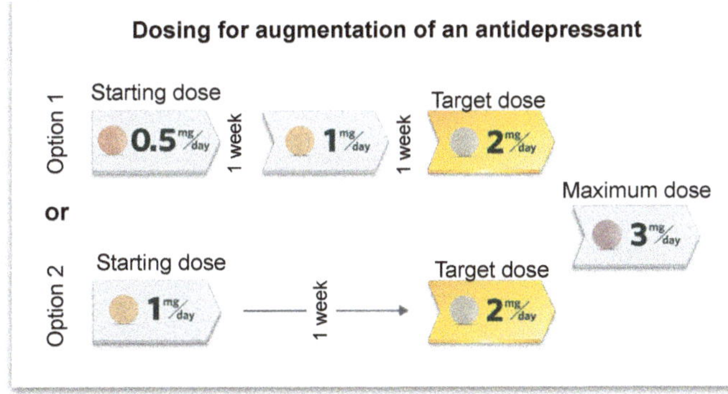

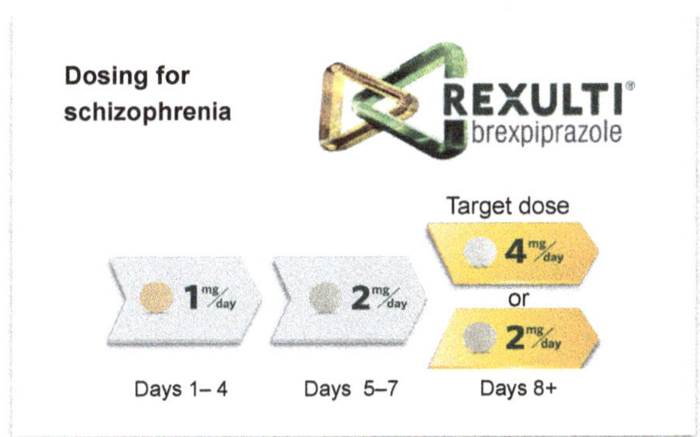

$5\text{-}HT_{1A}$ serotonin receptor agonists:

- Trazodone - antidepressant
- Nefazodone - antidepressant
- Flibanserin - libido enhancer

$5\text{-}HT_{1A}$ serotonin receptor partial agonists:

- Buspirone - anxiolytic
- Aripiprazole - antipsychotic
- **Brexpiprazole** - antipsychotic
- Cariprazine - antipsychotic
- Vilazodone - antidepressant
- Vortioxetine - antidepressant

Dynamic interactions:

- Antidopaminergic (balanced)
- EPS (low)
- CNS depression (minimal)
- Hypotensive effects (mild)
- Hyperglycemia (possible)
- Weight gain (possible)

Kinetic interactions:

- 2D6 substrate (major)
- 3A4 substrate (major)

When used to augment the strong 2D6 in**H**ibitors fluoxetine (Prozac) or paroxetine (Paxil), it is recommended brexpiprazole not exceed 2 mg.

page 16

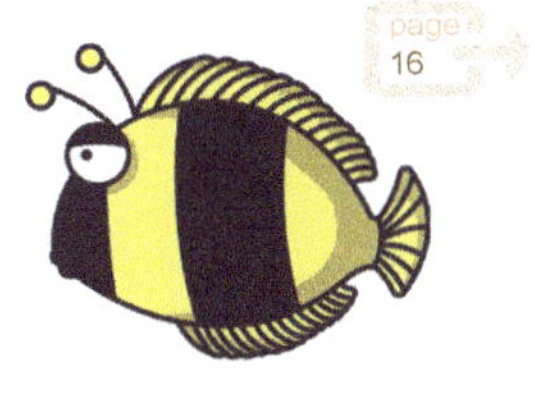

3A4 substrate

page 15

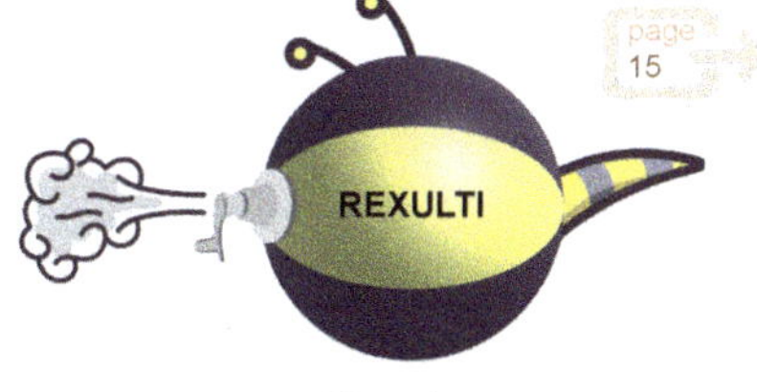

2D6 substrate

2016
$1,189–$1,452

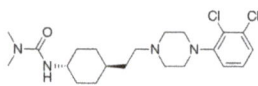

Cariprazine (VRAYLAR)

kar IP ra zeen / va RAY lar

"Car ripper seen (going) Vroom!"

- ❖ Antipsychotic (SGA)
- ❖ D2 partial agonist - ⇔ DA
- ❖ D3 partial agonist - ⇔ DA
- ❖ 5-HT_{1A} partial agonist - ⇔ DA
- ❖ 5-HT_{2A} antagonist - ⇧ DA

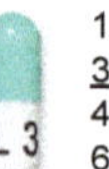

1.5
3
4.5
6
mg

Take your pick of mnemonics: *"Car ripper seen (going) Vroom!", "Car's V-rays", "Car ripper praising V-rays".*

Antipsychotics are represented with spooky mascots.

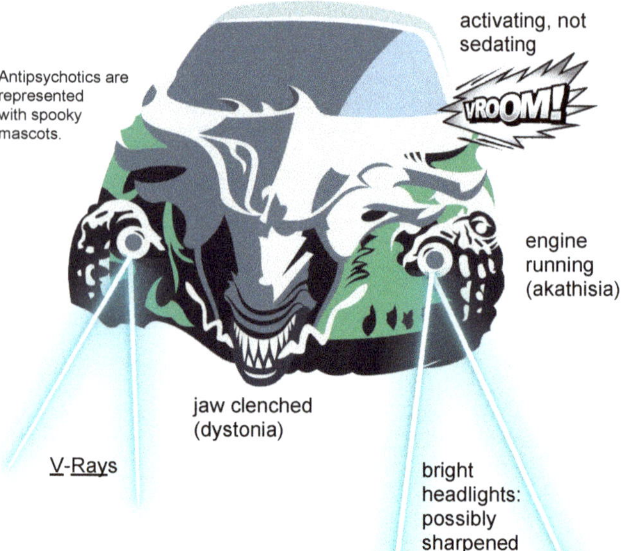

activating, not sedating

engine running (akathisia)

jaw clenched (dystonia)

V-Rays

bright headlights: possibly sharpened cognition

FDA-approved for
- ❖ Schizophrenia
- ❖ Bipolar I Disorder, manic/mixed episode
- ❖ Bipolar I Disorder, depressive episode

Used off-label for:
- ❖ Bipolar maintenance

Vraylar, released in 2016, is the third D2 partial agonist, after Abilify (aripiprazole) and Rexulti (brexpiprazole). Vraylar causes more EPS than Abilify and Rexulti, with 25% incidence of dystonia and 15% akathisia. It is more likely to cause nausea than other antipsychotics.

In addition to being a D2 partial agonist, Vraylar is D3 partial agonist, a unique property which may improve negative symptoms of schizophrenia (diminished emotional expression and avolition). Vraylar has a 5-fold selectivity for D3 over D2. Dopamine D3-preferring agents may provide cognitive benefits, although it may be too early to tell.

Dosing: For schizophrenia or mania, the label recommends 1.5 mg QD x 1 day, then 3 mg PO QD; May then adjust dose in 1.5 mg or 3 mg increments with max of 6 mg QD. Although higher doses were tested, no additional benefit was found at doses exceeding 6 mg; Because of the probability of akathisia, Dr. Tammas Kelly (Carlat Psychiatry Report, Aug 2019) recommends titrating more slowly, starting 1.5 mg QOD, increasing to 1.5 mg QD after a week. For bipolar depression the dose is 1.5 mg QD; At 14 days increase to the maximum dose for depression of 3 mg QD. However, the sweet spot for depression seems to be 1.5 mg, 3 mg causes more side effects without much additional benefit. As with most antipsychotics, discontinue if absolute neutrophil count (ANC) drops below 1,000.

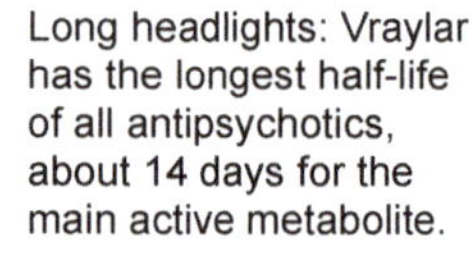

Long headlights: Vraylar has the longest half-life of all antipsychotics, about 14 days for the main active metabolite.

Akathisia is an uncomfortable feeling of internal motor restlessness with difficulty sitting still. The patient may fidget, pace, or rock back and forth.

Akathisia among SGAs (most to least):

- ❖ Cariprazine (Vraylar) - high
- ❖ Lurasidone (Latuda) - high
- ❖ Risperidone (Risperdal)
- ❖ Aripiprazole (Abilify)
- ❖ Paliperidone (Invega)
- ❖ Asenapine (Saphris)
- ❖ Ziprasidone (Geodon)
- ❖ Olanzapine (Zyprexa)
- ❖ Brexpiprazole (Rexulti) - low
- ❖ Pimavanserin (Nuplazid) - low
- ❖ Iloperidone (Fanapt)
  - marketed for those with akathisia
- ❖ Clozapine (Clozaril) - very low
- ❖ Quetiapine (Seroquel) - least

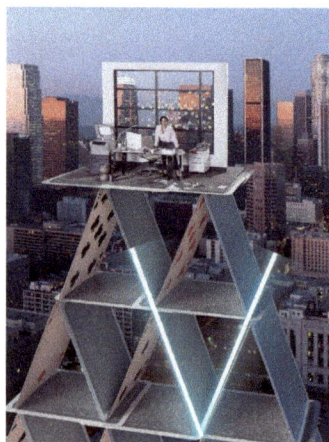

The Vraylar television ad showed a house of cards as a metaphor for mania, which may feel great to an individual with bipolar disorder until the inevitable crash to depression.

Side effect profile for D2 partial agonists:

Akathisia (common)	Vraylar > Abilify > Rexulti
Weight gain (minimal/ modest)	Rexulti > Abilify > **Vraylar**
Somnolence (minimal)	Abilify > Rexulti > Vraylar

Dynamic interactions:
- ❖ Antidopaminergic (balanced)
- ❖ EPS
- ❖ CNS depression (minimal)
- ❖ Hypotensive effects (mild)

Kinetic interactions:
- ❖ 3A4 substrate (major)
- ❖ The concentration of Vraylar is doubled by 3A4 inHibitors
- ❖ Avoid prescribing with 3A4 inDucers because Vraylar will be cleared too quickly

page 16

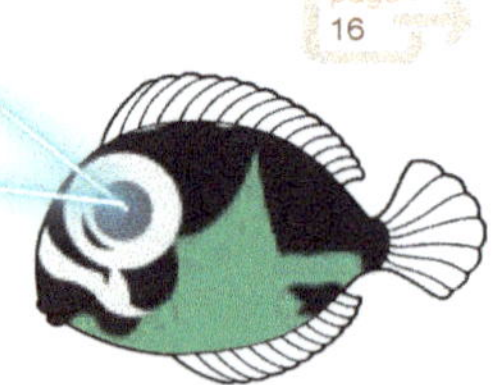

3A4 substrate (major)

2006
$224–$804

Paliperidone (INVEGA)

pal e PER i dohn / in VAY guh

"(Look what) Pale lips done In Vegas"

- ❖ Antipsychotic (SGA)
- ❖ D2 antagonist - ⇩ DA
- ❖ 5-HT_{2A} antagonist - ⇧ DA
- ❖ NE alpha-2 antagonist

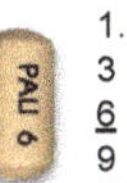

1.5
3
6
9
mg

FDA-approved for:
- ❖ Schizophrenia
- ❖ Schizoaffective disorder

Used off-label for:
- ❖ Bipolar disorder
- ❖ Aggression

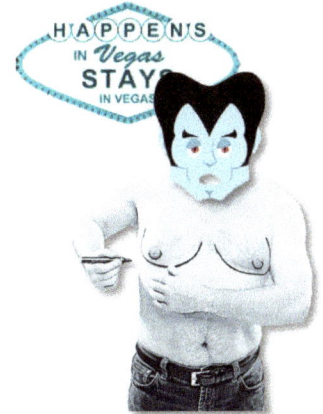

Antipsychotics are represented with spooky mascots.

Paliperidone (Invega) is the active metabolite of risperidone (Risperdal).

Paliperidone is cleared renally, so it is prefered over risperidone for those with hepatic insufficiency. Paliperidone has several other advantages to risperidone, including fewer interactions, slightly lower risk of EPS, and less sedation (although risperidone has relatively low sedation among antipsychotics). Paliperidone is one of the least sedating antipsychotics, allowing AM dosing. The only disadvantage of paliperidone is that, despite being available generically since 2015, it is > 10x more expensive than risperidone as of 2020. Refer to goodrx.com to see if this is still the case.

The tablet is extended-release, with a half-life of about 23 hours. The long-acting injectable (LAI) formulation (SUSTENNA) is given every 4 weeks. This is more convenient than the LAI version of risperidone (CONSTA), which is administered every 2 weeks. The monthly cost of Invega Sustenna and Risperdal Consta are equivalent, about $2,000 monthly.

Unfortunately paliperidone elevates prolactin to the same extent as risperidone. Either medication may cause gynecomastia, sexual dysfunction, and galactorrhea. With regard to prolactin elevation: risperidone = paliperidone >> all other second generation antipsychotics (SGAs).

Adult dosing: Start 6 mg PO q AM, which may be an effective target dose. If needed, may increase by 3 mg/day in intervals of ≥ 5 days. Max is 12 mg/day. See page 58 for dosing of long-acting injectable (LAI) formulations of paliperidone.

Equivalent dosing

PO risperidone	PO paliperidone
1 mg	3 mg
2 mg	
3 mg	6 mg 9 mg 12 mg
4 mg	
6 mg	

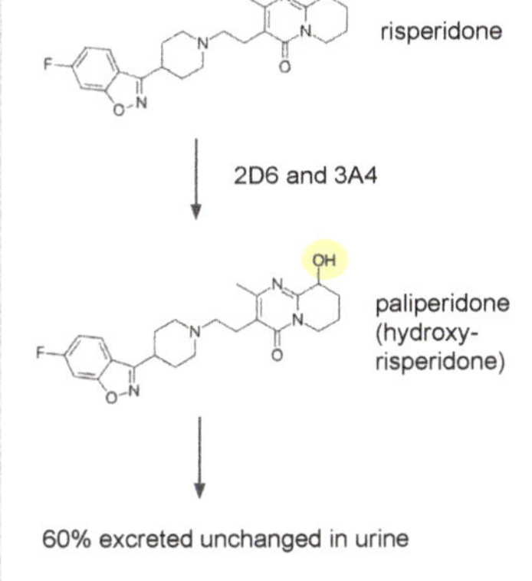

60% excreted unchanged in urine

Long-acting injectable (LAI) options with paliperidone palmitate:

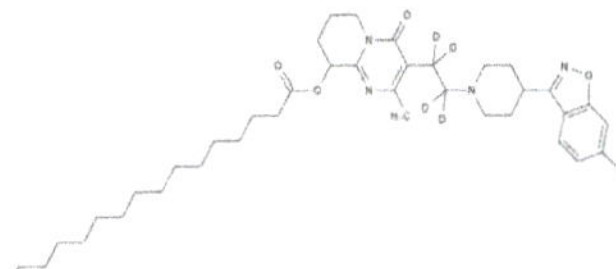

Invega SUSTENNA is q 4 weeks. No PO overlap is needed. This is a major advantage over the risperidone LAI (Risperdal Consta), which is q 2 weeks and requires a 3 week PO overlap.

Invega TRINZA, the q 3 month LAI, is available after 4 months of stability on Invega SUSTENNA.

Refer to page 58 for dosing.

Pill formulations (OROS and otherwise) with "ghost pill" shells passing in feces:

Antipsychotics
- ❖ Invega (paliperidone ER)

Antidepressants
- ❖ Wellbutrin XL (bupropion XL)
- ❖ Effexor XR (venlafaxine ER)
- ❖ Pristiq (desvenlafaxine ER)

Stimulants
- ❖ Concerta (methylphenidate ER)
- ❖ Ritalin SR (methylphenidate SR)
- ❖ Focalin XR (dexmethylphenidate ER)

Mood Stabilizer
- ❖ Tegretol XR (carbamazepine ER)

Opioids
- ❖ Oxycontin (oxycodone ER)
- ❖ Exalgo (hydromorphone ER)

Sources include: Tungaraza et al, 2003

The paliperidone tablet is an Osmotic controlled Release Oral delivery System (OROS). The drug is expelled through tiny holes in the coating, and empty "ghost capsules" are passed in feces.

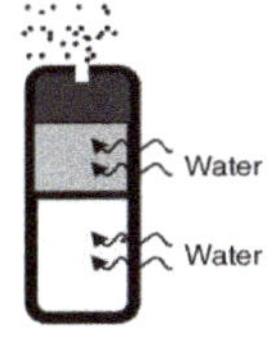

Dynamic interactions:
- ❖ Antidopaminergic (moderate)
- ❖ EPS (dose dependent)
- ❖ Sedation (mild)
- ❖ Hypotensive effects
- ❖ Prolactin elevation (strong)
- ❖ Hyperglycemia (moderate)
- ❖ Weight gain (moderate)
- ❖ QT prolongation (low risk)

Kinetic interactions:
- ❖ 60% of paliperidone is excreted unchanged in urine. CYP phase I metabolism accounts for less than 10% of paliperidone's clearance.

page 18

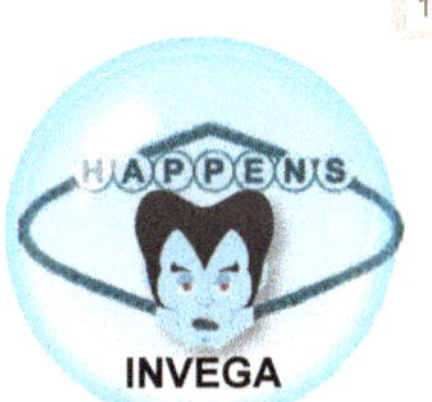

in a bubble - minimal clinically significant kinetic interactions

2009
$1,027–$1,116

Iloperidone (FANAPT)

eye loe PER i dohn / fan APT

"Fan Napped (with) Eye Opener"

- ❖ Antipsychotic (SGA)
- ❖ D2 antagonist - ⇩ DA
- ❖ 5-HT_{2A} antagonist - ⇧ DA

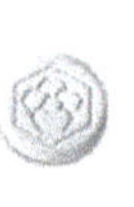

1
2
4
6
8
10
12 mg

FDA-approved for:
- ❖ Schizophrenia

Used off-label for:
- ❖ Bipolar disorder

"(Look what that) Eye Opener done (while that) Fan Napped."

Iloperidone (Fanapt), released in 2009, is marketed for patients taking antipsychotic medication who can't sit still, because it has low incidence of akathisia. Fanapt's only FDA-approved indication is schizophrenia.

The starting dose must be titrated to avoid orthostatic hypotension. Among antipsychotics, Fanapt has relatively high potential for weight gain, a distant #3 behind olanzapine and clozapine—*Fanapt gives you a fat fanny*.

Among available SGAs, Fanapt has a relatively high tendency to prolong QT interval, #2 behind ziprasidone (Geodon) among SGAs. Although the risk of clinically significant QT prolongation is minimal, advertisements for Fanapt caution "in choosing among treatments, prescribers should consider the ability of Fanapt to prolong the QT interval and the use of other drugs first".

Half-life is about 18 hours. It should be discontinued if absolute neutrophil count (ANC) drops below 1000 or if there is an unexplained drop in WBC.

As a point of trivia, iloperidone shares a mechanism of action with the rarely prescribed tricyclic antidepressant (TCA) trimipramine (Surmontil).

Iloperidone failed the approval process in Europe for treatment of schizophrenia, because risks of the drugs were deemed to outweigh potential benefits.

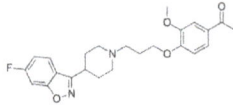

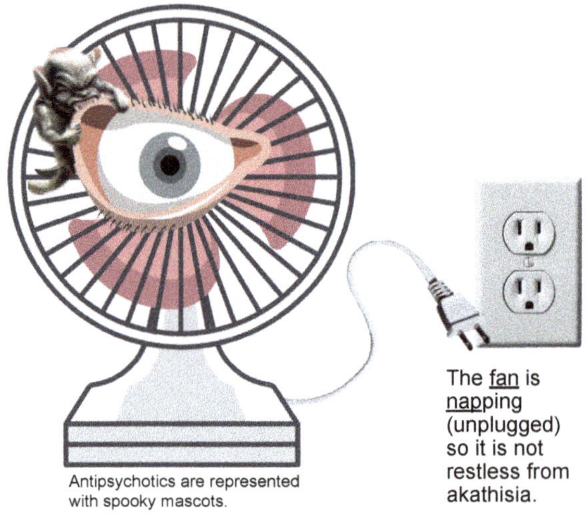

Antipsychotics are represented with spooky mascots.

The fan is napping (unplugged) so it is not restless from akathisia.

Dosing: See below for titration schedule. The titration pack contains #2 of 1 mg, #2 of 2 mg, #2 of 4 mg, and #2 of 6 mg tabs. The target dose for schizophrenia is 6–12 mg BID. Maximum 24 mg total daily dose. Adjust dose for kinetic interactions described below.

If started at 6 mg without titrating, the patient may pass out from hypotension.

Recommended titration:

Day one: 1 mg BID
Day two: 2 mg BID
Day three: 4 mg BID
Day four: 6 mg BID

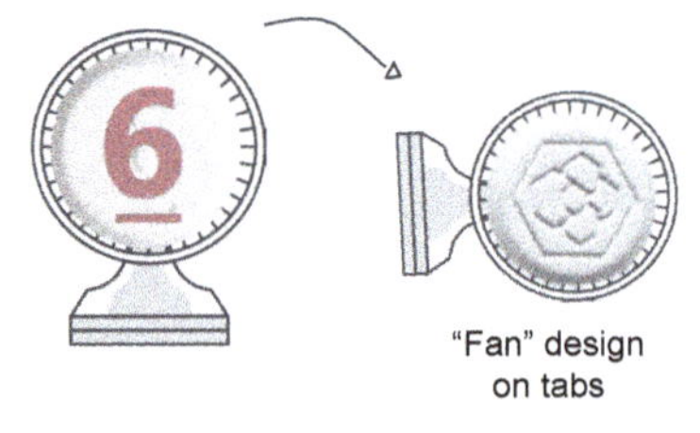

"Fan" design on tabs

Fanapt titration pack:

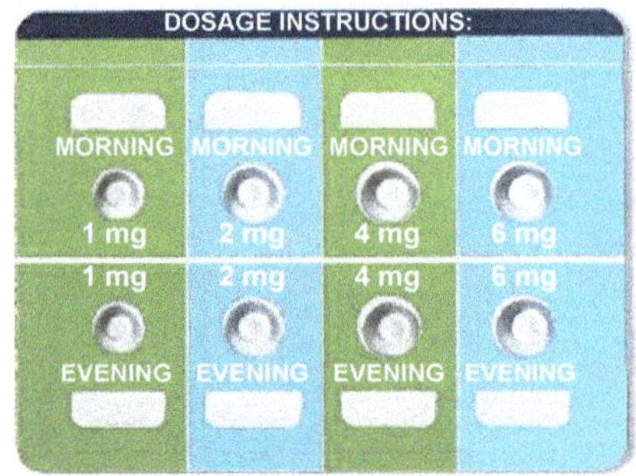

Dynamic interactions:
- ❖ Sedation
- ❖ Weight gain
- ❖ QT prolongation
- ❖ Dopamine antagonist
- ❖ Extrapyramidal effects
- ❖ Hypotensive effects
- ❖ Lowers seizure threshold

Kinetic interactions:
- ❖ 2D6 substrate
- ❖ 3A4 substrate

Levels of iloperidone are increased by 2D6 or 3A4 inHibitors, increasing the risk of QT prolongation. If a strong 2D6 or 3A4 inHibitor is in the pill box, use a ½ strength dose of iloperidone.

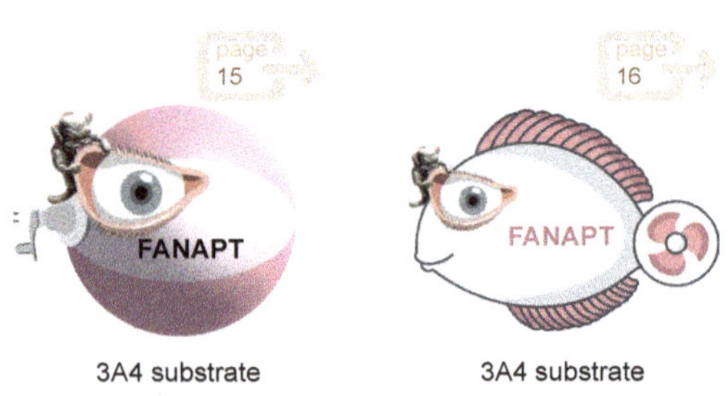

3A4 substrate

3A4 substrate

2009
$599–$728

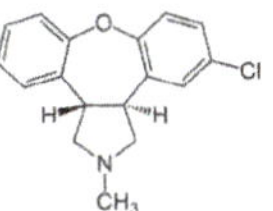

Asenapine (SAPHRIS)

a SEN a peen / SAFF ris

"Sapphire (for an) Ass in a pine"

- ❖ Antipsychotic (SGA)
- ❖ D2 antagonist - ⇩ DA
- ❖ 5-HT_{2A} antagonist - ⇧ DA
- ❖ Alpha-adrenergic antagonist

2.5
5
10
mg

FDA-approved for:
- ❖ Schizophrenia
- ❖ Bipolar disorder (ages 10+)
  - acute manic/mixed episode
  - maintenance

Used off-label for:
- ❖ Acute agitation

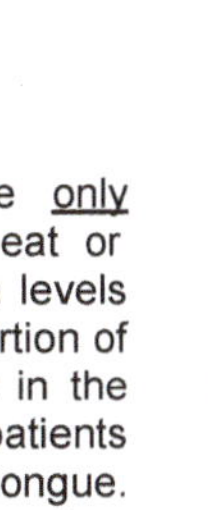

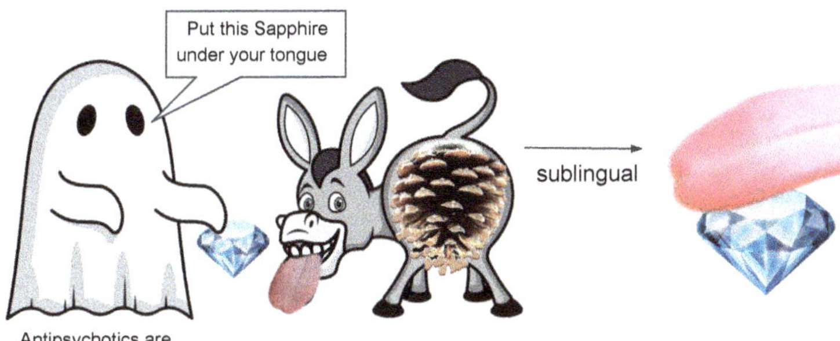

Antipsychotics are represented with spooky mascots.

Asenapine (Saphris), approved in 2009, is the only sublingual antipsychotic. The patient should not eat or drink for 10 minutes after taking it because serum levels will be decreased by about 15%. The swallowed portion of the medication is subject to first-pass metabolism in the liver before entering the general circulation. Some patients report lingering bad taste or numbing of the tongue. Patients complained about the original taste, so it now has a black cherry flavor. The patent for Saphris expires in 2021.

Asenapine can be used as a rapid-acting PRN for acute agitation. With sublingual administration it is absorbed directly into the bloodstream. Peak serum concentration is reached within 1 hour. The label recommends BID dosing, but half-life is 24 hours, so dosing it once daily at HS is a viable treatment option.

Asenapine is approved for schizophrenia and bipolar disorder. It is not a first-line choice for either condition due to cost, and rare idiopathic hypersensitivity reactions including anaphylaxis. Reactions may occur with the first dose.

Other side effects may include sedation, hypotension, and dose-related akathisia. Asenapine has little potential for causing weight gain. Oral ulcers are possible. Anticholinergic effects are minimal. It is contraindicated with severe hepatic insufficiency, because levels may increase 7-fold.

Dosing: The "minimal effective" daily dose for psychosis is 10 mg. The label recommends starting 5 mg BID, but to minimize sedation it is best given at night only (half-life is 24 hours). 10 mg HS is also a reasonable starting dose and target dose. Maximum dose is 20 mg/day. The 2.5 mg dose is for ages 10–17. Avoid rapid discontinuation. Taper over 2–4 weeks.

Saphris is a fluffy, white tablet that is too delicate for bottling, so it comes in a special case containing 10 tabs.

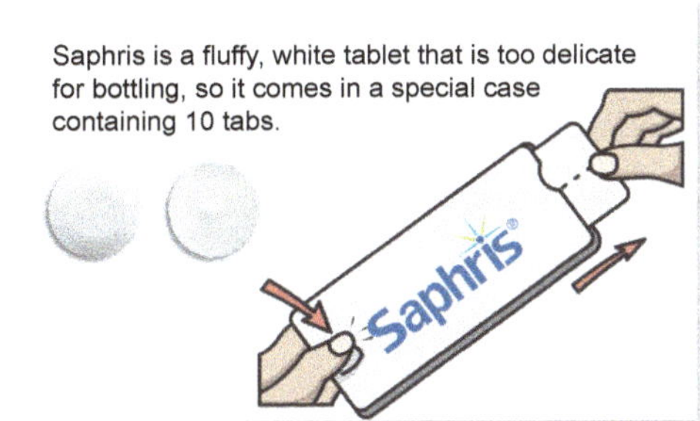

Dynamic interactions:
- ❖ Antidopaminergic (moderate)
- ❖ EPS (dose dependent)
- ❖ Sedation (mild)
- ❖ Hypotensive effects
- ❖ Prolactin elevation (strong)
- ❖ Hyperglycemia (moderate)
- ❖ Weight gain (moderate)
- ❖ QT prolongation (low/moderate)

Kinetic interactions:
- ❖ 1A2 substrate (major)
  - Smoking inDuces 1A2 and may lower levels of asenapine
  - 1A2 inHibitors increase levels of asenapine, and dose adjustment is recommended.

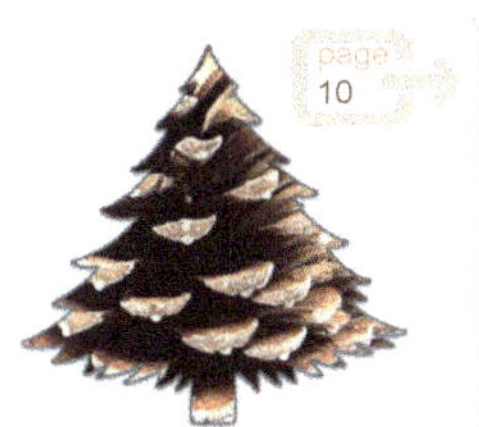

1A2 substrate (minor)

2019
$1,192

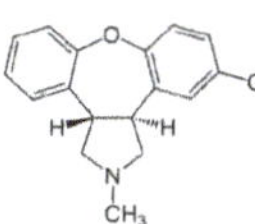

Asenapine transdermal (SECUADO)

a SEN a peen / seh kue AH doe

"See (the) caudal (end of an) Ass"

- ❖ Antipsychotic (SGA)
- ❖ D2 antagonist - ⇩DA
- ❖ 5-HT_{2A} antagonist - ⇧DA
- ❖ Alpha-adrenergic antagonist

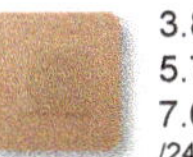

3.8
5.7
7.6
/24 hr

FDA-approved for:
- ❖ Schizophrenia

Secuado (asenapine) is a once daily "transdermal drug delivery system" approved in 2019 for schizophrenia. This is the only transdermal antipsychotic. The transdermal route bypasses "first-pass" metabolism through the liver that oral medications are subject to. Asenapine tablets are not subject to "first-pass" metabolism either, because they are administered sublingually.

Onset of effect is much more gradual than with sublingual asenapine. It takes 12–24 hours for serum levels to peak (versus 1 hour sublingually).

Side effects include skin irritation (15%) and those associated with sublingual asenapine. Avoid exposing the patch to external heat sources during wear because drug absorption will be increased.

There have been no head-to-head comparisons between sublingual Saphris and transdermal Secuado.

Dosing: Start with the 3.8 mg/24 hours patch; The dosage may be increased to 5.7 mg/24 hours or 7.6 mg/24 hours, if needed, after one week; In short-term trials, there were more side effects and no added benefit with the maximum dose of 7.6 mg/24 hours

Dose equivalents: 3.8 mg/24 hours patch = 5 mg BID of sublingual asenapine; 7.6 mg/24 hours = 10 mg twice daily.

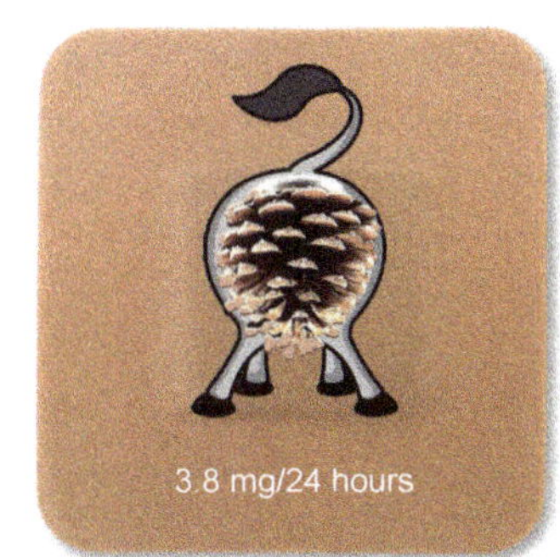

transdermal patch

2020
$1300

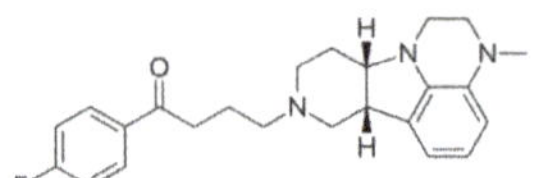

Lumateperone (CAPLYTA)

luma TEP er ohn / cap LIE ta

"'Luminated Cap lighter"

- ❖ Antipsychotic (SGA)
- ❖ D2 antagonist - ⇩ DA
- ❖ 5-HT_{2A} antagonist - ⇧ DA
- ❖ Glutamate modulator

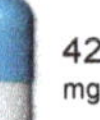

42 mg

FDA-approved for:
- ❖ Schizophrenia

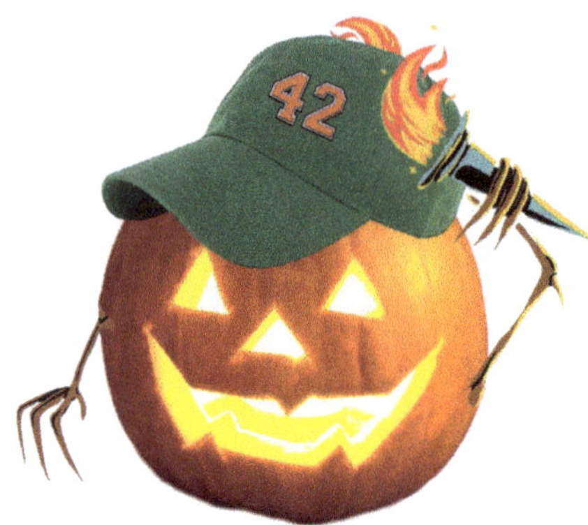

Antipsychotics are represented with spooky mascots.

42 On Jackie Robinson Day (April 15), all players in Major League Baseball wear Robinson's uniform number, 42. For lumateperone, 42 mg is the only recommended dose.

Lumateperone is typically administered at night, which is also the time of day to illuminate a Jack-o'-lantern.

To improve tolerability, "take lumateperone with a bag of candy" (food) to delay peak blood levels.

Lumateperone (Caplyta) is a new antipsychotic that purportedly modulates glutamate in addition to the usual SGA mechanism of blocking D2 and 5-HT_{2A} receptors. However, the official prescribing information does not mention glutamate, suggesting the FDA saw insufficient evidence for lumateperone being a first-in-class novel antipsychotic. It appears to be equally effective as risperidone (Risperdal) with fewer side effects other than sedation (Citrome, 2016). Caplyta's effectiveness head-to-head with other antipsychotics is to be determined.

Lumateperone's D2 receptor occupancy is lower than most other antipsychotics. This means extrapyramidal side effects are unlikely. The other antipsychotics with low D2 occupancy are quetiapine (Seroquel) and clozapine (Clozaril).

Lumateperone is also a weak D2 receptor partial agonist. The stronger D2 partial agonists are aripiprazole (Abilify), brexpiprazole (Rexulti), and cariprazine (Vraylar).

Lumateperone has a favorable side effect profile. In clinical trials no single adverse effect led to > 2% discontinuation. The main side effects are somnolence/sedation (24% vs 10% placebo) and dry mouth (6% vs 2% placebo). At one year, lumateperone caused a modest weight loss of 3.2 kg (7 pounds) but a modest elevation in A1c and lipids. It does not appear to cause hypotension, prolactin elevation, or QT prolongation.

Lumateperone is extensively metabolized, resulting in more than twenty metabolites. It is a highly susceptible 3A4 substrate, making it contraindicated in combination with the medications listed below.

Because lumateperone can be highly sedating, it is typically administered at night. Taking lumateperone with food improves tolerability by delaying peak blood levels. This is more relevant if dosed during the day. Unlike ziprasidone (Geodon) and lurasidone (Latuda), taking lumateperone with food is not required for GI absorption.

Dosing: 42 mg is the only recommended dose, typically given at bedtime; Titration is not necessary (nor possible); No dose adjustment is required for renal impairment; Avoid with moderate/severe hepatic insufficiency.

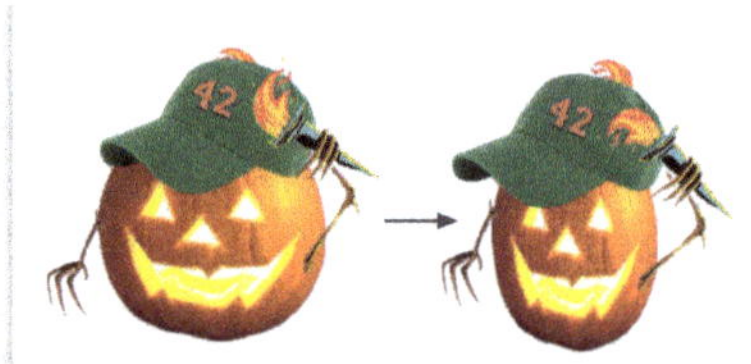

Lumateperone is associated with a loss of 3.2 kg (7 pounds) at one year.

Dynamic interactions:
- ❖ Antidopaminergic
- ❖ Extrapyramidal effects (mild)
- ❖ Sedation (high/moderate)
- ❖ Hypotensive effects (minimal)
- ❖ Prolactin elevation (minimal)

Kinetic Interactions:
- ❖ 3A4 substrate
- ❖ UGT substrate

The fish (our symbol for a 3A4 substrate) is big because with lumateperone 3A4 interactions are a very big deal.

Lumateperone is contraindicated with 3A4 inDucers due to rapid clearance. Levels will be decreased up to 20-fold, rendering lumateperone useless when given concomitantly with:

- ❖ Carbamazepine (Tegretol)
- ❖ Modafinil (Provigil)
- ❖ Phenytoin (Dilantin)
- ❖ Phenobarbital (Luminal)
- ❖ Oxcarbazepine (Trileptal)
- ❖ St. John's wort
- ❖ Rifampin (20-fold decrease)

Lumateperone should also be avoided with moderate-to-strong 3A4 inHibitors which can dramatically increase blood levels. Strong 3A4 inhibitors include:

- ❖ Fluconazole and other -azole antifungals
- ❖ Clarithromycin (antibacterial)
- ❖ Ritonavir (antiretroviral, HIV treatment)

Lumateperone is a UGT substrate, which should not be combined with valproic acid (Depakote, Depakene)—a UGT inHibitor that dramatically increases lumateperone blood levels.

page 16

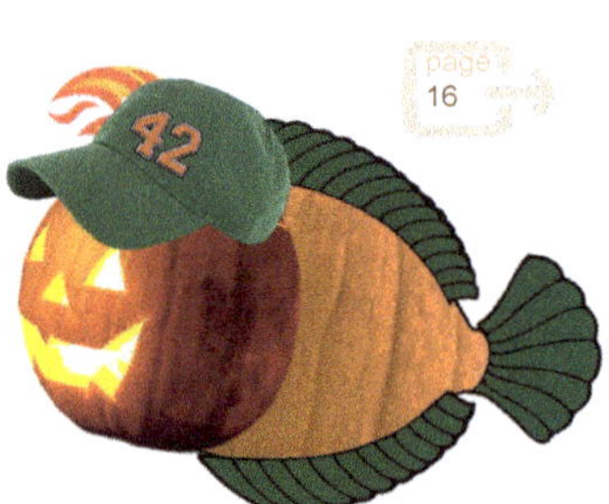

3A4 substrate (major)

page 17

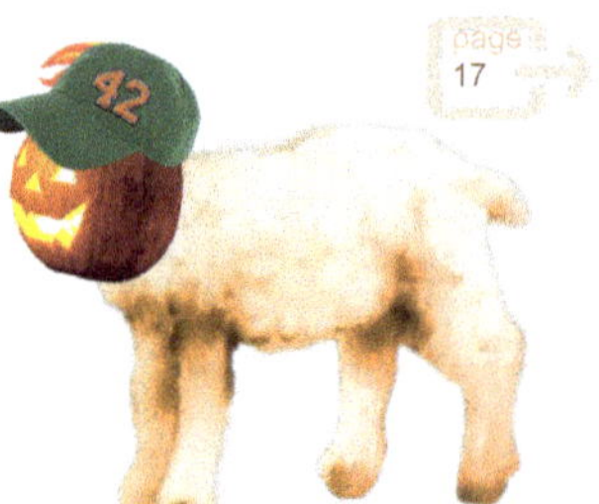

UGT1A4 substrate

2017
$2,741–$3,097

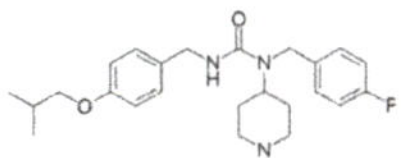

Pimavanserin (NUPLAZID)

PIM a VAN ser in / Nu PLAHZ id

"Pima van (New plaster)"

- ❖ Novel antipsychotic
- ❖ Nondopaminergic
- ❖ 5-HT_{2A} inverse agonist

10 tab
17 tab
34 cap
mg

FDA-approved for:

- ❖ Psychosis associated with Parkinson's disease

Pimavanserin (Nuplazid), released in 2017, is FDA-approved for hallucinations and delusions associated with Parkinson's disease. Up to 50% of patients with Parkinson's disease develop these problems. Some sources refer to pimavanserin as a second generation antipsychotic (SGA), but its antipsychotic mechanism is entirely different from other medications in this class.

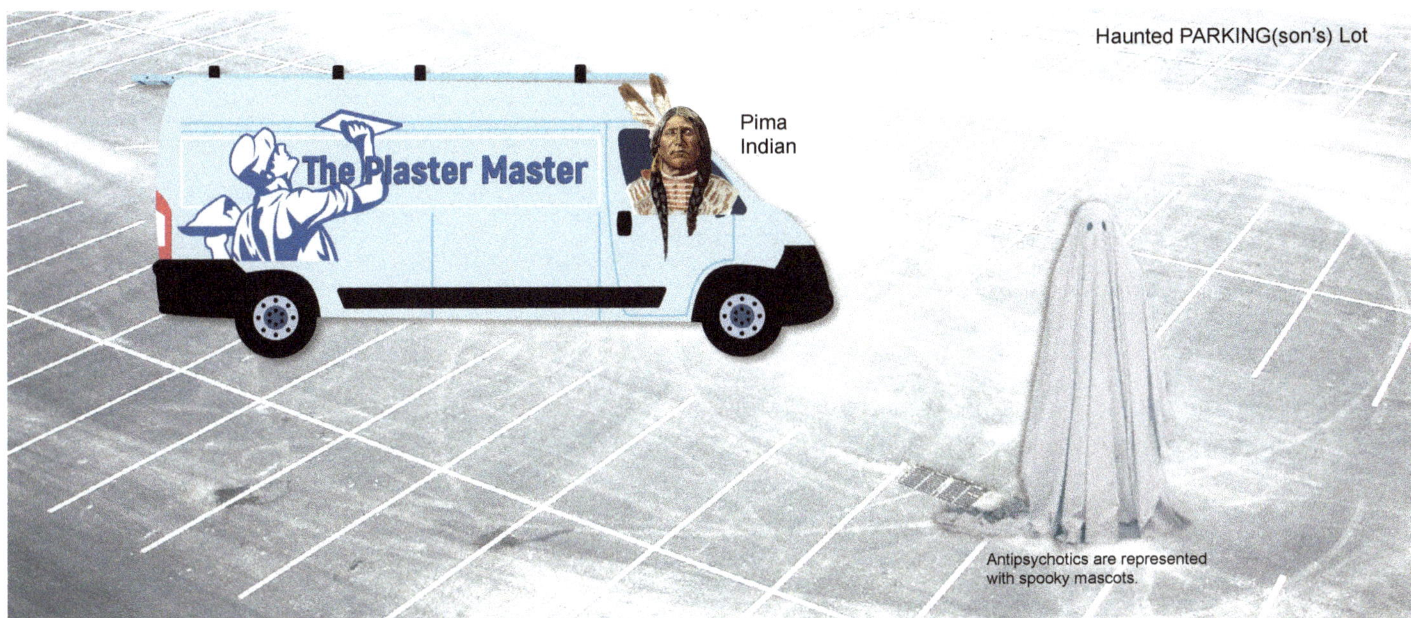
Haunted PARKING(son's) Lot
The Plaster Master
Pima
Indian
Antipsychotics are represented
with spooky mascots.

Pimavanserin is the only available antipsychotic that does not act on dopamine receptors (unless you count cannabidiol). This makes pimavanserin ideal for Parkinson's disease, which is aggravated by dopamine blockade. Pimavanserin has a relatively unique mechanism as a selective serotonin inverse agonist that preferentially targets 5-HT_{2A} receptors. By definition, an inverse agonist binds to a receptor and produces effects opposite to those of an agonist. The effect of the inverse agonist can be blocked by an antagonist. A few other medications in this book are inverse agonists (among other mechanisms) but we refer to them as antagonists for simplicity.

Prior to pimavanserin the antipsychotic of choice for individuals with Parkinson's disease was quetiapine (Seroquel), which causes little to no extrapyramidal symptoms (EPS). Clozapine (Clozaril), which does not cause EPS, would be a good choice for this population if not for its numerous health risks and lab monitoring requirements.

Side effects of pimavanserin include peripheral edema (7%) and nausea (7%). It can cause angioedema, i.e., localized non-pitting edema of deep dermis and subcutaneous tissue. Pimavanserin may modestly prolong QT interval, but otherwise does not have side effects associated with other antipsychotics such as sedation, weight gain, constipation, gynecomastia or neutropenia.

All antipsychotics, pimavanserin included, carry a **black box warning** of increased mortality in elderly patients with dementia-related psychosis. For pimavanserin, the warning reads "not approved for dementia-related psychosis unrelated to the hallucinations and delusions associated with Parkinson's disease psychosis". Over the course of a 10-week controlled trial for the intended population, the rate of death was 4.5%, compared to a 2.6% in placebo-treated patients. Most of the deaths appeared to be either cardiovascular (e.g., heart failure, sudden death) or infectious (e.g., pneumonia). Exercise caution

in patients with uncorrected electrolyte abnormalities or any type of heart condition (recent heart attack, congestive heart failure, arrhythmia, bradycardia, etc.)

Nasrallah et al (2019) demonstrated successful treatment of clozapine-resistant psychosis with pimavanserin in individuals without Parkinson's disease. It appears to improve negative symptoms of schizophrenia (diminished emotional expression and avolition). Pimavanserin has potential for treatment-resistant depression as an adjunct to an SSRI or SNRI (Fava et al, 2019).

Oddly, the 10 mg and 17 mg pills are tablets while the 34 mg pill is a capsule.

Dosing: Start at 34 mg once daily, which is the target dose. Titration is unnecessary. In the presence of a strong 3A4 inhibitor, use a half strength dose of pimavanserin. With a strong 3A4 inducer, monitor for efficacy and exceed 34 mg if necessary.

Dynamic interactions:

- ❖ QT prolongation (low risk)

Kinetic interactions:

- ❖ 3A4 substrate (major)
  - dose adjustments apply (see above)

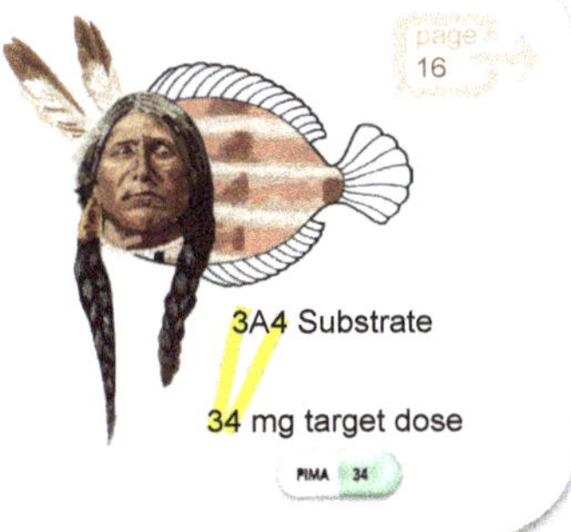

Long-Acting Injectable (LAI) antipsychotics

Although patients with schizophrenia are more likely to adhere to taking antipsychotics than placebo, compliance in the community is still less than 50%. To address this problem, several antipsychotics are available as long-acting injectables (LAIs). There are no LAI mood stabilizers, antidepressants, or stimulants. The older antipsychotics (haloperidol and fluphenazine) are "decanoate" formulations, which means the drug is in a sesame oil suspension. Decanoate injections are painful (*decan-OWW!-ate)* and can leave a tender bump under the skin that may take weeks to resolve. For decanoate shots, the Z-track injection technique is used. Confirm that the nurse will be injecting into the correct muscle (deltoid vs gluteal). With deltoid injections (smaller muscle), medication will be distributed more quickly and have a shorter half-life than with gluteal injections (larger muscle). The patient must first take the oral medication prior to receiving the LAI to establish tolerability, typically for at least 2 days. Tolerability to PO risperidone is sufficient to start LAI paliperidone, which is the active metabolite of risperidone. It is not advisable to give any LAI to someone with a history of neuroleptic malignant syndrome (NMS). Rather than being aggressive with the LAI dose, it may be a good strategy to go light on the LAI and supplement with a low PO dose that can be easily adjusted based on response and side effects. It is OK to give injections more frequently than the listed intervals if serum drug levels are monitored. Serum drug levels are worth following with LAIs in any event. Refer to official prescribing information for guidance on missed/late/early doses.

Medication	Strength	Given	PO overlap	Pain	Max	Info
HALDOL DECANOATE (haloperidol)	Usually 100 mg or 200 mg but can customize dose from vial	q 4 wk (q 3–4 wk) IM	1–3 wk	Yes	450 mg monthly (too high)	Traditionally given with 1–3 wk PO overlap, with a maximum of 100 mg for the first injection. If > 100 mg is needed, give the balance in 3–7 days if no EPS. According to Ereshefsky (1993) it can be given without a PO overlap if the loading dose of the LAI equals 20x the total daily PO dose. Subsequent monthly injections are typically 10–15 x the oral daily dose. 200 q 4 wk is equivalent to 14–20 PO QD, which is anticipated to produce a serum haloperidol level of 5–12 ng/mL. The FDA max of 450 mg/mo (equivalent to 30–45 mg PO daily) carries significant risk of tardive dyskinesia, so try not to exceed 200 mg of the LAI monthly (unless serum levels are lower than anticipated). Consider 25% dose decrease about every 3 months because it tends to accumulate. Gluteal is preferable, but deltoid is acceptable.
PROLIXIN DECANOATE (fluphenazine)	12.5 mg 25 mg 50 mg 100 mg	q 3–6 wk IM or SC	0–7 days	Yes	100 mg q 3 wk (too high)	Start 12.5 mg q 3 wk (roughly equivalent to 10 mg PO daily) or 25 mg q 3 wk. Onset of effect is within 24–72 hours. A realistic max dose is 50 mg q 3 wk or 100 mg q 6 wk, either of which is roughly equivalent to 40 mg PO daily. Since fluphenazine is a high potency typical antipsychotic (like haloperidol), there is significant risk of tardive dyskinesia. Gluteal is preferred, but deltoid is acceptable.
RISPERDAL CONSTA (risperidone)	12.5 mg 25 mg 37.5 mg 50 mg	q 2 wk IM	3 wk	No	50 mg q 2 wk	Rarely used because Risperdal Consta must be given every 2 weeks—*you're getting shots Constantly.* Also a 3-week PO overlap is required which is the time needed for microspheres to hydrolyze—so you are still taking pills past the 2nd injection. Must be refrigerated. Usual starting and maintenance dose is 25 mg q 2 wk. FDA max is 50 mg q 2 wk. May be given in gluteal or deltoid.
PERSERIS (risperidone)	90 mg 120 mg	q 4 wk SC	None needed	No	120 mg q 4 wk	Approved in 2018. Given subcutaneously (SC) in the abdomen. No loading dose or supplemental PO risperidone is recommended (after PO tolerability established). To be administered by a healthcare professional.
INVEGA SUSTENNA (paliperidone palmitate)	39 mg 78 mg 117 mg 156 mg 234 mg	q 4 wk IM	None needed	No	234 mg monthly	Onset within a few hours, no PO overlap required. Prefilled syringes, which do not need to be reconstituted or refrigerated. Standard dose is 234 mg once, then 156 mg on day 8 (with window of day 4 – day 12), then 117 mg monthly thereafter (equivalent to about 6 mg PO QD). Although not ideal, you can give the first dose (234 mg) on Monday and the second (156 mg) on Thursday to expedite a hospitalization. The q 4 wk injections can be +/- 7 days. PO risperidone is sufficient for establishing tolerability. First 2 injections in deltoid for faster distribution, with subsequent injections deltoid or gluteal.
INVEGA TRINZA (paliperidone palmitate)	273 mg 410 mg 546 mg 819 mg	q 3 mo IM	N/A—transition from Sustenna	No	819 mg q 3 mo	To use Trinza, the patient must first have received 4 monthly Sustenna injections, and the last two Sustenna doses must be the same strength. See dose conversion table below. The q 3 mo injections can +/- 14 days because medication release continues for up to 4.5 months. May be given gluteal or deltoid.
ABILIFY MAINTENA (aripiprazole)	300 mg 400 mg	q 4 wk IM	2 wk	No	400 mg monthly	The label recommends starting a maintenance dose of 400 mg/mo unless this patient is a 2D6 poor metabolizer (10% of population), then start 300 mg. It is recommended to back down to 300 mg if side effects occur. It is possible to give only 200 mg from the vial. Minimal pain with injection, certainly less painful than Aristada. Deltoid or gluteal.
ARISTADA (aripiprazole lauroxil)	441 mg 662 mg 882 mg 1064 mg	q 4–8 wk* IM	3 wk (unless started with Initio)	Yes	882 mg monthly	Prefilled syringes requiring no reconstitution. Must shake forcefully and inject immediately and rapidly so microcrystals do not clog the needle. *Given q 4 wk, other than the 882 mg strength which is q 4–6 wk, or the 1064 mg which is q 8 wk (equivalent to 882 mg q 6 wk). If changing from Maintena to Aristada, give the first Aristada injection 2 to 3 wk after the last Maintena injection. When transitioning from PO aripiprazole to Aristada, the 3 wk PO overlap can be replaced with a single 30 mg PO dose plus an Aristada Initio injection. The 441 mg strength may be given deltoid or gluteal. Higher strengths should be gluteal.
ARISTADA INITIO (aripiprazole)	675 mg	once	Single 30 mg PO dose	Yes	675 mg once	Aristada Initio is a one-time injection in the deltoid. It lets you start the q 4–8 wk Arista injections (see above) without a 3 wk PO overlap. On the same day, give aripiprazole 30 mg PO x 1, Initio injection x 1, and the first Aristada injection (or within 10 days). Tolerability to aripiprazole must first be established—in clinical trials this was done with aripiprazole 5 mg PO x 2 days, then on day three, 30 mg PO + Initio 675 mg in deltoid (preferably for quicker absorption) + Aristada 1064 mg in gluteal (to repeat Aristada 1064 mg q 2 mo). Initio must be given in deltoid.
ZYPREXA RELPREVV (olanzapine)	150 mg 210 mg 300 mg	q 2–4 wk IM	None needed	No	300 mg q 2 wk	Rarely prescribed due to black box warning of post-Injection delirium/sedation syndrome (PDSS) of olanzapine overdose which can lead to coma, likely due to intravascular injection. Restricted distribution program. Patients must be observed for at least 3 hours post-injection in a registered facility. Risk of PDSS is about 0.07% (about 1 in 1400 injections), with patients recovering within 72 hours. Deep intramuscular gluteal injection only. See package insert.

Dose conversions for risperidone/paliperidone products

PO risperidone	PO paliperidone	Risperdal Consta	Perseris	Invega Sustenna	Invega Trinza
1 mg	3 mg	12.5 mg q 2 wk	–	39 mg q 4 wk	–
2 mg		25 mg q 2 wk	–	78 mg q 4 wk	273 mg q 3 mo
3 mg	6 mg 9 mg 12 mg	37.5 mg q 2 wk	90 mg q 4 wk	117 mg q 4 wk	410 mg q 3 mo
4 mg		50 mg q 2 wk	120 mg q 4 wk	156 mg q 4 wk	546 mg q 3 mo
6 mg		–	–	234 mg q 4 wk	819 mg q 3 mo

Aripiprazole dose conversions

PO aripiprazole	Abilify Maintena	Aristada q 4 wk	Aristada q 6 wk	Aristada q 2 mo
10 mg	300 mg q 4 wk	441 mg q 4 wk	–	–
15 mg	400 mg q 4 wk	662 mg q 4 wk	882 mg q 6 wk	1064 mg q 2 mo
20 mg	–	882 mg q 4 wk**	–	–

**Note that Aristada 882 mg has been shown to be no more effective than lower doses (for q 4 week dosing).

Muscarinic (cholinergic) effects – everything wet

Before we discuss anticholinergic toxicity, let's discuss the opposite, for the sake of context. SLUDGE syndrome is a mnemonic for the result of overload of muscarinic acetylcholine receptors, as caused by poisoning with pesticide or nerve gas.

Signs of cholinergic overload:

S – Salivation
L – Lacrimation (also lactation)
U – Urination
D – Diaphoresis (also diarrhea)
G – Gastrointestinal upset (including diarrhea)
E – Emesis

Miosis (constricted pupils) and bradycardia would also be expected.

The treatment for SLUDGE poisoning is atropine, which is the strongest anticholinergic (antimuscarinic).

Anticholinergic toxicity, described below, is the opposite of SLUDGE. With cholinergic overload, everything is wet, filling the SLUDGE buckets. With anticholinergic toxicity, everything is "dry as a bone".

There could also be a bucket labeled Breast Milk, because cholinergic drugs can stimulate lactation for breastfeeding women.

Brady(cardia) Bunch SLUDGE buckets filled with fluids produced in excess with cholinergic toxicity

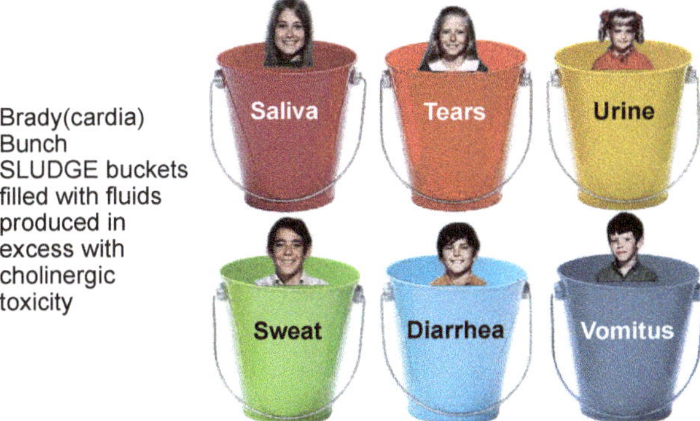

Cholinergic Alzheimer's medications such as donepezil (Aricept) can cause SLUDGE effects including nausea, vomiting, diarrhea, hypersalivation, miosis and bradycardia.

Sudden withdrawal of a high-dose anticholinergic medication such as benztropine (Cogentin) can cause SLUDGE symptoms by cholinergic rebound.

Anticholinergic (antimuscarinic) effects – everything dry

When we refer to "anticholinergic", we actually mean antimuscarinic. We're talking about blocking the action of the neurotransmitter acetylcholine at muscarinic receptors, not at nicotinic receptors. Anticholinergic side effects are especially problematic for older adults. Ongoing use of strong anticholinergic medication can increase risk of dementia by 50%.

Tacky (tachycardia) Auntie Choli is...

"Dry as a bone"
- Constipation (risk of ileus, bowel rupture)
- Urinary retention
- Decreased sweating; flushing—"Red as a beet"
- Dry mouth (risk of sublingual adenitis)
- Dry nasal mucus membranes
- Dry eyes
- Inhibition of lactation

"Mad as a hatter"
- Confusion, memory problems
- 50% increased risk of developing dementia
- Delirium with visual hallucinations

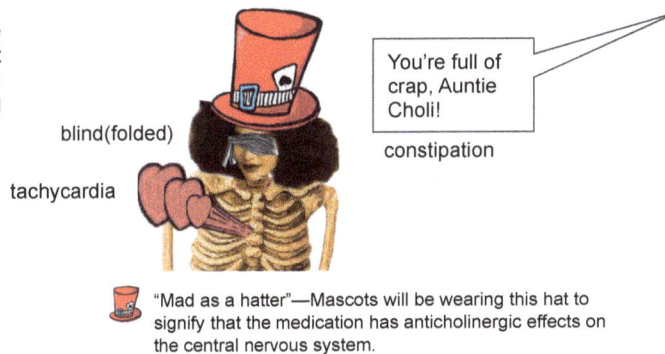

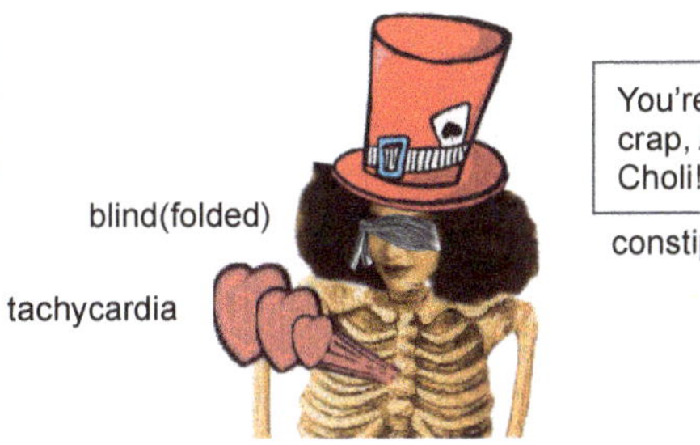

 "Mad as a hatter"—Mascots will be wearing this hat to signify that the medication has anticholinergic effects on the central nervous system.

"Blind as a bat"
- Cycloplegia (loss of accommodation)—lens cannot focus on near objects
- Photophobia due to mydriasis (dilated pupils)
- Increased intraocular pressure; contraindicated in angle-closure glaucoma (unless already treated by laser iridotomy)

Anticholinergic Drugs

Anticholinergic (antimuscarinic) agents block muscarinic acetylcholine receptors. Atropine is the strongest anticholinergic. They are used to treat:
- **Parkinsonism, EPS** - benztropine (Cogentin), trihexyphenidyl (Artane), diphenhydramine (Benadryl) are given for dystonic reactions
- **Overactive bladder (OAB)** - oxybutynin (Ditropan), tolterodine (Detrol), etc decrease premature detrusor contractions
- **Irritable bowel syndrome (IBS)** - dicyclomine (Bentyl) and hyoscyamine (Levsin) slow GI transit time
- **To decrease secretions and spasms** of rhinorrhea, hypersalivation, hyperhidrosis, diarrhea, peptic ulcers, biliary colic, and renal colic
- **Vertigo and motion sickness** - meclizine (Antivert), scopolamine (Transderm Scōp)
- **Asthma and COPD** - inhaled ipratropium (Atrovent) works as a bronchodilator
- **Bradycardia** - injections of atropine increase heart rate; In cardiac arrest, atropine is given to reverse asystole and severe bradycardia.
- **Cycloplegia** - Atropine eye drops are used to paralyze the accommodation reflex and produce mydriasis (pupil dilation) for procedures
- **Nerve agent poisoning** - Atropine is used to counteract poisoning by pesticides and other agents that block the action of acetylcholinesterase

Anticholinergics should not be routinely coadministered with high potency antipsychotics. Although some psychiatrists automatically add benztropine to haloperidol, this is not recommended, at least for long-term use. Anticholinergics do not prevent, but rather increase risk of tardive dyskinesia. Also, anticholinergics exacerbate the underlying cognitive impairment in patients with schizophrenia.

Anticholinergic Cognitive Effects

The elderly are especially susceptible to cognitive side effects of anticholinergic (antimuscarinic) medications. These "mad as a hatter" cognitive impairments may include:

- Memory problems
- Increased risk of developing dementia
- Delirium

Delirium is an acute confusional state that develops over a short period of time, typically hours to days. It tends to fluctuate from hour to hour. Classically, delirium is worse in the evening, a phenomenon colloquially referred to as "sundowning". Delirium involves impaired attention and disorientation. Visual hallucinations are common in the delirious state (as opposed to psychosis, which is more likely to manifest as auditory hallucinations). Medications that can contribute to delirium in elderly patients are listed below as 2 to 3 points on the anticholinergic burden scale. Most episodes of delirium are multifactorial, brought about by a combination of medications (anticholinergics, opioids, benzodiazepines, corticosteroids) and medical conditions. Delirium is very common among medically hospitalized elderly patients.

Treatment of acute delirium includes a short-term course of an antipsychotic, one with minimal anticholinergic properties. Antipsychotics scoring 0 or 1 points on the anticholinergic burden scale are suitable. For acute agitation associated with delirium, IM ziprasidone (Geodon) is a good choice. Benzodiazepine use should be minimized, unless the delirium is caused by withdrawal from benzodiazepines or alcohol (delirium tremens).

The anticholinergics that impair cognition:

- Block the M1 muscarinic receptor subtype
- Get past the blood brain barrier (BBB) by
  - being a small molecule
  - being lipid soluble (i.e., lipophilic, not hydrophilic)
  - having a neutral charge
  - not being a P-gp substrate

P-glycoprotein (P-gp) is an efflux transporter that pumps substances out of the CNS, back into systemic circulation. P-gp works as a component of the BBB, preventing the accumulation of certain drugs (P-gp substrates) in the brain.

P-gp

Pumpers gonna pump

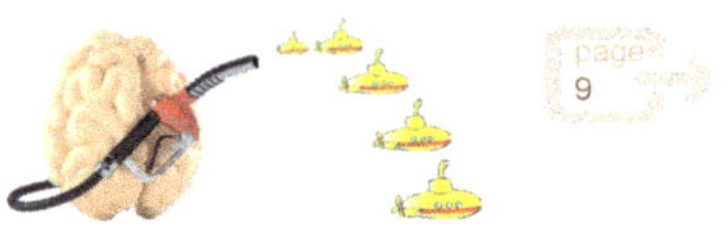

page 9

Anticholinergic Burden Scale (Risk of CNS impairment/dementia) – "mad as a hatter"

Anticholinergic load should be minimized with older adults. Dose should be taken into consideration when estimating risk.

	3 Points (worst)	2 points	1 point (mild)	0 points
TCA Antidepressants	Amitriptyline, Clomipramine, Doxepin ≥ 50 mg, Imipramine, Maprotiline, Protriptyline, Trimipramine	Desipramine (Norpramin) Doxepin ≤ 25 mg (Sinequan) Nortriptyline (Pamelor)	Amoxapine (Asendin) Doxepin ≤ 10 mg (Sinequan)	Doxepin ≤ 6 mg (Silenor)
Other Antidepressants	N/A	Paroxetine (Paxil) - *"Paxil packs it in"* (constipation as a peripheral anticholinergic effect)	Citalopram (Celexa) Fluoxetine (Prozac) MAOIs Mirtazapine (Remeron) Sertraline (Zoloft)	SNRIs, Other SSRIs, Bupropion (Wellbutrin), Trazodone, Nefazodone, Vilazodone (Viibryd), Vortioxetine (Trintellix)
Antipsychotics (and other D2 blockers)	Low potency FGAs: Chlorpromazine (Thorazine) Promethazine (Phenergan) Thioridazine (Mellaril)	Intermediate potency FGAs: Loxapine (Loxitane) Molindone (Moban) Perphenazine (Trilafon) SGAs: Clozapine (Clozaril) Olanzapine (Zyprexa)	High potency FGAs: Fluphenazine (Prolixin) Haloperidol (Haldol) Pimozide (Orap) Prochlorperazine (Compazine) Thiothixene (Navane) Trifluoperazine (Stelazine) SGAs: Pimavanserin (Nuplazid) Quetiapine (Seroquel)	SGAs: Aripiprazole (Abilify) Asenapine (Saphris) Brexpiprazole (Rexulti) Cariprazine (Vraylar) Iloperidone (Fanapt) Lurasidone (Latuda) Paliperidone (Invega) Risperidone (Risperdal) Ziprasidone (Geodon)
Antihistamines	Cyproheptadine (Periactin) Diphenhydramine (Benadryl) Doxylamine (Unisom) Meclizine (Antivert) Hydroxyzine (Vistaril)	Chlorpheniramine (Chlor-Trimeton),	Cetirizine (Zyrtec) Cimetidine (Tagamet) Fexofenadine (Allegra) Loratadine (Claritin) Ranitidine (Zantac)	Levocetirizine (Xyzal)
Anticholinergics for OAB	Oxybutynin (Ditropan)	Tolterodine (Detrol)	Fesoterodine (Toviaz) Solifenacin (Vesicare)	Darifenacin (Enablex) Trospium (Sanctura)
Other Anticholinergics	Atropine (injected) Benztropine (Cogentin) Dicyclomine (Bentyl) Hyoscyamine (Levsin) Scopolamine (Transderm Scōp) Trihexyphenidyl (Artane)	Amantadine (Symmetrel) Atropine eye drops	Ipratropium inhaler (Atrovent) Note that ipratropium is like an inhaled form of atropine (the strongest anticholinergic)	Glycopyrrolate (Robinul)* *Strong anticholinergic but does not cross blood-brain barrier; Therefore it causes constipation but not cognitive problems.
Muscle relaxants	Carisoprodol (Soma) Orphenadrine (Norflex)	Cyclobenzaprine (Flexeril) Baclofen (Lioresal)	Methocarbamol (Robaxin)	Metaxalone (Skelaxin) Tizanidine (Zanaflex)
Sedatives	See antihistamines	See antihistamines	Diazepam (Valium) Temazepam (Restoril)	**Other benzodiazepines Z-drugs; barbiturates; melatonin
Mood stabilizers; Antiepileptics	N/A	Carbamazepine (Tegretol)	Lithium Oxcarbazepine (Trileptal)	All other anticonvulsants
Other	N/A	Cimetidine (Tagamet) Codeine Metoclopramide (Reglan) Pseudoephedrine (Sudafed)	Buspirone (Buspar) Pramipexole (Mirapex)	All antihypertensives, cognitive enhancers and ADHD stimulants; atomoxetine, ondansetron, tramadol, ropinirole

Compiled from many sources. There are at least 10 published anticholinergic risk/burden scales (including Beers criteria) which differ substantially in the estimation of anticholinergic load for certain medications.

**These sedatives may impair cognition, but not by anticholinergic effect.

1st generation H_1 antihistamines

All are sedating and highly anticholinergic.

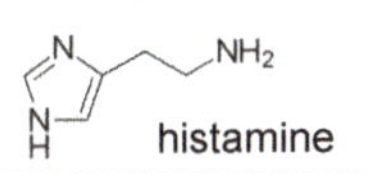

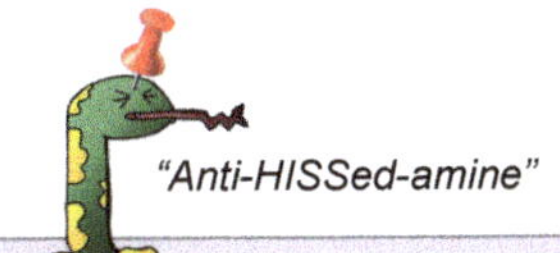

Antihistamine	~ monthly cost	Uses (*off-label)	Anti-cholinergic	Anti-serotonin	Comments
Diphenhydramine (BENADRYL)	$5	Allergy symptoms Urticaria/Pruritus Allergic reactions (IM) Extrapyramidal symptoms (EPS) Insomnia (short-term) Sedation Motion sickness prevention	+++	no	PO Benadryl is available over the counter (OTC). IV or IM diphenhydramine is highly effective for the treatment of an acute dystonic reaction. In treatment of EPS, it is more effective for dystonia than for akathisia.
Doxylamine (UNISOM)	$10	Insomnia Allergy symptoms	+++	no	Available OTC. Nearly identical to Benadryl.
Hydroxyzine (VISTARIL, ATARAX)	$15	Anxiety Urticaria/Pruritus Sedation Nausea Insomnia	+++	no	Generally less sedating than Benadryl. Commonly used PRN as an anxiolytic. Those accustomed to benzodiazepines often report hydroxyzine is useless for anxiety. Hydroxyzine is metabolized to the 2nd generation antihistamine cetirizine (Zyrtec).
Cyproheptadine (PERIACTIN)	$20	Allergic rhinitis Urticaria *Appetite stimulation *Serotonin syndrome *Nightmares *Akathisia *Female anorgasmia (PRN) *SSRI-induced night sweats	+++	yes	May lead to large weight gain; Prescribed off-label to stimulate appetite. Due to anti-serotonergic properties, cyproheptadine can make antidepressants ineffective.
Meclizine (ANTIVERT, "DRAMAMINE LESS DROWSY")	$10	Motion sickness Vertigo *Nausea	+++	no	Similar to hydroxyzine with a shorter half-life. Less sedating than the 1st generation antihistamine. Available Rx and OTC.
Dimenhydrinate (DRAMAMINE original)	$10	Motion sickness Nausea	+++	no	Available OTC, more sedating than meclizine
Orphenadrine (NORFLEX)	$20	Musculoskeletal pain	+++	no	Structure similar to diphenhydramine
Promethazine (PHENERGAN)	$10	Nausea/vomiting Motion sickness Allergic conditions Urticaria Sedation	+++	no	Used mostly as an antiemetic. It has a phenothiazine structure like several first generation antipsychotics and is a weak D2 blocker. Monograph on page 40.

Diphenhydramine (BENADRYL)

#210
1946
$2 - $8

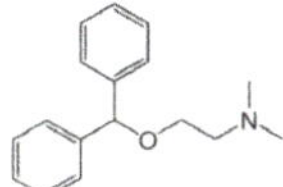

DYE fen HYE dra meen / BEN uh dril

"Dippin' hydra's Bean drill"

- 1st Generation antihistamine
- Anticholinergic
- Over-the-counter

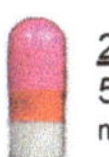

25
50
mg

FDA-approved for:

- Allergy symptoms
- Urticaria/pruritus
- Allergic reactions (IM, IV)
- Extrapyramidal symptoms (EPS)
- Insomnia (short-term)
- Sedation
- Motion sickness prevention

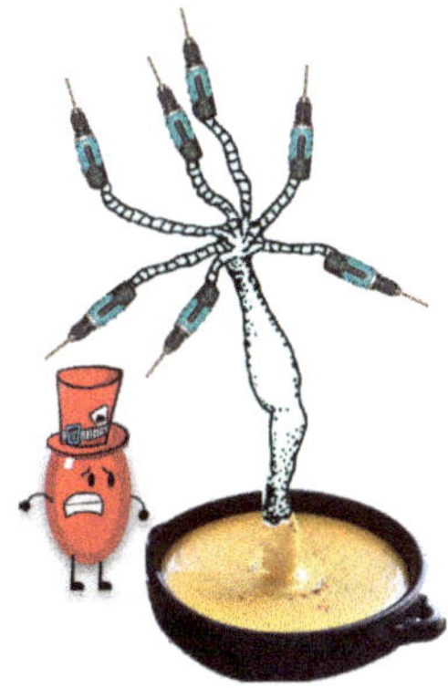

Anticholinergic with CNS effects—"mad as a hatter"

Benadryl is an effective OTC sleep aid with a duration of action of about 4–6 hours. It is a strong antihistamine and strong anticholinergic. Compared to other sleep medications, it may cause a bit more grogginess or "hangover" in the morning due to its half-life of 9 hours. Since long-term use of anticholinergics may lead to dementia, Benadryl is not recommended for long-term daily use. For insomnia, trazodone is a better choice.

Diphenhydramine is considered safe for children and during pregnancy and breastfeeding.

Intravenous or intramuscular diphenhydramine is classically used to treat severe allergic reactions as an antihistamine. IV or IM diphenhydramine is also a fast-acting and effective treatment for an acute dystonic reaction, due to anticholinergic effect. Another option for acute dystonia is benztropine (Cogentin).

Dosing: For most indications, a single dose is 25–50 mg, with a maximum of 100 mg/dose and 300 mg/day. For insomnia, take 30 minutes before bedtime PRN. For acute dystonia, use 25–50 mg IM or IV.

In the treatment of EPS, diphenhydramine is more effective for dystonia than for akathisia.

IM Benadryl is also useful for acute agitation. For extreme agitation with aggression (in a patient with high tolerance to sedatives) a "B-52" may be administered. This is slang for Benadryl 50 mg, haloperidol (Haldol) 5 mg, plus lorazepam (Ativan) 2 mg IM. The B-52 is two injections, the Haldol plus Ativan mixed in one syringe, and the Benadryl alone in the other.

If an antihistamine sleep medication is needed, a small dose of the TCA doxepin is a better choice. At 10 mg doxepin is antihistaminergic without much anticholinergic burden. At higher doses, doxepin is highly anticholinergic.

Tylenol PM is a combination of acetaminophen and diphenhydramine.

Dynamic interactions:

- Sedative
- Anticholinergic
  - constipation
  - confusion
  - urinary retention
  - dry mouth

Kinetic interactions:

- None significant

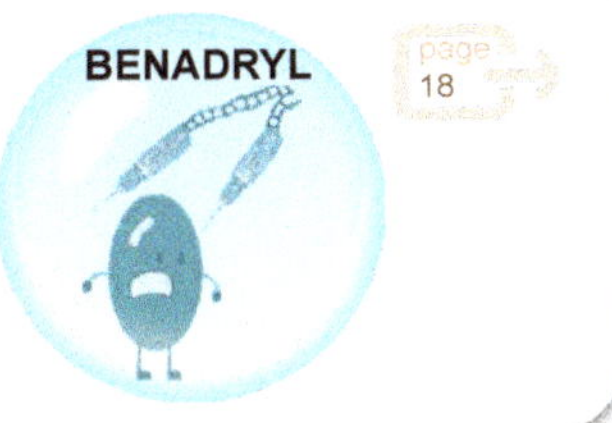

page 18

1949
$4–$17

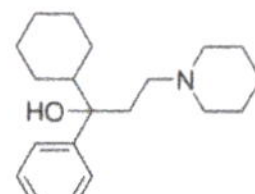

Trihexyphenidyl (ARTANE)

try hex e FEN id il / AR tane

"Triangle hexagon Art"

- ❖ Anticholinergic
- ❖ Possibly dopaminergic

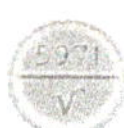

2
5
mg

FDA-approved for:

- ❖ Parkinson's disease
- ❖ Extrapyramidal symptoms (EPS)

Used off-label for:

- ❖ Sialorrhea (hypersalivation)
- ❖ Hyperhidrosis (sweating)

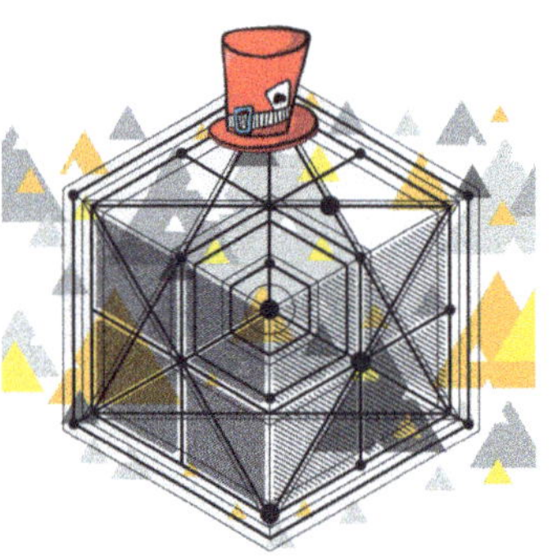

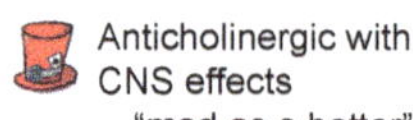

Anticholinergic with CNS effects —"mad as a hatter"

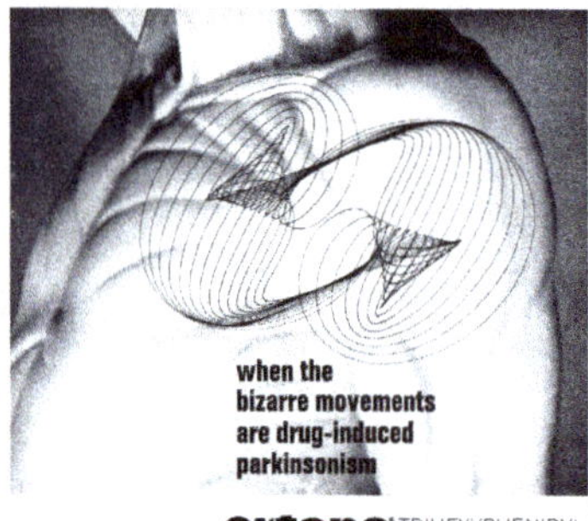

For treatment of EPS, Artane (trihexyphenidyl) is considered second-line to benztropine (Cogentin). Artane is dosed TID, while Cogentin is generally BID. Half-life is about 7 hours. It is only available orally.

Artane is not a controlled substance, but it is used recreationally as a hallucinogen, in large amounts. Artane is considered the most stimulating anticholinergic drug, possibly due to dopaminergic effect. It may produce euphoria. Although benztropine can also cause anticholinergic delirium at high dose, benztropine is not sought by recreational users.

As with any strong anticholinergic, long-term use may increase risk of dementia.

Dosing: Start 1 mg QD and increase to 2 mg TID over a few days. Standard maintenance dose is 2–5 mg TID, maximum of 15 mg/day. Discontinue by tapering to avoid cholinergic rebound (SLUDGE, page 59).

Dynamic interactions:

- ❖ Sedative (minimal)
- ❖ Anticholinergic
  - constipation
  - confusion
  - urinary retention
  - dry mouth

Kinetic interactions:

- ❖ None significant

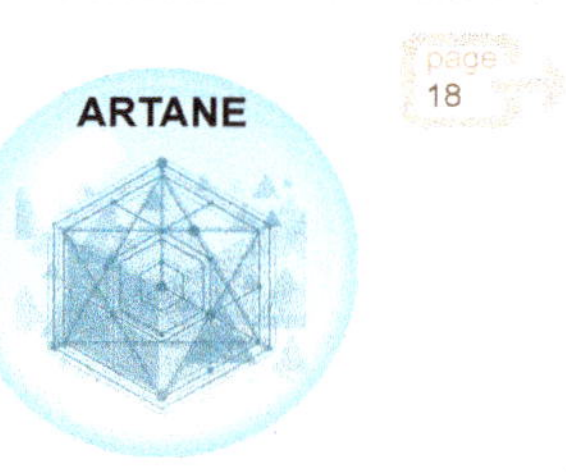

page 18

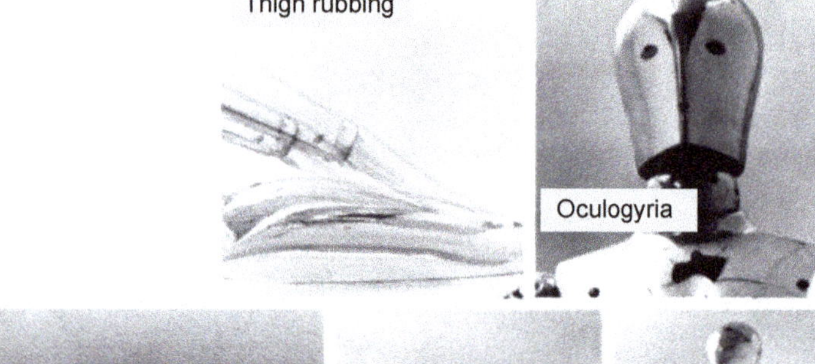

Propulsive gait

Choreoathetosis

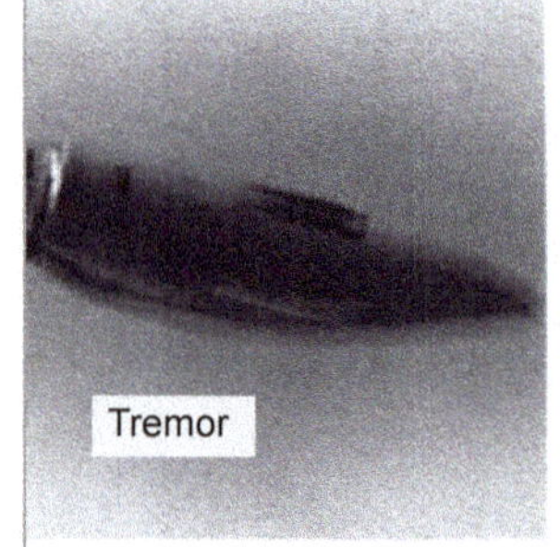

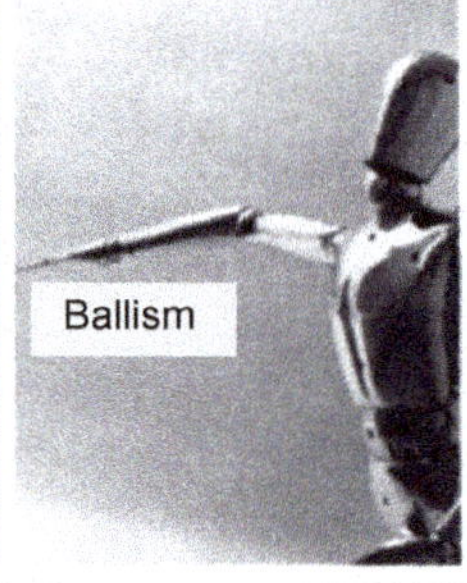

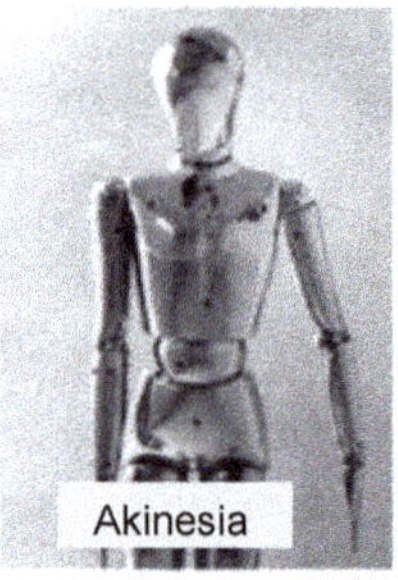

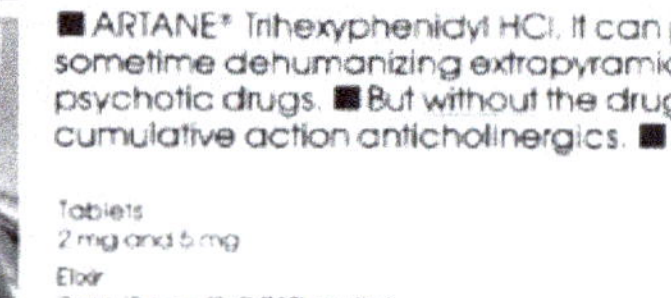

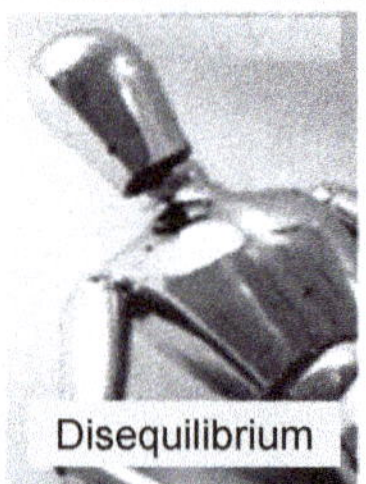

Rigidity

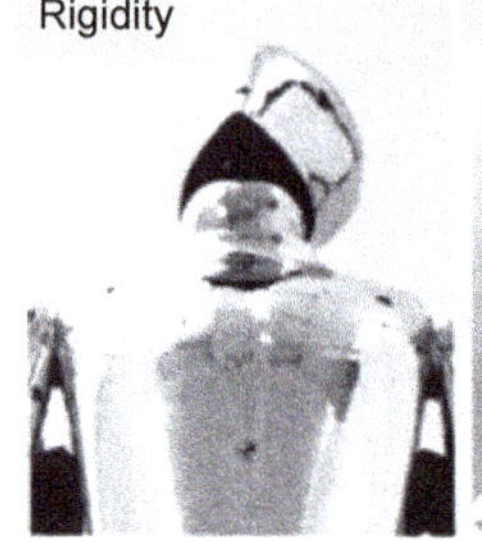

Torticollis

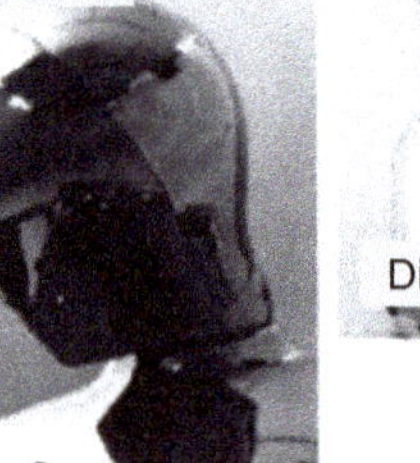

■ ARTANE* Trihexyphenidyl HCl. It can prevent or reverse the sometime dehumanizing extrapyramidal effects of the anti-psychotic drugs. ■ But without the drug buildup potential of cumulative action anticholinergics. ■ And at lower cost.

Tablets
2 mg and 5 mg
Elixir
2 mg/5 cc with 0.08% methylparaben, 0.02% propylparaben and 5% Alcohol as preservatives
SEQUELS*
Sustained Release Capsules 5 mg

ARTANE®

TRIHEXYPHENIDYL HCl

TO REMOVE THE "CHEMICAL STRAITJACKET"

LEDERLE LABORATORIES, A Division of American Cyanamid Co. Pearl River, N.Y 10965

#211
1954
$12–$26

Benztropine (COGENTIN)

BENZ tro peen / co GENT in

"Benz Cog"

❖ Anticholinergic

0.5
1
2
mg

FDA-approved for:
- ❖ Parkinson's disease
- ❖ Extrapyramidal symptoms

Used off-label for:
- ❖ Sialorrhea (hypersalivation)
- ❖ Hyperhidrosis (sweating)

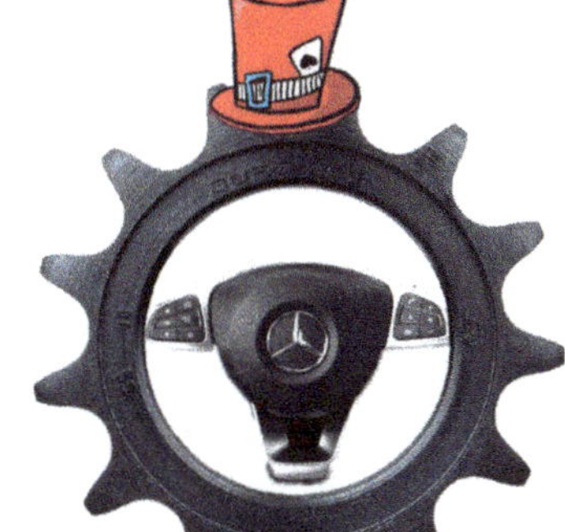

Mercedes Benz steering wheel inside a cogwheel

Anticholinergic with CNS effects—"mad as a hatter"

Benztropine (Cogentin) is an anticholinergic (antimuscarinic) frequently prescribed by psychiatrists as an add-on to high potency first generation antipsychotics to counter extrapyramidal symptoms (EPS), especially dystonia. Benztropine is not very effective for akathisia and can worsen tardive dyskinesia. Half-life is at least 12 hours.

Some prescribers, when starting haloperidol (Haldol), routinely start benztropine concurrently to prevent dystonia. However, benztropine does not prevent tardive dyskinesia (TD). If tardive dyskinesia develops, anticholinergics should be stopped because they may exacerbate TD.

Antipsychotics lower dopamine activity by blocking D2 receptors. Extrapyramidal symptoms are due to a relative deficiency of DA and an excess of acetylcholine in the nigrostriatal pathway. EPS can be relieved by increasing the availability of dopamine and/or blocking acetylcholine.

Intramuscular benztropine is available for treatment of an acute dystonic reaction such as oculogyric crisis or torticollis. IM diphenhydramine (Benadryl) is equally effective. Oculogyric crisis is a prolonged upward deviation of the eyes bilaterally. Torticollis is a dystonic reaction with the head persistently turned to one side, often associated with painful muscle spasms.

Laryngeal dystonia is also responsive to benztropine. This is a type of tardive dystonia occuring after prolonged antipsychotic use. The condition is caused by periodic spasms of the larynx (voice box) manifested by hoarseness or difficulty speaking.

Cognitive impairment ("mad as a hatter") from benztropine is a bigger problem than commonly appreciated (Lupu et al, 2017). As with any strong anticholinergic, long-term use may increase risk of dementia.

Dosing: A typical dosage of PO benztropine is 0.5–1 mg BID, with a maximum total daily dose of 4–6 mg. A reasonable PRN dosage is 1 mg q 8 hr. For acute dystonia, give 2 mg IM x 1. Discontinue by tapering to avoid cholinergic rebound (SLUDGE, page 59).

Cogwheeling - physical exam finding indicative of Parkinson's disease in which passive movement of an arm elicits ratchet-like start-and-stop movements.

Here are the high potency 1st generation antipsychotics (FGAs). They have the highest incidence of EPS and are therefore the most likely culprits to need an anticholinergic add-on:

- ❖ Haloperidol (Haldol)
- ❖ Fluphenazine (Prolixin)
- ❖ Pimozide (Orap)
- ❖ Thiothixene (Navane)
- ❖ Trifluoperazine (Stelazine)

Cogentin is rarely, if ever, needed in combination with these low EPS antipsychotics:

- ❖ Clozapine (Clozaril)
- ❖ Olanzapine (Zyprexa)
- ❖ Quetiapine (Seroquel)
- ❖ Aripiprazole (Abilify)
- ❖ Iloperidone (Fanapt)
- ❖ Pimavanserin (Nuplazid)

Cogentin is not needed if the patient is already taking a highly anticholinergic drug like diphenhydramine (Benadryl). Refer to the anticholinergic burden scale on page 60.

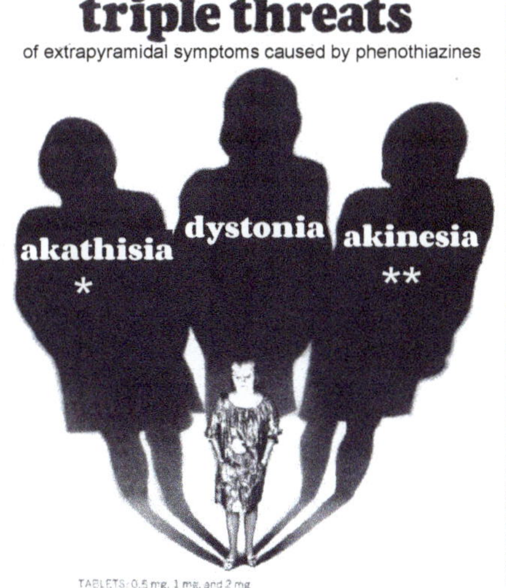

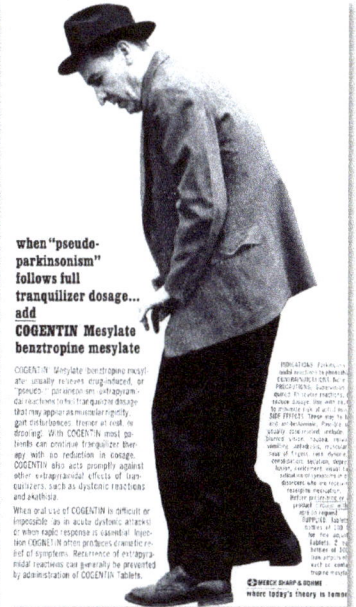

when "pseudo-parkinsonism" follows full tranquilizer dosage... add COGENTIN Mesylate benztropine mesylate

MERCK SHARP & DOHME where today's theory is tomorrow's therapy

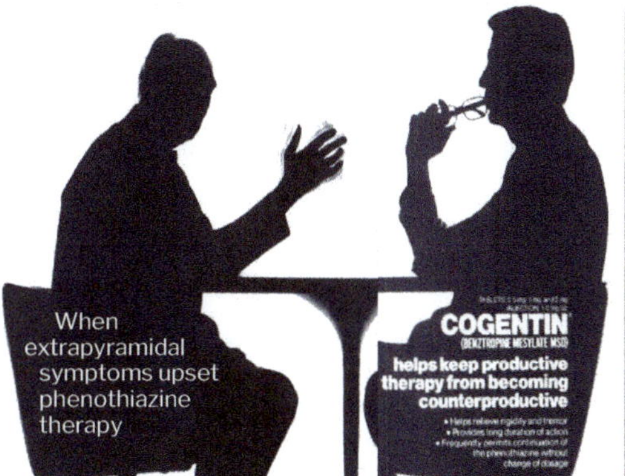

When extrapyramidal symptoms upset phenothiazine therapy
COGENTIN
(BENZTROPINE MESYLATE MSD)
helps keep productive therapy from becoming counterproductive

* Anticholinergics are not first-line treatment for akathisia. More effective treatments for akathisia include the beta blocker propranolol (Inderal) or benzodiazepines.

** Akinesia is another term for pseudo-parkinsonism, including the "Thorazine shuffle".

Dynamic interactions:
- ❖ Sedative (mild)
- ❖ Anticholinergic
  - constipation
  - confusion
  - urinary retention
  - dry mouth

Kinetic interactions:
- ❖ None significant

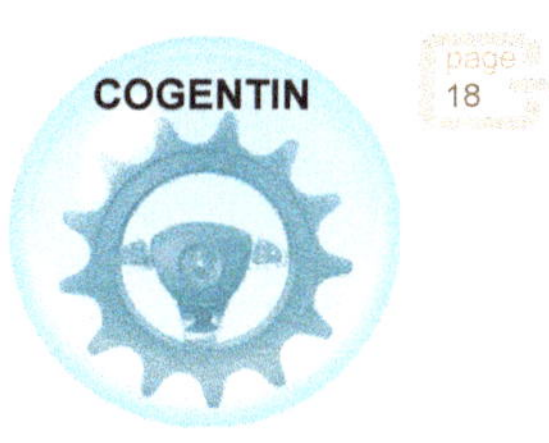

page 18

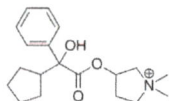

1961
$14 - $63

Glycopyrrolate (ROBINUL)

GLY koe PIE roe late/ ROB in ol

"Robbin' all Glad cops"

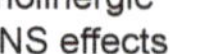

❖ Anticholinergic
❖ No CNS effects

1 mg

FDA-approved for:
❖ Peptic ulcer disease
❖ COPD (inhaler)
❖ Anesthesia adjunction (IV, IM)

Used off-label for
❖ Sialorrhea (hypersalivation) - 1st line PO
❖ Hyperhidrosis (sweating) - 1st line

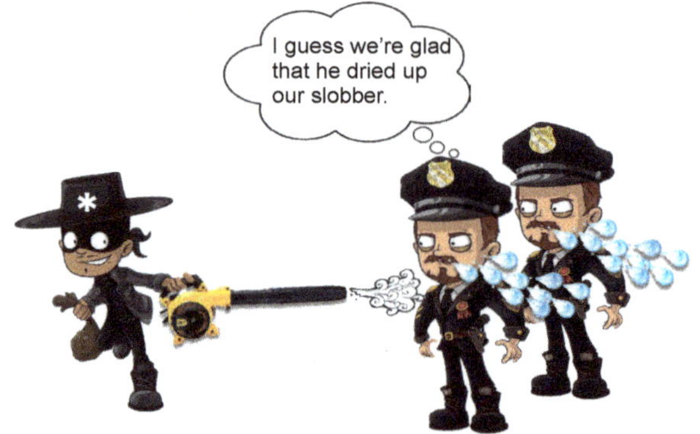
I guess we're glad that he dried up our slobber.

✱ The Mad-Hatter hat is not depicted for glycopyrrolate because it does not cross the blood-brain barrier.

The anticholinergic medication glycopyrrolate (Robinul), also known as glycopyrronium, is the preferred (oral) antisialagogue for clozapine-induced hypersalivation (drooling). Glycopyrrolate dries the mouth without causing cognitive impairment because it does not cross the blood-brain barrier (BBB). "Mad as a hatter" does not apply. However, addition of an anticholinergic can exacerbate clozapine-induced constipation, which can be severe—potentially leading to bowel rupture. Inability to cross the BBB also makes glycopyrrolate useless for treatment of EPS. An alternative that can treat both sialorrhea and EPS is benztropine (Cogentin). To avoid constipation, a topical alternative for clozapine-induced hypersalivation is atropine ophthalmic (Atropisol) 1–3 drops sublingually at bedtime (shown below).

Glycopyrrolate is the preferred treatment of hyperhidrosis (sweating). It works well as an add-on to address antidepressant-induced sweating (Mago, 2013). A topical form of glycopyrrolate called glycopyrronium (Qbrexza) is approved as an expensive underarm wipe for axillary hyperhidrosis (excessive underarm sweating). Glycopyrrolate and glycopyrronium are the same molecule.

As with most anticholinergics, there are no CYP interactions to worry about.

The inhaled formulation of glycopyrrolate is called Seebri Neohaler. For context, there are several more popular anticholinergic inhalers for COPD, including tiotropium (Spiriva), ipratropium (Atrovent), and umeclidinium (Incruse Ellipta).

Dosing: For drooling or sweating (off-label), give 1–2 mg PO q 6 hr PRN; Max is 8 mg/day; For peptic ulcer disease, give on a scheduled basis, 1–2 mg PO BID–TID Start: 1 mg PO tid; Max is 8 mg/day.

Dynamic interactions:
❖ Anticholinergic (peripheral effects)
- constipation
- urinary retention
- dry mouth

Kinetic interactions:
❖ None significant

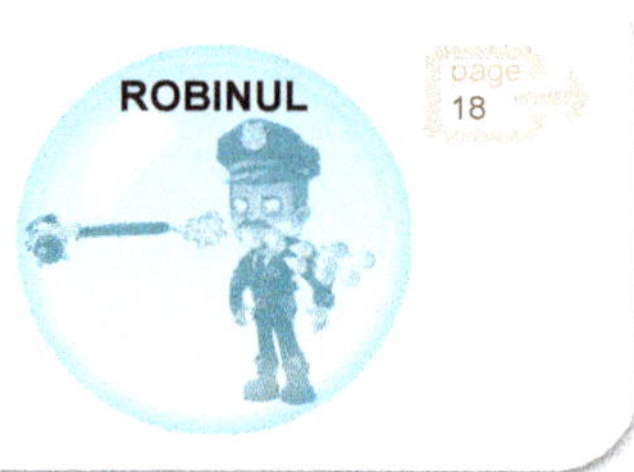
ROBINUL

#298
1960
$25 - $67

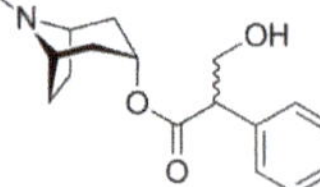

Atropine

AT roe peen

"AT-AT dropping"

❖ Anticholinergic

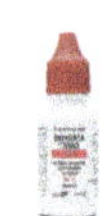

1% eye drops

FDA-approved for:
❖ See below

Used off-label for:
❖ Clozapine-induced hypersalivation (eye drops applied sublingually)

"Atropine is anticholinergic". Atropine, first isolated in 1833, is the strongest anticholinergic. It occurs naturally in a number of plants including deadly nightshade, Jimson weed, and mandrake. These plants are powerful hallucinogens and deliriants due to anticholinergic chemicals including atropine, hyoscyamine, and scopolamine.

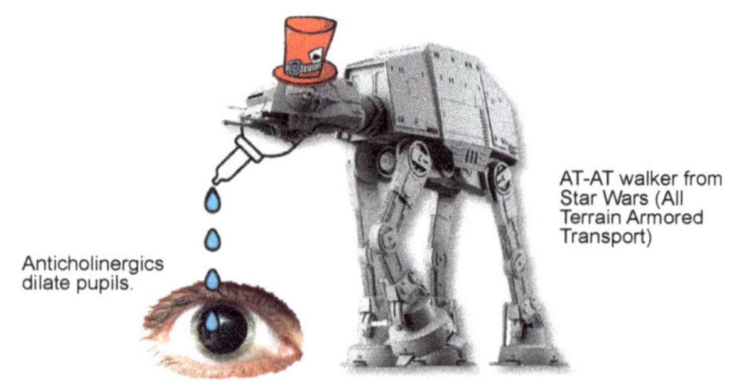
AT-AT walker from Star Wars (All Terrain Armored Transport)
Anticholinergics dilate pupils.

Uses of parenteral (SC, IM or IV) atropine:
❖ ATROPEN auto-injector for organophosphate poisoning (insecticides, nerve agents)
❖ ACLS protocol for bradycardia, to increase heart rate
❖ Anesthesia adjunct to decrease saliva

Uses of atropine ophthalmic drops (ATROPISOL):
❖ Dilation of pupils before eye exams to better visualize the retina
❖ To paralyze the ciliary muscle in order to determine the true refractive error of the eye (cycloplegic refraction)
❖ Treatment of amblyopia (lazy eye) by blurring the better-seeing eye as an alternative to wearing an eyepatch
❖ Treatment of uveitis (inflammation of iris, choroid, and ciliary body)
❖ Off-label treatment of clozapine-induced hypersalivation, given sublingually. Some systemic absorption is expected, and pupils may dilate to some extent. An alternative is ipratropium nasal spray given sublingually (Atrovent nasal, approved for rhinorrhea), which has less systemic absorption than atropine. For ipratropium, give 1–3 sprays SL at HS (not intranasal) up to 3x daily.

Oral atropine:
❖ In combination with the opioid diphenoxylate (LOMOTIL) for treatment of diarrhea. The atropine component contributes in small part to the antidiarrheal effect, included primarily as a determent to consuming large amounts of Lomotil to get high.

Dosing: For clozapine-induced hypersalivation: Atropine ophthalmic (Atropisol) 1–3 drops sublingually HS. Watch for possible daytime rebound salivation. May be used up to TID.

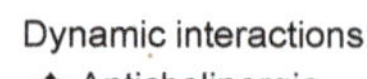

Dynamic interactions:
❖ Anticholinergic

Kinetic interactions:
❖ None significant

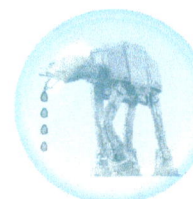

Tardive dyskinesia (TD) is a potentially irreversible movement disorder caused by dopamine D2 receptor-blocking medications taken for 6 months or longer. TD almost never occurs before 3 months on an antipsychotic. Haloperidol (Haldol) and metoclopramide (Reglan) are the most common culprits, because other medications with high risk of TD are rarely prescribed. The yearly incidence of developing TD is about the same throughout the course of treatment with a D2 blocker. In other words, the risk of developing TD during the first year on haloperidol is about the same as during the fifth year or the tenth year. Older adults are at higher risk.

First generation antipsychotics (FGAs) with strong affinity for D2 receptors (high potency FGAs) pose the highest risk of tardive dyskinesia. Second generation antipsychotics (SGAs) generally pose less of a risk because they block 5-HT_{2A} serotonin receptors with greater affinity than they block D2 receptors. Blocking 5-HT_{2A} receptors (on dopamine neurons) increases the release of dopamine in the basal ganglia, thereby preventing development of D2 receptor hypersensitivity, which leads to TD.

According to the maladaptive synaptic plasticity hypothesis, D2 receptor hypersensitivity and neuronal damage caused by oxidative stress can result in the formation of abnormal new connections between the basal ganglia and the cerebral cortex, leading to involuntary movements that persist even after the offending drug is removed. It stands to reason that general neuroprotectants (e.g., antioxidants) may improve or prevent TD (Deardorff et al, 2019).

Treatment of TD consists of tapering off the offending medication over a few weeks and, if necessary, replacing it with an antipsychotic with negligible D2 blocking potency such as clozapine (Clozaril), quetiapine (Seroquel), or pimavanserin (Nuplazid). Abruptly stopping the D2 blocker can worsen TD by suddenly exposing hypersensitive D2 receptors to more dopamine. TD caused by abruptly stopping a D2 blocker is called withdrawal-emergent dyskinesia.

If TD emerges, you should taper off of anticholinergics such as benztropine (Cogentin), diphenhydramine (Benadryl), and trihexyphenidyl (Artane). Although helpful for other types of extrapyramidal symptoms (EPS), anticholinergics worsen TD. It may take several months for TD movements to improve.

Medications proven to improve TD:

Medication	Class	Comments
Clonazepam (KLONOPIN)	Benzodiazepine	Consider for first-line treatment of TD
Amantadine (SYMMETREL)	NMDA antagonist and dopaminergic	FDA-approved for parkinsonism
Valbenazine (INGREZZA)	Dopamine depleting agent	The first FDA-approved TD treatment, 2017
Deutetrabenazine (AUSTEDO)	Dopamine depleting agent	The second FDA-approved TD treatment, 2018
Tetrabenazine (XENAZINE)	Dopamine depleting agent	Approved as orphan drug for Huntington's in 2008, used off-label for TD
Reserpine (SERPASIL)	Dopamine depleting agent	Reserpine depletes the reserves of dopamine in presynaptic neurons It was used for treatment of psychosis prior to modern antipsychotics. It is also used for HTN. Not recommended due to too many side effects, including hypotension
Ginkgo biloba extract	Antioxidant	"EGb-761" brand, 240 mg daily is well tolerated but risk of bleeding
Botulinum toxin (BOTOX)	Neurotoxin that inhibits acetylcholine release from nerve endings	Botox is effective for localized tardive dystonia that may accompany tardive dyskinesia. The most common location is the neck (cervical dystonia). Not for injection into the tongue

Note that the dopamine depleting agents (VMAT2 inhibitors) may induce parkinsonism as an adverse effect.

Less proven TD treatments:

Medication	Class	Comments
Melatonin	Neuroprotectant	10 mg decreases symptoms 24–30% by 6 weeks. Benign,cheap, neuroprotective, and may help cognition; There is no reason not to try melatonin if tardive dyskinesia is a concern.
N-Acetylcysteine (NAC)	Neuroprotectant	Benign treatment with no expected risks, side effects, or interactions; Inexpensive; No reason not to try it
Vitamin B6 (Pyridoxine)	Vitamin	400–1200 mg daily (high dose). 1200 mg may be effective even 8 weeks after cessation. Neuropathy (reversible) may occur at doses over 200 mg.
Vitamin E	Vitamin	Previously recommended but larger studies found it to be ineffective for TD. May increase risk of prostate cancer
Propranolol	Beta blocker	Also helps essential tremor and akathisia. Contraindicated with bradycardia or asthma
Buspirone (BUSPAR)	Anxiolytic	Very high doses have been used, up to 180 mg/day (60 mg TID). FDA max is 60 mg/day.
Mirtazapine (REMERON)	Antidepressant	20 of 22 cases of movement disorder (including TD) improved on mirtazapine 30 mg (Alarcón et al, 2003).

Other medications that may potentially improve TD include baclofen (Lioresal), valproate (Depakote), zolpidem (Ambien), donepezil (Aricept), zonisamide (Zonegran), and omega-3 fatty acids.

Principal sources:
Forgotten but not gone: new developments in the understanding and treatment of tardive dyskinesia; Jonathan Meyer; CNS Spectrums (2016).
An update on tardive dyskinesia: From phenomenology to treatment; Wain and Jankovic; Tremor and Other Hyperkinetic Movements journal (2013).

VMAT Inhibitors (dopamine depleting agents) for treatment of chorea

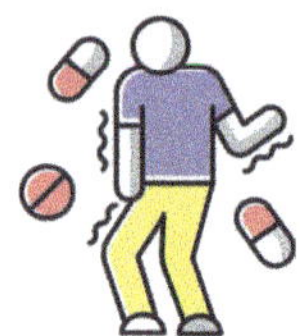

The involuntary movements of tardive dyskinesia (TD) and Huntington's disease (HD) are described as chorea (choreiform movements) derived from the Greek word for "dance". Chorea involves irregular movements (as opposed to repetitive movements) that appear to flow from one muscle to the next. Choreiform movements occur both at rest and with action. The patient may attempt to disguise chorea by incorporating involuntary movements into a purposeful activity such as adjusting clothes. A common example of chorea is "milkmaid's grip"—hand muscles squeezing and releasing as if milking a cow.

For context: Parkinson's disease (PD) does not manifest as chorea, but levodopa (PD treatment) can cause choreiform movements. For context, a parkinsonian tremor is a slow repetitive tremor. Characteristic of parkinsonism is the "pill rolling" tremor that looks like the individual is a rolling a pill between the thumb and other fingers. parkinsonian tremor is unique as a resting tremor that disappears with movement. With parkinsonism, the patient has no problem bringing a cup or soup spoon to their mouth but may spill the liquid while resting the cup/spoon on the lips.

Chorea of tardive dyskinesia: Only severe cases of tardive dyskinesia manifest as choreiform movements of the arms. TD is more likely to involve tongue movements, lip smacking, excessive blinking, grimacing or raising of eyebrows. Often the patient with TD will be unaware of orofacial movements. When TD affects the upper extremities, it starts as irregular finger movements—as if the patient is playing an invisible piano or air guitar (fretting hand, not strumming hand).

Vesicular monoamine transporter (VMAT) is a protein that transports monoamines (dopamine, serotonin, norepinephrine, epinephrine, and histamine) into synaptic vesicles of presynaptic neurons. By depleting dopamine from synaptic vesicles (and thereby depleting dopamine in the synapse), VMAT inhibitors have antipsychotic properties. The original VMAT inhibitor, reserpine, was used as an antipsychotic. In contrast to modern antipsychotics that block dopamine receptors, dopamine depleting drugs pose little to no risk of causing tardive dyskinesia. However, VMAT inhibitors can cause akathisia (restlessness) and parkinsonism.

Nowadays VMAT inhibitors are used to treat tardive dyskinesia (TD) and Huntington's disease. In both conditions, choreiform movements are caused by excessive dopamine activity in the areas of the brain that control movement. TD is caused by dopamine D2 receptor hypersensitivity on postsynaptic neurons, resulting from prolonged exposure to a D2 blocking medication such as haloperidol (Haldol) or metoclopramide (Reglan). Huntington's disease is an autosomal dominant disease that causes death of neurons. In the early stages of HD, chorea results from excessive activity of (presynaptic) dopaminergic neurons. Chorea diminishes at advanced stages of HD, at which time dystonia emerges.

Vesicular monoamine transporter inhibitors may cause depression and suicidal ideation by depleting serotonin, which is also a monoamine neurotransmitter.

In the early stages of Huntington's disease, neurons release an excessive amount of dopamine, resulting in choreiform involuntary movements. VMAT inhibitors decrease the amount of dopamine available for release.

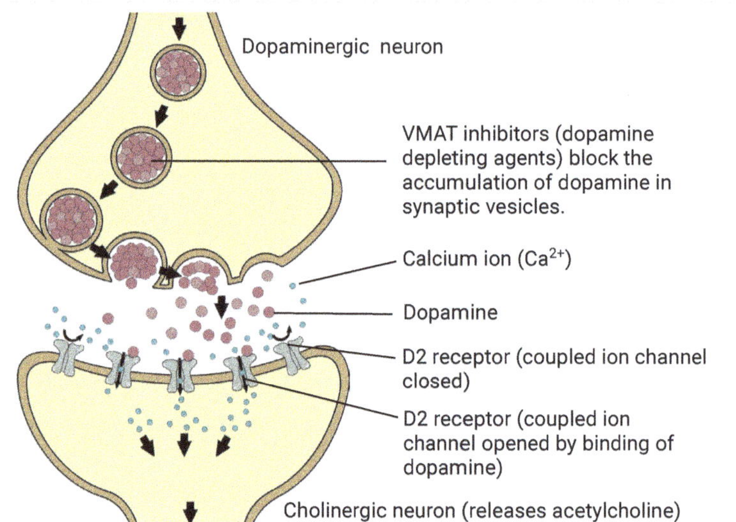

With tardive dyskinesia (TD), D2 receptors are hypersensitive to stimulation by dopamine. VMAT inhibitors alleviate TD by decreasing the amount of DA available to bind hypersensitive receptors.

VMAT Inhibitors (dopamine depleting agents)

Drug	Year	Cost	Inhibitor of	Reversibility	FDA-approved for
Tetrabenazine (XENAZINE)	2008	$1,000	VMAT2	Reversible	Huntington's
Deutetrabenazine (AUSTEDO)	2017	$3,000	VMAT2	Reversible	Huntington's & TD
Valbenazine (INGREZZA)	2018	$10,000	VMAT2	Reversible	Tardive dyskinesia (TD)
Reserpine (SERPASIL)	1955	$30	VMAT2 > VMAT1	Irreversible	Hypertension

2008
$362–$2,300

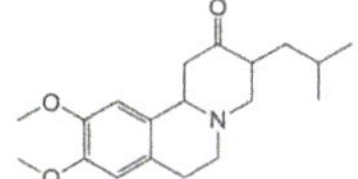

Tetrabenazine (XENAZINE)

tet ra BEN uh zeen / ZEN uh zeen

"Xena's Tetris bin"

- ❖ VMAT2 Inhibitor
- ❖ Dopamine depleting agent
- ❖ Anti-chorea medication

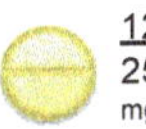

12.5
25
mg

FDA-approved for:
- ❖ Huntington's disease

Used off-label for:
- ❖ Tardive dyskinesia
- ❖ Tic disorders including Tourette's
- ❖ Hemiballismus due to subthalamic nucleus damage
- ❖ Treatment-resistant schizophrenia

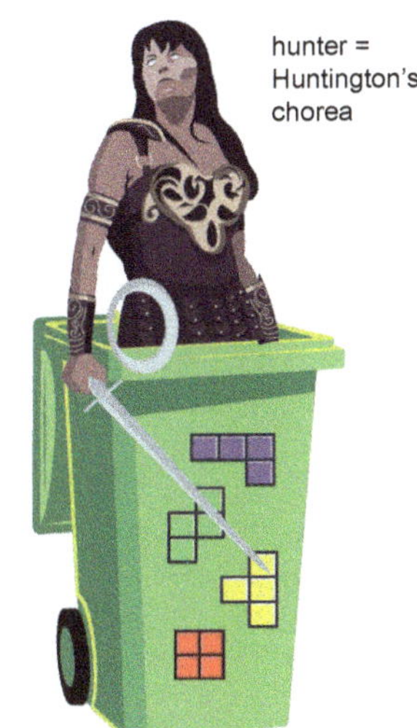

Xena: Warrior Princess was a television series running from 1995 to 2001 as a spin-off from *Hercules: The Legendary Journeys*

Tetrabenazine (Xenazine) is a presynaptic monoamine-depleting agent that can dampen abnormal dopamine release. Tetrabenazine was developed as a treatment for schizophrenia over 50 years ago.

Tetrabenazine was the first FDA-approved treatment for Huntington's chorea (2008), after it had been available in other countries for decades. Unlike subsequent VMAT inhibitors, tetrabenazine is not FDA-approved for tardive dyskinesia (TD), although it is effective for TD, off-label.

Psychiatric side effects of VMAT inhibitors are of major concern. Behavior change, depression, and suicide are possible with these medications. Per black box warning, VMAT inhibitors are contraindicated for Huntington's patients who are actively depressed. VMAT inhibitors may also cause cognitive deficits.

In addition to relieving tardive dyskinesia caused by antipsychotics, tetrabenazine has antipsychotic properties of its own. It has been used off-label for treatment-resistant schizophrenia, augmenting a modern antipsychotic.

Tetrabenazine can greatly increase prolactin levels by decreasing dopamine release. Dopamine, also known as "prolactin-inhibiting factor", inhibits release of prolactin from the pituitary gland.

In treatment of Huntington's disease it may be difficult to distinguish between adverse drugs reactions and progression of the underlying disease. There have been cases of neuroleptic malignant syndrome associated with tetrabenazine, caused by decreased dopamine transmission.

Dosing: Maintenance range is 25–100 mg/day in divided doses; Start at 12.5 mg q AM x 1 week, then 12.5 mg BID x 1 week; Then may increase by 12.5 mg/day in weekly intervals; Divide to TID if > 37.5 mg/day. Consider 2D6 genotyping if planning to exceed 50 mg/day, which is the maximum dose for patients who are 2D6 poor metabolizers or those taking a strong 2D6 inHibitor such quinidine, fluoxetine (Prozac), paroxetine (Paxil), or bupropion (Wellbutrin).

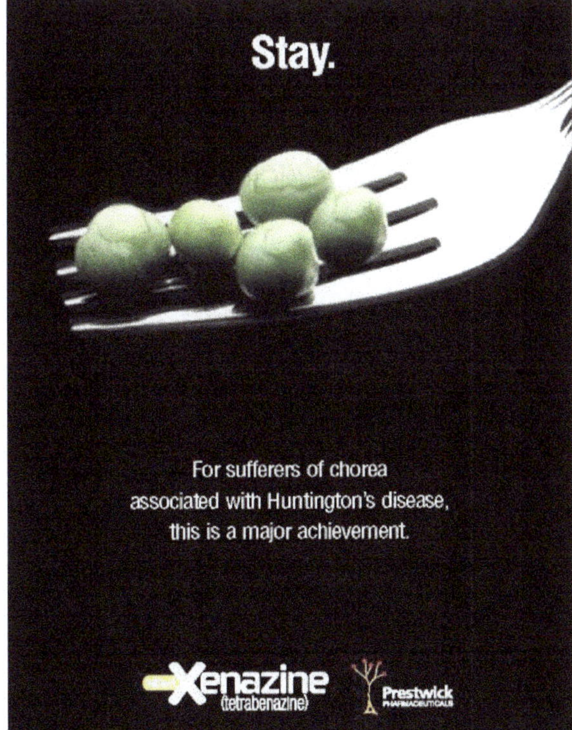

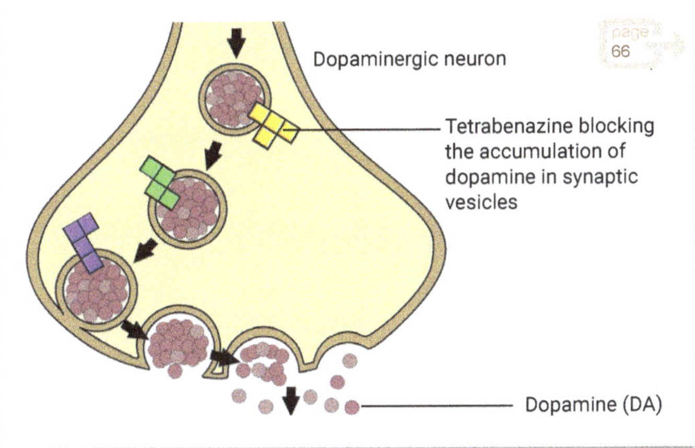

page 66

Dynamic interactions:
- ❖ CNS depression
- ❖ Prolactin elevation (strong)
- ❖ QT prolongation

Kinetic interactions:
- ❖ Exposure to tetrabenazine is significantly increased in 2D6 poor metabolizers or if co-administered with a strong 2D6 inhibitor.

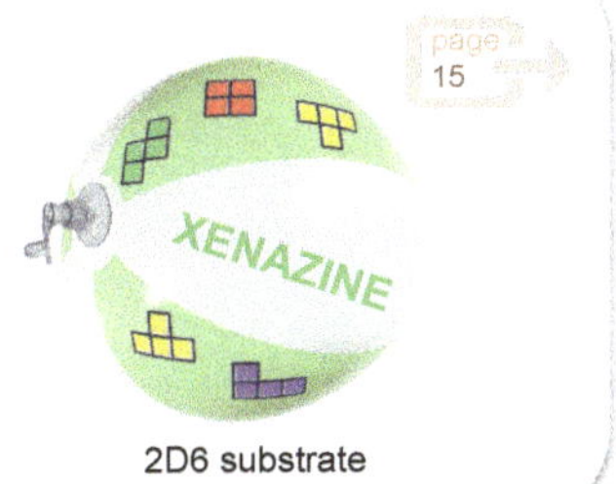

2D6 substrate

page 15

2017
$5,399–$5,725

Deutetrabenazine (AUSTEDO)

[du tet ra BEN uh zeen / ah STED oh

"Dueling tetris bins (to) Oust TD"

- VMAT2 Inhibitor
- Dopamine depleting agent

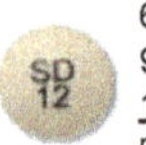

6
9
12
mg

FDA-approved for:

- Tardive dyskinesia
- Huntington's chorea

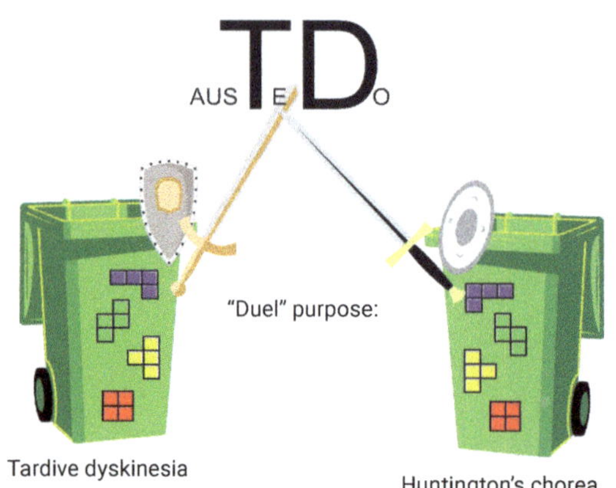

Deutetrabenazine (Austedo) is the VMAT inhibitor FDA-approved for both tardive dyskinesia (TD) and chorea of Huntington's disease. Compare this to tetrabenazine (Xenazine) which is only approved for Huntington's, and valbenazine (Ingrezza) which is only approved for TD.

Deutetrabenazine was the first drug containing deuterium, aka "heavy hydrogen" (an extra neutron), to receive FDA approval. Deuterated drugs take longer for the body to clear. Hence, deutetrabenazine has a longer duration of action than tetrabenazine, allowing for less frequent dosing.

Psychiatric side effects of VMAT inhibitors are a major concern when used for treating Huntington's chorea. Black box warnings state that VMAT inhibitors are contraindicated for Huntington's patients who are actively depressed due to risk of suicide.

TD patients tend to experience fewer psychiatric side effects than Huntington's patients, possibly because TD patients are also taking an antipsychotic. The incidence of somnolence was 11% (versus 4% placebo) for Huntington's patients. Somnolence was not an issue with TD patients. A few patients experienced insomnia.

Dosing: For TD, the initial dose is 12 mg/day, with recommended range of 12–48 mg/day. Divide doses to BID if total daily dose is above 12 mg. The recommended dose range for Huntington's chorea is slightly lower. Titrate at weekly intervals by 6 mg/day based on reduction of involuntary movements and tolerability. Consider checking an EKG for QT prolongation prior to exceeding 24 mg/day. Consider 2D6 genotyping prior to exceeding 36 mg/day (18 mg BID), which is the maximum dose for patients who are 2D6 poor metabolizers or those taking a strong 2D6 inHibitor.

Dynamic interactions:

- Prolactin elevation (strong)
- CNS depression
- QT prolongation

page 15

Kinetic interactions:

- Exposure to tetrabenazine is significantly increased in 2D6 poor metabolizers or if co-administered with a strong 2D6 inhibitor.

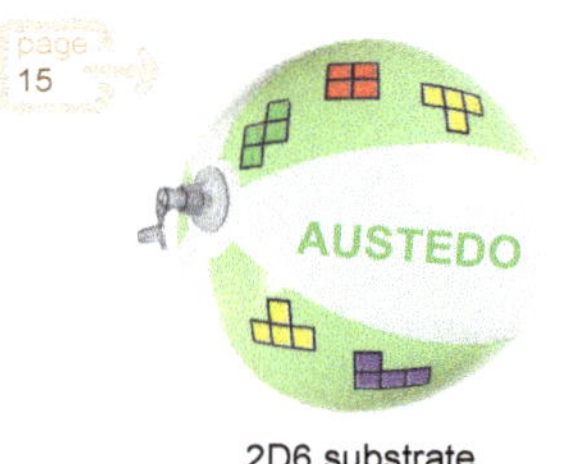

2D6 substrate

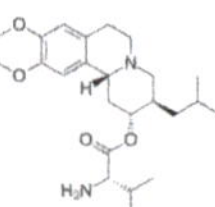
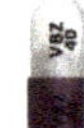

2018
$10,000

Valbenazine (INGREZZA)

val BEN uh zeen / in GREH zah

"Valved bin In grease"

- VMAT2 Inhibitor
- Dopamine depleting agent

40
80
mg

FDA-approved for:

- Tardive dyskinesia

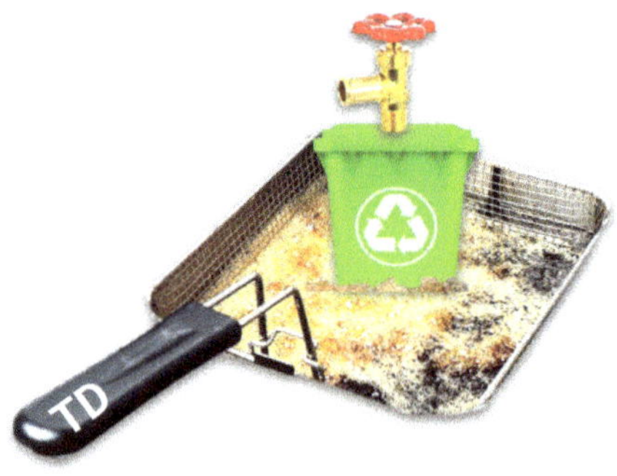

Valbenazine (Ingrezza) is the VMAT inhibitor FDA-approved for tardive dyskinesia but not for Huntington's. The active metabolite of valbenazine is one of the four stereoisomers of tetrabenazine (Xenazine). Prolactin elevation is less pronounced with valbenazine compared to the other VMAT inhibitors. Ingrezza can be titrated more quickly than Austedo and has a longer half-life, allowing QD dosing rather than BID (as with Austedo) or TID (as with Xenazine).

Valbenazine does not have the black box warning seen with other VMAT inhibitors (those approved for Huntington's) concerning risk of depression, behavioral change, and suicide. However, patients at risk for suicide or violent behavior were excluded from clinical trials.

The most common side effect is somnolence (11% vs 4% placebo). Otherwise, incidence of side effects is low, but some patients experience balance problems, dizziness, akathisia/restlessness, and arthralgia. As with other VMAT inhibitors, QT prolongation may occur at high doses.

Dosing: Start: 40 mg QD x 1 week, then increase to 80 mg QD (maintenance dose). Dose should not exceed 40 mg/day if taken with a strong 3A4 inHibitor. Concomitant use with a strong 3A4 inDucer is not recommended because valbenazine levels will be too low. Consider decreasing the dose for a 2D6 poor metabolizer, guided by tolerability.

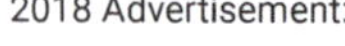

2018 Advertisement:

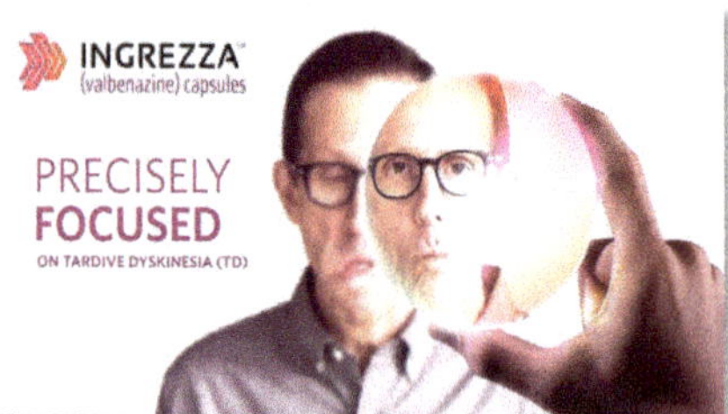

Dynamic interactions:

- Prolactin elevation
- CNS depression
- QT prolongation

Kinetic interactions:

- 3A4 substrate (major)
- 2D6 substrate

page 15

2D6 substrate

page 16

3A4 substrate (major)

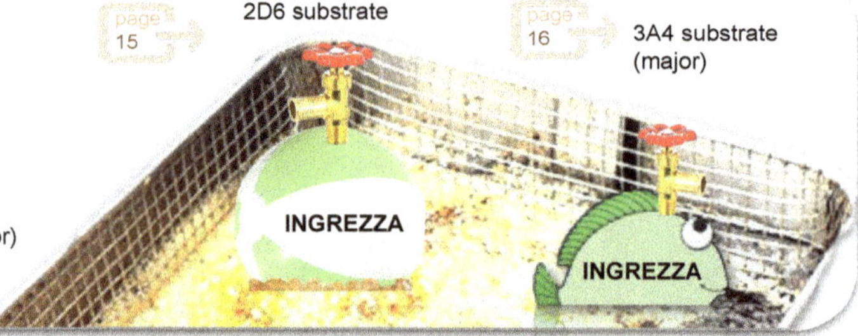

1955
$20–$37

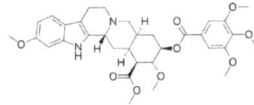

Reserpine (SERPASIL)

re SER pine / SIR pa sil

"serpent re-slurping (dopamine)"

❖ Nonselective, irreversible VMAT Inhibitor
❖ Dopamine depleting agent

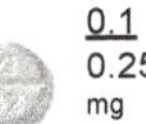

0.1
0.25
mg

FDA-approved for:
❖ Hypertension

Used off-label for:
❖ Refractory schizophrenia (rarely)
❖ Huntington's chorea
❖ Thyrotoxicosis (thyroid storm)

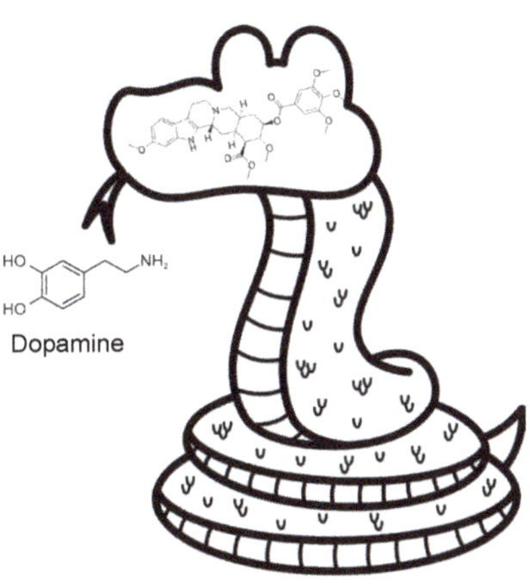

Reserpine depletes the reserves of dopamine in presynaptic neurons. Reserpine (Serpasil) is a nonselective vesicular monoamine transporter (VMAT) inhibitor, binding both VMAT1 and VMAT2. VMAT1 is mostly expressed in neuroendocrine cells. VMAT2 is mostly expressed in neurons. The newer VMAT inhibitors tetrabenazine (Xenazine), deutetrabenazine (Austedo), and valbenazine (Ingrezza) selectively block VMAT2.

Reserpine blocks VMAT irreversibly, so its effects are long lasting. It takes days to weeks for neurons to replenish the depleted transporters.

Reserpine was isolated in 1952 from Indian snakeroot (*Rauwolfia serpentina*) which had been used for centuries in India for the treatment of insanity. Reserpine is generally categorized as an antihypertensive, which is its only FDA-approved indication. A reserpine-hydrochlorothiazide combo pill is available for treatment of refractory high blood pressure. The reserpine-thiazide diuretic combination is one of the few hypertension treatments shown to reduce mortality in randomized controlled trials (JAMA, 1979).

Reserpine was used to treat schizophrenia prior to the arrival of chlorpromazine (Thorazine), which was more effective. The use of reserpine as an antipsychotic has largely been abandoned, but rarely psychiatrists will use it as an adjunct to a modern antipsychotic (dopamine D2 receptor blocker) for refractory cases.

Reserpine was the first compound shown to be an effective antidepressant in a randomized placebo-controlled trial, but it may be more likely to cause depression because it depletes serotonin. Reserpine's antihypertensive effect is mostly due to depletion of norepinephrine.

Reserpine was used to treat dyskinesia of Huntington's disease prior to arrival of the selective VMAT2 inhibitors, which are less likely to drop blood pressure and heart rate. Consider reserpine for treatment of tardive dyskinesia when comorbid with severe hypertension. Low dose reserpine is fairly well tolerated, with nasal congestion being the most common side effect.

Dosing: The usual dose for hypertension is 0.5 mg QD x 1–2 weeks, with maintenance dose of 0.1–0.25 mg QD. For schizophrenia it was dosed 0.1–1 mg QD, with the usual dose of 0.5 mg QD.

This American Journal of Psychiatry ad from 1955 describes reserpine as a "nonhypnotic tranquilizing agent" that "produces remissions in severe neuropsychiatric states".

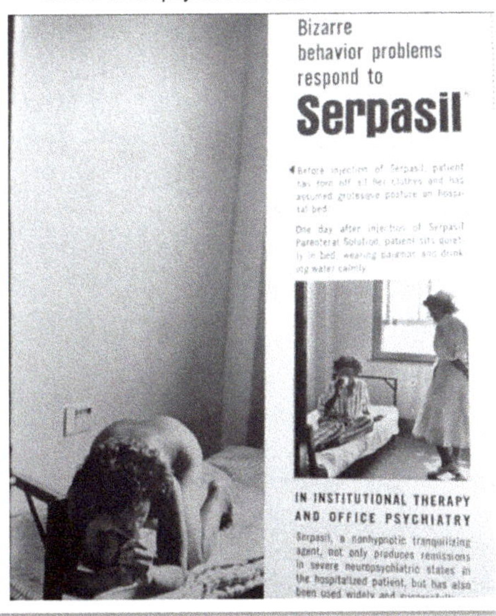

Low dose reserpine was promoted as a "gentle mood-leveling agent" for patients who are "incapable of dealing calmly with a daily pile-up of stressful situations".

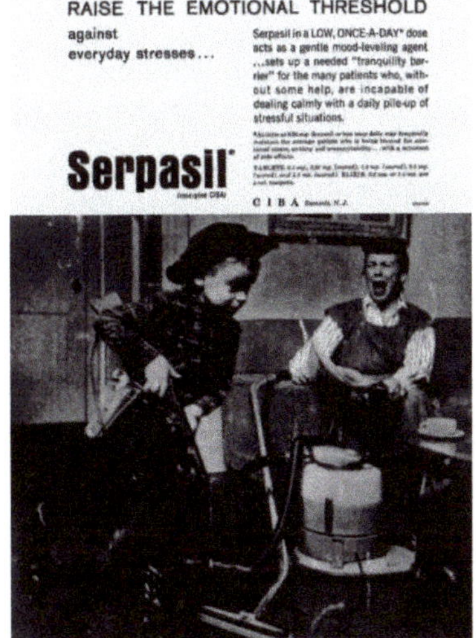

Serpatilin, the combination of reserpine with the stimulant methylphenidate (Ritalin), is no longer available nor advisable.

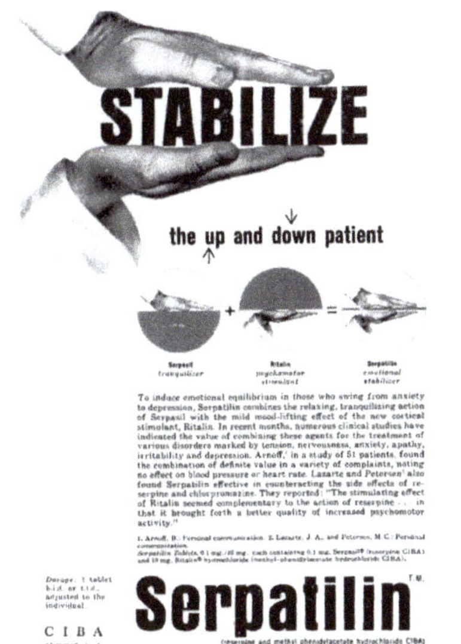

Dynamic interactions:
❖ Antidopaminergic
❖ Antiserotonergic
❖ Hypotensive

Kinetic interactions:
❖ P-gp inhibitor

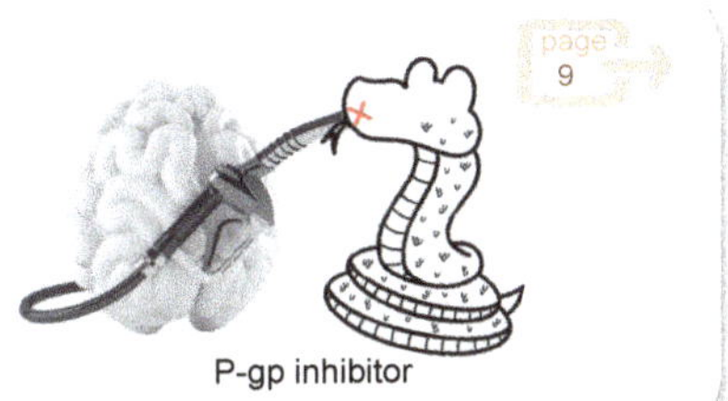
P-gp inhibitor

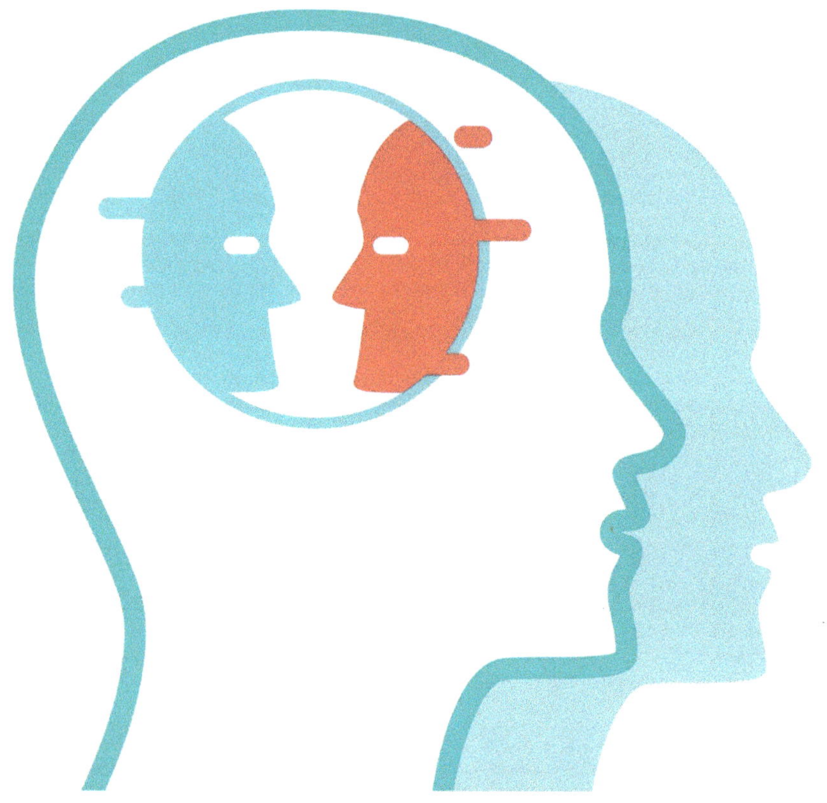

#4
1995
IR $4–$22
ER $4–$32

Metformin (GLUCOPHAGE)

met FORM in / GLU co faahj

"Mr. Met formin' Glucose fudge"

❖ Biguanide anti-hyperglycemic

ER: 500 750 mg

500 850 1000 mg

FDA approved for:
- ❖ Diabetes mellitus, type 2

Used off-label for:
- ❖ Adjunct to 2nd gen antipsychotics
- ❖ Polycystic ovary syndrome (PCOS)
- ❖ Weight loss
- ❖ Longevity

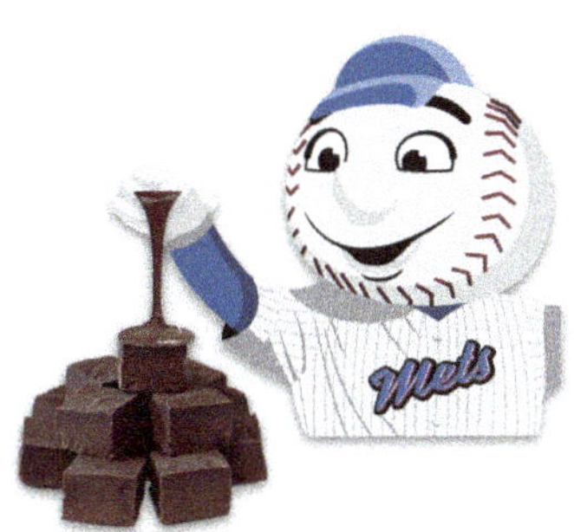

Dosing: Starting dose for the IR formulation is 500 mg BID with meals. If treating diabetes, increase the dose in increments of 500 mg weekly. The maximum total daily dose is 2550 mg per day, which would be prescribed as 850 mg TID with meals. If gastrointestinal side effects with IR, change to ER. For the ER formulation start 1000 mg q PM with the evening meal, with maximum 2000 mg/day. Off-label treatment or prevention of antipsychotic-induced weight gain is dosed similarly to diabetes.

Hemoglobin A1c

Normal .... 4.0–5.6 %
Prediabetes .... 5.7–6.4 %
Diabetes .... ≥ 6.5 %

Average glucose of 100 .... 5.1 %
Average glucose of 200 .... 8.6 %
Average glucose of 300 .... 12.1 %

The diabetic patient needs more than just metformin if A1c ≥ 9.0%.

Metformin (Glucophage) is the first line medication for prevention and treatment of type II diabetes. It works by decreasing glucose production by the liver and increasing insulin sensitivity of body tissues. Metformin reduces hunger and promotes fat loss. Since metformin is renally excreted, unmetabolized, it is not involved in CYP interactions.

Metformin is the preferred medication to prevent or reverse weight gain caused by second generation antipsychotics (SGAs). If a patient on an SGA gains > 5 pounds in first month or > 10 pounds from baseline, consider adding metformin. Many psychiatrists use topiramate (Topamax) as their go-to weight loss medication, but metformin is probably a better choice (see table below). Obese patients (diabetic or otherwise) taking metformin typically lose about 7 kg (15 pounds). It could be argued that metformin should be given to most patients starting olanzapine (Zyprexa) or clozapine (Clozaril), the antipsychotics most likely to cause significant weight gain and diabetes. Refer to Maayan et al, *Neuropsycho-pharmacology*, 2010.

Metformin has been demonstrated to reduce inflammation and slow the aging process in several lab critters. It is possible that metformin can prevent cancer and promote longevity in humans (Barzilai et al, 2016). A large study called Targeting Aging with Metformin (TAME) is in progress. Metformin appears to prevent cognitive decline with aging (Ng et al, 2014).

Metformin does not cause hypoglycemia. Fingerstick glucose monitoring at home is unnecessary when metformin is prescribed to non-diabetics. Even in overdose, only 10% of individuals develop hypoglycemia. Side effects are gastrointestinal including diarrhea (50%), nausea (25%), and flatulence (10%). GI side effects are less problematic with the ER formulation (10% diarrhea). There is a black box warning of the possibility of lactic acidosis, which is very rare at standard doses in healthy individuals. Do not prescribe metformin to patients with serious medical illness. Risk of acidosis with a large overdose is about 33%. A metabolic panel should be checked yearly. This would reveal acidosis as low bicarbonate (listed as CO_2). Signs of acidosis are nonspecific with subtle onset, including malaise, myalgias, abdominal pain, respiratory distress, or somnolence. Metformin has a 3% risk of contributing to Vitamin B12 deficiency due to malabsorption. Consider checking B12 levels at one year and then every 2 or 3 years.

Initiation of metformin is not recommended for patients with eGFR under 45 (renal insufficiency). Discontinue metformin if eGFR falls below 30. Temporarily discontinue metformin prior to iodinated contrast imaging procedures and restart in 48 hours if eGFR is normal.

Metformin blunts muscle growth from resistance exercise training in older adults (Walton et al, 2019).

Adjuncts to ameliorate antipsychotic-induced weight gain

Medication	Metformin (GLUCOPHAGE)	Topiramate (TOPAMAX)
Class	Diabetes medication	Antiepileptic
Site of action	Periphery	CNS
Benefits	Weight loss Prevention of diabetes Decreased lipids Possible anti-aging Possible cancer prevention	Weight loss Headache prevention
Risk of acidosis	Rare lactic acidosis	Relatively common metabolic acidosis
Other risks	Vitamin B12 deficiency (3%)	Kidney stones (15% with long-term use)
Most common side effects	Diarrhea and GI distress (tolerance usually develops)	Cognitive impairment, especially > 200 mg; Weight loss dose is 25 mg BID x 1 week then 50 mg BID which is unlikely to impair cognition.
Contraindications	Renal insufficiency	None
Cost	$4–$32	$4–$82

A 2010 meta-analysis of medication for antipsychotic-associated weight gain found metformin slightly more effective than topiramate (Maayan, et al, *Neuropsychopharmacology*).

Dynamic interactions:
- ❖ Black box warning for risk of lactic acidosis, which is increased by carbonic anhydrase inhibitors such as topiramate (Topamax), zonisamide (Zonegran), acetazolamide (Diamox), and dichlorphenamide (Keveyis)
- ❖ Heavy alcohol consumption increases the risk of acidosis with metformin

Kinetic interactions:
- ❖ Cimetidine (Tagamet) may compete with metformin for urinary excretion

"in a box" - clinically significant kinetic interactions are possible but unlikely

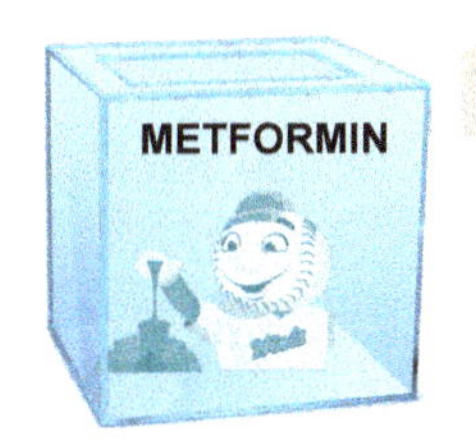

2018
$1,290–$3,041

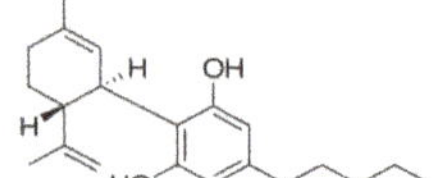

Cannabidiol (CBD; EPIDIOLEX)

can na bi DI ol / e pid e oh LEX

"Cannabis B.I.D. oil"

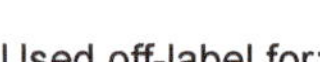

- ❖ Cannabinoid
- ❖ Antiepileptic
- ❖ Antipsychotic
- ❖ Neuroprotectant
- ❖ Non-controlled

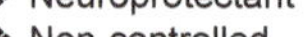

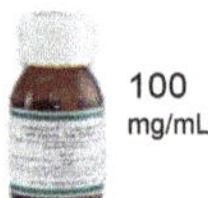

100 mg/mL

FDA-approved for:
- ❖ Lennox-Gastaut syndrome
- ❖ Dravet syndrome

Used off-label for:
- ❖ Schizophrenia
- ❖ Anxiety

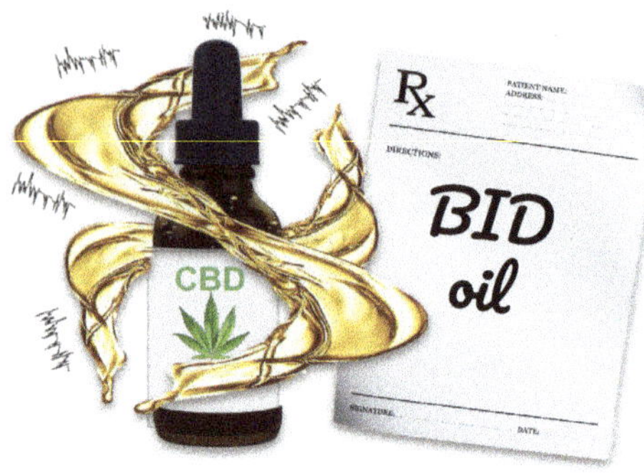

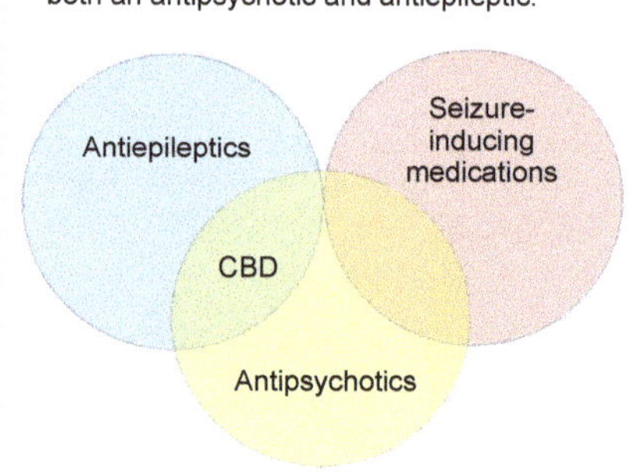

Epidiolex, pharmaceutical grade cannabidiol (CBD), was FDA-approved in 2018 for treatment of seizures associated with Lennox-Gastaut syndrome (LGS) and Dravet syndrome in children (age 2 and older). Lennox-Gastaut syndrome (LGS) is a type of childhood-onset epilepsy starting between 2–6 years of age. LGS is characterized by a triad of multiple seizure types, intellectual impairment, and characteristic EEG findings.

CBD is one of over 100 cannabinoids contained in marijuana. It should not be confused with "medical marijuana". In 2018 the DEA labeled Epidiolex as having low potential for abuse, classifying it as a Schedule V (five) controlled substance (lowest level of restriction). In 2020 the DEA dropped the restriction, so Epidiolex is no longer a controlled substance.

In clinical trials for schizophrenia, the subjects themselves were unable to tell whether they were in the treatment or placebo group.

CBD is an indirect antagonist of CB1 and CB2 cannabinoid receptors. CBD is an antipsychotic, neuroprotectant, and appetite suppressant which does not get the consumer "high". In many ways it is the opposite of tetrahydrocannabinol (THC), the main psychoactive component of cannabis. THC is a CB1 and CB2 agonist which makes it "The High Causer" in marijuana. Pure CBD is **not** likely to cause a false positive drug screen for marijuana (THC).

Epidiolex is an oral solution that (thankfully for the purpose of this mnemonic) is dosed BID. Somnolence is the main side effect of CBD. It has a good safety profile, but hepatotoxicity is possible.

CBD appears to work as an antiepileptic by inactivating voltage-gated sodium channels of the neuronal cell membrane.

CBD has demonstrated efficacy for schizophrenia at high dose. It is postulated to work as an antipsychotic through the endocannabinoid system. It is not FDA-approved for schizophrenia, but the future is promising. CBD may also be effective for social anxiety (Blessing EM et al, 2015).

Over-the-counter CBD oil is legal in all 50 states as long as it is extracted from the hemp plant, a variety of cannabis containing minimal THC. Of 84 online products tested, only 30% contained the advertised amount of CBD, and 21% contained THC (Boon-MIller et al, 2017).

Dosing: The dose for schizophrenia is 800–1,200 mg daily, which is at least $1,000 of the OTC product monthly. For anxiety, 25–200 mg daily is a reasonable dose. Reputable CBD products include Elixinol, Encore Life and Bluebird Botanicals.

	Tetrahydrocannabinol (THC)	Cannabidiol (CBD)
Pure Rx form	Dronabinol (Marinol), nabilone (Cesamet) - Schedule III	Epidiolex
Psychoactive?	The High Causer in marijuana; cognitive impairment	No "high" feelings, but may reduce anxiety
Psychosis	Cannabis use in adolescence triples the risk of psychotic disorders (Jones HJ et al, 2018)	Antipsychotic properties
Seizure	Epileptogenic (lowers seizure threshold)	Anticonvulsive (raises seizure threshold)
Neurotoxicity	Likely neurotoxic	Likely neuroprotective (antioxidant and cholinergic)
Munchies?	Yes. The Hunger Causer.	No; May cause weight loss.
FDA approval	Dronabinol (Marinol) to stimulate appetite (1985)	Epidiolex for pediatric seizures (2018)
Mechanism	CB1 and CB2 agonist	Indirect antagonist of CB1 and CB2 receptors
Drug interactions	Pure THC has few clinically significant interactions	Substrate of 3A4 and 2C19. InHibitor of 2C9, 2C19, UGT enzymes and others.

Dynamic interactions:
- ❖ Sedation/CNS depression

Kinetic interactions:
- ❖ 2C19 inHibitor (strong) - CBD may increase levels of 2C19 substrates such as diazepam (Valium) and clobazam (Onfi). Clobazam, a benzodiazepine approved for Lennox-Gastaut syndrome, is increased 3-fold by CBD.
- ❖ CYP3A4 substrate (minor)
- ❖ UGT inhibitor

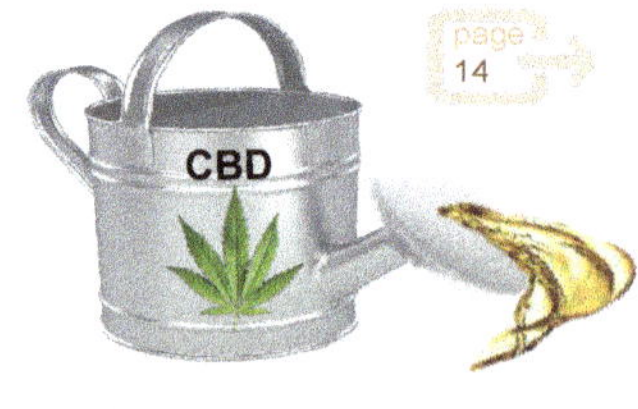

page 14

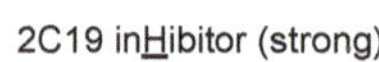

2C19 inHibitor (strong)

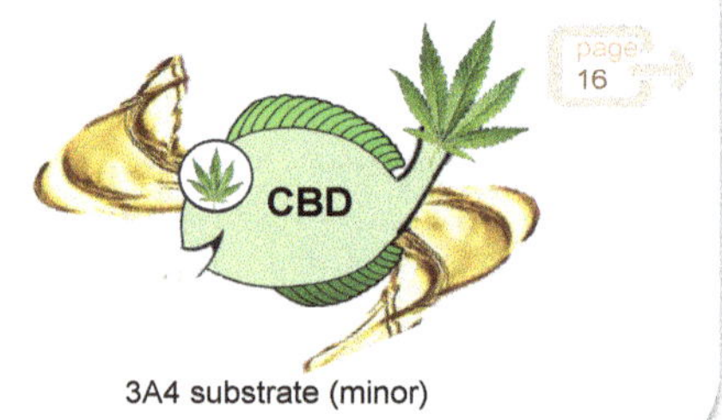

page 16

3A4 substrate (minor)

1966
$11–$75

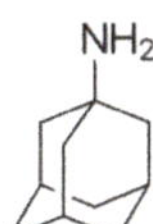

A<u>man</u>tadine (SYMMETREL)

a MAN ta deen / SIM i trel

"Symmetrical man to dine"

- Anti-Parkinson agent
- NMDA antagonist
- Dopaminergic

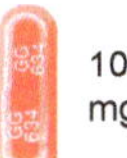

100 mg

FDA-approved for:

- Extrapyramidal symptoms (EPS)
- Parkinsonism
- Influenza A (not used because most strains are resistant)

Used off-label for:

- Fatigue of multiple sclerosis
- Cognitive problems post brain injury
- Neuroleptic malignant syndrome (NMS)
- Sexual dysfunction
- Antipsychotic-associated weight gain
- Antipsychotic-induced hyperprolactinemia
- Treatment-resistant depression
- ADHD
- OCD

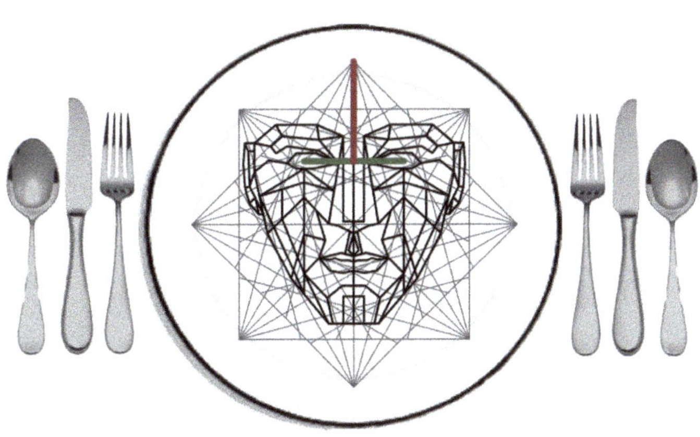

Antipsychotics lower dopamine (DA) activity. Extrapyramidal symptoms are caused by a relative deficiency of DA and an excess of acetylcholine in the nigrostriatal pathway. The anticholinergics diphenhydramine (Benadryl), benztropine (Cogentin), and trihexyphenidyl (Artane) relieve EPS by opposing acetylcholine activity. By contrast, amantadine (Symmetrel) primarily <u>relieves EPS by enhancing DA activity</u>. Although the mechanism is not well understood, amantadine probably increases synthesis and release of DA.

While anticholinergics worsen tardive dyskinesia (TD), amantadine has been shown to <u>improve TD</u>. Amantadine is useful for treatment of EPS when the anticholinergic side of effects of Benadryl, Cogentin, or Artane cannot be tolerated (e.g., due to dry mouth, constipation, confusion, or vision problems). Amantadine is only <u>moderately anticholinergic</u>. The other three choices for treatment of EPS are highly anticholinergic. Amantadine has the added benefit of <u>countering antipsychotic-induced weight gain and hyperprolactinemia</u>. Theoretically, amantadine could worsen psychosis by dopaminergic effects, but this problem is rarely encountered.

Amantadine is used as monotherapy in early Parkinson's disease (PD) and as an adjunct in later stages, usually for patients with levodopa-induced dyskinesia. Amantadine may be effective in controlling PD tremor, which is often resistant to levodopa. Unfortunately, for some PD patients the benefit lasts only a few weeks.

Amantadine is structurally related to me<u>mant</u>ine (Namenda). Both may enhance cognition, but a<u>mant</u>adine has more potential risks and side effects. Amantadine may cause loss of appetite, nausea, dizziness, insomnia, confusion, hallucinations, <u>edema</u>, and livedo reticularis (purplish red, net-like, blotchy spots on skin). <u>Congestive heart failure</u> is possible with chronic therapy.

Like memantine, amantadine is a weak NMDA receptor antagonist. Additionally, amantadine increases dopamine (DA) release. It is the dopaminergic effect that makes amantadine useful for treatment of parkinsonism, EPS, and NMS (all of which are caused by DA deficiency or DA blockade). Dopaminergic side effects of amantadine can include hallucinations and <u>compulsive behaviors</u> such as gambling, spending sprees, or sexual indiscretions. Theoretically, amantadine could induce mania or psychosis. <u>Sudden withdrawal of amantadine may cause NMS</u>.

Dosing: To <u>treat EPS</u>, the recommended dose is 100 mg BID. The maximum dose for EPS is 300 mg total daily dose; It is dosed similarly for <u>Parkinson's disease</u>, with a maximum of 400 mg/day; <u>To counter prolactin elevation from antipsychotic medication</u>, 100 mg BID has been used; Taper gradually to discontinue to avoid NMS. Use lower dose if renal insufficiency.

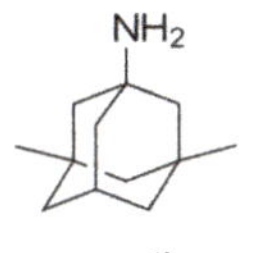

memantine

Note the structural similarity to memantine (Namenda), which is FDA-approved for moderate to severe Alzheimer's dementia.

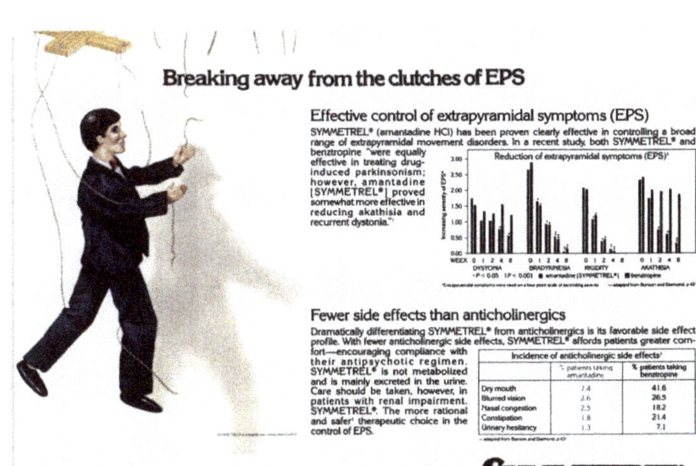

Dynamic interactions:

- Dopaminergic
- Anticholinergic (moderate)

Kinetic interactions:

- Amantadine is not metabolized. It is excreted primarily through the kidneys. Hence, minimal drug-drug interactions.

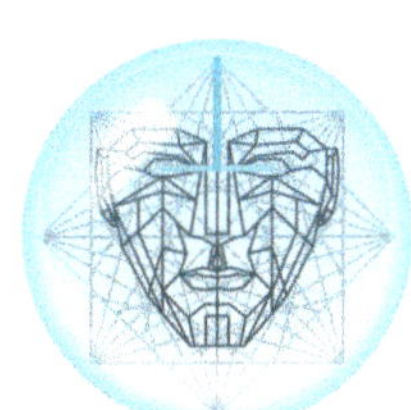

in a bubble - minimal clinically significant kinetic interactions

About the author:

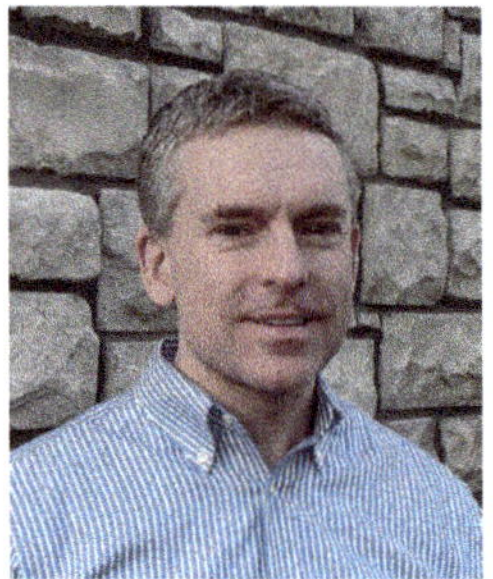

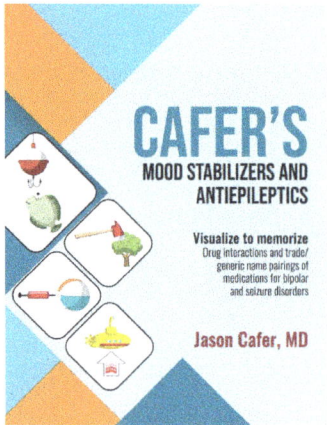

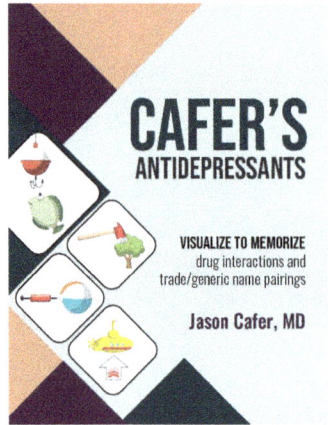

Dr Jason Cafer is Medical Director for Behavioral Health Services at SSM Health/St. Mary's Hospital in Jefferson City, Missouri where he serves as attending physician for a bustling 20-bed acute inpatient psychiatric ward. He graduated from University of Missouri-Columbia School of Medicine in 2003 and completed Psychiatric Residency at the same institution in 2007. He is a diplomate of the American Board of Psychiatry and Neurology and is also board-certified in Addiction Medicine by the American Board of Preventive Medicine. Prior to St. Mary's, he practiced inpatient psychiatry at Fulton State Hospital and outpatient at Comprehensive Health Systems. In 2007 he founded Iconic Health, a medical informatics startup that obtained angel round funding. He was Principal Investigator for Phase I and II Small Business Innovation Research (SBIR) grants for "Online Rural Telepsychiatry Platform" (2007-2009) funded by the United States Department of Agriculture. He is the inventor of United States Patent US8255241B2 which was the subject of an SBIR grant awarded by the Department of Health and Human Services for "Medication IconoGraphs: Visualization of Complex Medication Regimens". He completed *Cafer's Psychopharmacology* while serving as preceptor for Stephens College Master of Physician Assistant Studies program. Dr. Cafer aspires to provide an online Continuing Medical Education course for psychiatrists and other medical professionals.

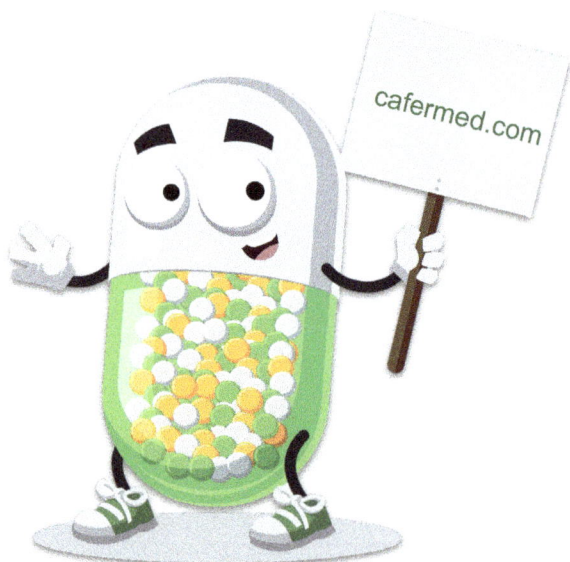

www.ingramcontent.com/pod-product-compliance
Lightning Source LLC
Chambersburg PA
CBHW042356030426
42336CB00030B/3498
* 9 7 8 1 7 3 5 0 9 0 1 1 5 *